Breast Reconstruction with Autologous Tissue

Hisham Fansa
Christoph Heitmann

Breast Reconstruction with Autologous Tissue

With Contributions by Onno Frerichs

Springer

Hisham Fansa
Department of Plastic, Reconstructive
and Aesthetic Surgery
Klinikum Bielefeld, Germany

Center for Aesthetic Plastic Surgery
and Reconstructive Breast Surgery
Munich, Germany

Center for Aesthetic Plastic Surgery
and Reconstructive Breast Surgery
Zurich, Switzerland

Christoph Heitmann
Practice for Plastic Surgery
Munich, Germany

ISBN 978-3-319-95467-7 ISBN 978-3-319-95468-4 (eBook)
https://doi.org/10.1007/978-3-319-95468-4

Library of Congress Control Number: 2018961211

This Springer imprint is published by the registered company Springer Nature Switzerland AG
The registered company address is: Gewerbestrasse 11, 6330 Cham, Switzerland

Preface

As plastic surgeons breast surgery is our passion. The last 25 years, we have concentrated on breast surgery and reconstructive breast surgery. This book is a result of our experience in breast reconstruction. It focuses on autologous breast reconstruction. We wanted to describe the techniques we are familiar with and that have proven to lead to safe oncologic and satisfying aesthetic results. In our breast centre, we are in a unique position to perform the oncological and the reconstructive part of surgery ourselves. We have determined that understanding of the oncological and the reconstructive needs offers better results for the patients. Reconstructive breast surgery should always be embedded in the multidisciplinary approach of breast cancer treatment, especially as the paradigm shift from secondary reconstructions to primary reconstructions has taken place.

We aimed to outline the necessary anatomy, the basics of breast-conserving therapy (BCT) and the oncoplastic surgery that is becoming more and more popular. Especially free microvascular flaps are described in detail and as instructive as possible. We understand microsurgical flaps to be the best kind of reconstructive procedure that offers long-lasting and best aesthetic results without the drawbacks of foreign body surgery. In the hand of the dedicated surgeon, autologous microsurgical breast reconstruction is fast and reliable and offers the best possible outcome.

We were lucky that our colleagues at our practice supported us enthusiastically. We would like to thank them, especially Dr. Irene Richter-Heine, Dr. Felix Vollbach and Dr. Maria Wetzel, from Munich. Dr. Onno Frerichs, Bielefeld, gave special input to the FCI flap chapter. A special thanks goes to our Team at our office, Kathrin Ascher, Christina Püls and Verena Vilgertshofer, and, of course, to Prof. Dr. Axel-Mario Feller who popularized many of the presented techniques in the German-speaking countries.

Hisham Fansa
Munich, Germany

Christoph Heitmann
Munich, Germany

Contents

Surgical Anatomy

H. Fansa, C. Heitmann, *Breast Reconstruction with Autologous Tissue*,
https://doi.org/10.1007/978-3-319-95468-4_1

1

The female breast has three functions: (1) the “technical” function is production of breast milk to allow breastfeeding. (2) In our society the breast also defines femininity; and in the opposite gynaecomastia is regarded as undesirable. (3) Aesthetic function of the breast always also includes symmetry of the breasts.

In the following we will concentrate on the anatomic details which are of interest for surgery.

1.1 Breast

The breast develops subcutaneously and is an appendix of the skin. Generally it develops over the fourth intercostal space (ICS). The breast consists of lobular units which drain the produced milk via the lactiferous ducts to the nipple. The nipple is surrounded by the areola. Sebaceous glands, raised above the surface of the areola, are named areolar glands or Montgomery’s glands. The nipple and areola are named nipple-areola complex (NAC).

In childhood injuries to the skin or the gland can interfere with the development and lead to malformation or aplasia. For example, surgical incisions in the heart or thoracic surgery can injure the gland, or inner scaring can prevent normal development and lead to asymmetry. Burn injuries can also obstruct breast development in puberty due to skin contracture resulting in dysplasia and asymmetry.

The suspensory Cooper’s ligaments hold the breast. However they do not attach the breast to the thoracic wall. The breast is relatively mobile and only attached to the skin of the thoracic wall medially (sternum) and at the inframammary fold (IMF). Additional attachments are observed around the areola. These zones of adherence are cutaneous structures and do not belong to the glandular tissue. They act like adherence zones in the abdomen or gluteal fold. There are no significant adherence zones cranially or laterally. The absent cranial fixation allows to use “push-up” bras that push the breast tissue into the décolleté. In the supine position, the breast moves laterally. Upright, the IMF is fixed, and the breast can only move caudally above the IMF. The superficial and deep breast fascia sheathes the breast, but do not contribute to the fixation.

> The breast can move on the thoracic wall. It is only fixed at the sternum, the IMF and the areola. The IMF is stronger than the medial adherence. There are no adherence zones cranially or laterally.

1.1.1 Accessory Glands

In rare cases accessory glands can be found in the axilla, subcutaneously, in deep planes or in the upper arm. Usually the additional breast tissue is only noted in the menstrual cycle. They can be removed if they cause discomfort. In the so-called carcinoma of unknown primary (CUP), they can be the origin of the cancer. Especially after involution the primary cancer is difficult to locate.

1.2 Arterial Supply

The arteries of the breast run together with the veins. However the main drainage is subcutaneous. The nerves also run with the vascular bundles. The breast is supplied by a *deep* (▫ Fig. 1.1) and *superficial* (▫ Fig. 1.2) arterial system.

The internal mammary artery (IMA, correctly: internal thoracic artery) mainly supplies the deep system. Others are the lateral thoracic artery and the thoracoacromial artery that supplies the pectoralis major muscle. The deep branches of the IMA perforate the intercostal muscles between the fourth and sixth ICS and then perforate the pectoralis major muscle and enter the breast. The main branch is mostly found above the fourth rib. A septum is located around the vessels, the so-called *Würinger septum* (▫ Fig. 1.3), named after Elisabeth Würinger. The septum and the vessels within can be of different characters: multiple small vessels within the entire septum or centrally located strong vessels that are immediately seen in surgery (▫ Fig. 1.4). The different structures of the septum are some reason why this important anatomical tissue has been noted too late. The Würinger septum is the base for the central pedicle in breast reduction and mastopexy. It allows safe perfusion of the breast and the NAC.

The superficial system also originates from the IMA. The branches leave the IMA in the second to

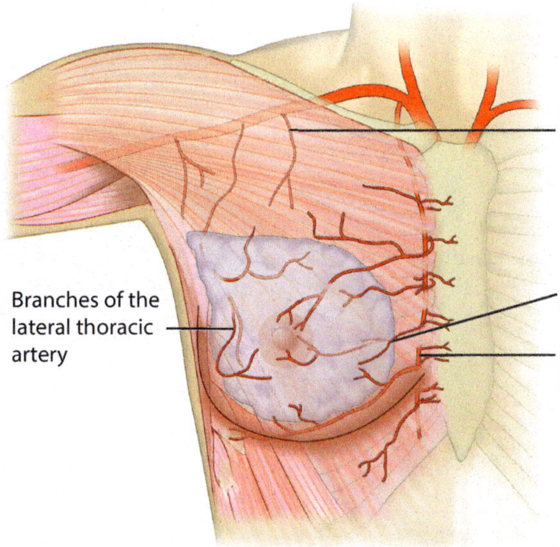

Fig. 1.1 The deep system originates from the IMA. Other branches arise from the lateral thoracic and the thoracoacromial artery that supplies the pectoralis major muscle. The deep branches from the IMA perforate the intercostal muscles. The main branch is mostly located above the fourth rib. They run within the Würinger septum. The central vessels allows a safe pedicle in reduction surgery

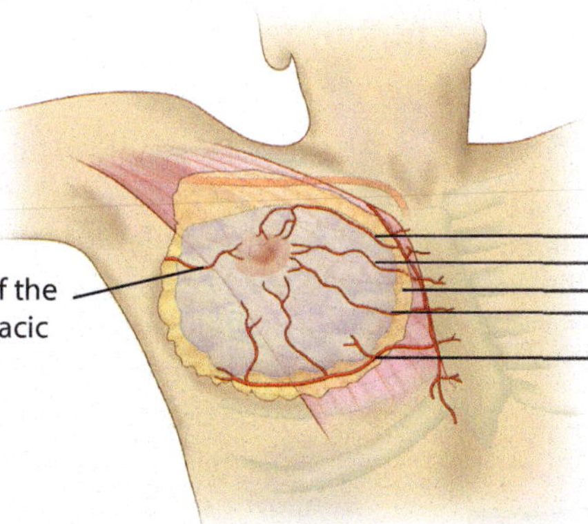

Fig. 1.2 In the superficial system, the perforators from the IMA supply the breast and the skin. These perforators are also named IMA perforators, IMAP. The strongest perforators are located in the second and third ICS. They secure the superior/medial pedicle of the breast in mastopexy or reduction. The lateral thoracic artery is located at the lateral border of the pectoralis major muscle. Cranially the thoracoacromial artery supplies the breast from the pectoralis major muscle

fifth ICS, perforate the intercostal muscles in the direction of the sternum, perforate the pectoralis major and then enter the breast. These perforators are also named IMA perforators, IMAP. They supply the skin (including the NAC) and the breast in a subcutaneous plane. The strongest perforators are located in the second and third ICS. They secure the superior/medial pedicle of the breast in mastopexy or reduction. In light-skinned patients, the course of the concomitant veins can offer information on the course of the IMAP. The terminal IMAP branches of the fifth ICS supply the inferior parts of the breast and the IMF (Fig. 1.5).

The lateral thoracic artery is located at the lateral border of the pectoralis major muscle. There are branches into the terminal lateral vessels to the breast. Cranially the thoracoacromial artery supplies the breast from the pectoralis major muscle. These branches are not very strong but add to the superior pedicle in reduction surgery.

The superficial system is dominant in the medial and superior breast supply, where it allows

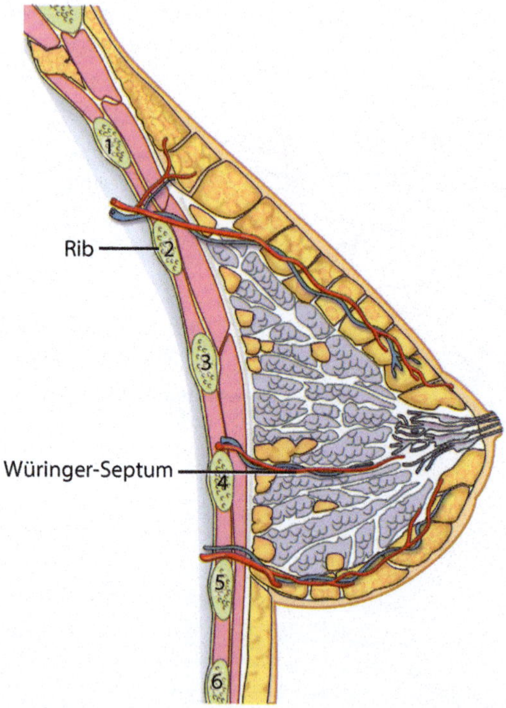

Fig. 1.3 Transverse section of the breast. The main branch of the Würinger septum is located above the fourth rib in most cases. The septum and the vessels within can be of different characters: multiple small vessels within the entire septum or centrally located strong vessels that are immediately seen in the surgery. The Würinger septum is the base for the central pedicle in breast reduction and mastopexy. It allows safe perfusion of the breast and the NAC

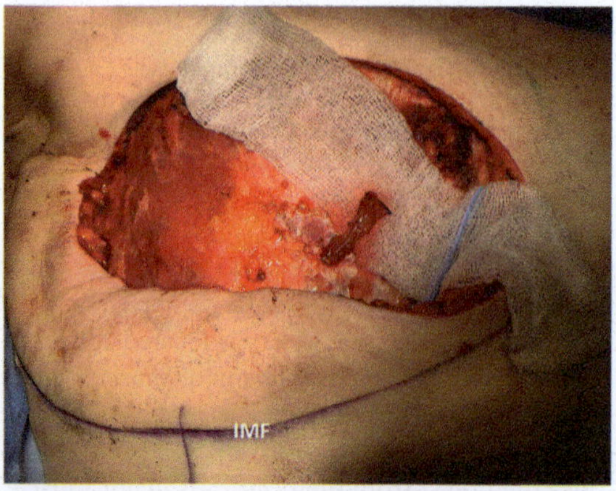

Fig. 1.4 Strong perforator from the Würinger septum in a mastectomy and immediate reconstruction. The perforators are not always so strong but present in most cases

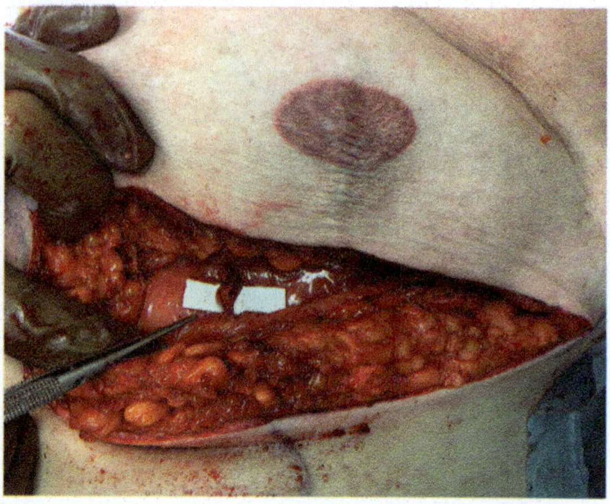

Fig. 1.5 Strong perforator in the IMF in a conversion from implant to autologous tissue after a prophylactic mastectomy

a safe pedicle for the breast and the NAC. The deepithelializing technique preserves the superficial vessels; however, the corium does not add perfusion.

The vascular supply to the breast is the base for vascular pedicles in reduction/mastopexy, for oncoplastic techniques and for the recipient vessels in breast reconstruction. It consists of the following:

- Deep system: branches from the IMA supply the breast centrally via the Würinger septum in the fourth ICS. These branches allow a central pedicle. Together with superficial branches from the fifth ICS, they supply the inferior pedicle.
- Superficial system: IMA perforators supply the breast and skin.
  - The strongest are located in the second and third ICS; they allow a superior and medial pedicle.
  - The vessels from the fifth ICS supply the IMF and the lower breast pole.
  - Superficial branches from the lateral thoracic artery supply the lateral parts of the breast; they support a lateral pedicle for the NAK.
  - Terminal branches from the thoracoacromial artery supply the cranial breast.

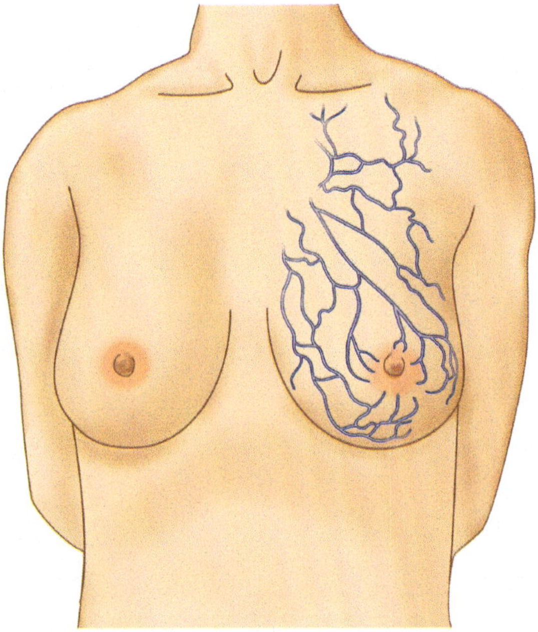

Fig. 1.6 The main venous drainage runs via the subcutaneous veins that close to the sternum run with their concomitant arteries but further branch in the periphery. Superiorly and medially they drain into the internal mammary vein (IMV). Due to their superficial course, the veins can offer information on the course of the IMAP in light-skinned patients. This can be used for planning the recipient vessels in autologous reconstruction

1.3 Veins

The venous drainage is together with the arterial supply. The main drainage runs via the subcutaneous veins that close to the sternum run with their concomitant arteries but further branch in the periphery (Fig. 1.6). Superiorly and medially they drain into the internal mammary vein (IMV). Due to their superficial course, the veins can offer information on the course of the IMAP in light-skinned patients. This can be used for planning the recipient vessels in autologous reconstruction. Superficial veins have more valves than the IMV. This has to be respected when used in reconstruction.

1.4 Lymphatics

Lymphatic drainage of the breast is mainly to the axilla and less parasternally and infraclavicularly. Few lymph nodes are located submammary; however in most cases they drain to the axilla. The lymphatic anatomy is very variable. The introduction of the sentinel lymph node concept revealed that lymphatic drainage is very individual and therapy should follow the anatomy.

Lymphatic metastasis is found mostly in the axilla. The axilla also drains the arm and the lateral thoracic wall. The amount of lymph nodes is very variable. Some note 20–30 nodes, while others describe 60–70. Due to the narrow situation in the axilla and the fact that lymphatics are a low-pressure system already, little scarring can cause a lymph oedema of the arm and breast.

Three levels are determined with regard to the pectoralis minor muscle: level 1 includes the nodes inferior and lateral to the muscle; level 2 includes the nodes below/posterior to the muscle, thus the central and apical nodes; and level 3 includes the nodes above the muscle, thus apical and below the clavicle. Axillary lymphadenectomy usually includes removal of nodes of levels 1 and 2.

> Lymphatic drainage is mainly to the axilla and to a lesser extent parasternal and infraclavicular. Clinically there are three distinct levels in the axilla.

1.5 Sensitivity

Due to a "multiple" innervation, there is no one nerve that supplies the NAC. Lateral as well as medial pedicles in reduction surgery show adequate NAC sensitivity.

Sensitive nerves supply the breast from medial intercostal nerves to supraclavicular and thoracoacromial branches. The fourth intercostal nerve supplies the breast with a deep and superficial branch. The latter is considered to innervate the NAC.

Literature

1. van Deventer PV, Graewe FR. The blood supply of the breast revisited. Plast Reconstr Surg. 2016;137:1388–97.
2. Würinger E, Mader N, Posch E, Holle J. Nerve and vessel supplying ligamentous suspension of the mammary gland. Plast Reconstr Surg. 1998;101:1486–93.

General

H. Fansa, C. Heitmann, *Breast Reconstruction with Autologous Tissue*,
https://doi.org/10.1007/978-3-319-95468-4_2

The breast is an individual organ which changes over the years due to gravity, pregnancy, lactation and menopause. In addition to the individual shape, the shape of the thorax and the position on the thorax influence the breast. The term *breast footprint* describes the position and base of the breast.

2.1 Breast Footprint

The upper breast border, the IMF and the medial and lateral breast border define the breast footprint. These borders determine the base but are individually positioned on the thorax. Some breasts, for example, have a wider distance from the sternum than others. In addition the position of the IMF is variable, leading to interindividual differences in horizontal and vertical dimensions.

2.1.1 Upper Breast Border

The upper breast border is the transition between the thoracic wall and the breast. This curved line is visible in most cases or can be made visible by lifting the breast. It starts laterally under the preaxillary fullness. The upper border has no adherence zone. Patients with a low border have less volume in the décolleté; patients with a high upper border have a more bouffant décolleté. Implants or lipofilling can push the upper border cranially. A permanent fixation with sutures, for example, in a mastopexy is not possible. In an autologous reconstruction, however, the transition zone can be reconstructed with sutures. The upper border can also be lowered in reduction surgery. Basically a cranialization of the upper border as demanded by many patients appears unnatural and not aesthetically pleasing.

Based on the fact that the NAC should be placed at the midpoint or slightly below the breast centre, the upper border can help to position the new NAC position in reduction surgery. It should be placed in the upper third or midway of the new breast.

Tip

The upper border can be used to avoid a high riding NAC when planning a breast reduction or mastopexy.

2.1.2 Inframammary Fold (IMF)

The IMF is an adherence zone. Its position is individual and develops from the connection of the superficial and the deep fascia. Lifting the arms can lift the IMF by 1–2 cm. However, in an upright position, the IMF does not lower and stays fixed. Only in some post-bariatric patients or patients with a loose adherence a loss of fixation is evident. In these patients the breast can be moved caudally over the IMF. The IMF can be asymmetrical in both breasts. This should be addressed with the patients before surgery because in some cases they do not notice this fact before surgery but complain after.

The IMF is an important border that can only be moderately changed. The IMF can be fixed to the thorax, but lifting the IMF is only possible if the weight on the IMF is significantly reduced. Otherwise the breast will slide down. A lifting of the IMF using inferior breast pedicles is very difficult.

In some primary augmentations or in tuberous breast deformities, a lowering of the IMF is necessary to adjust breast volume and NAC position. The new IMF should be fixed in these cases. A very firm IMF can remain if a lowering is planned. The IMF then acts as constriction ring on the implant resulting in a double bubble.

An unintended lowering of the IMF can take place in the reduction or augmentation/augmentation-mastopexy. The breast volume drops under the IMF, and the scar that was positioned in the IMF travels onto the breast. This phenomenon is more often found in inferior breast reduction pedicles, too large implants or saline implants.

! A firm IMF can remain if a lowering is planned. The IMF then acts as constriction ring on the implant resulting in a double bubble.

2.1.3 Medial Border

Like the IMF the medial border is an adherence zone. This border determines the cleavage. A change of the medial border is only moderately possible. It can be tried in asymmetries. If the medial breast distance is wide, it is difficult to correct without the danger of causing medial deformities such as symmastia.

> The medial border is an adherence zone and determines the cleavage. A change of the medial border is only moderately possible.

2.1.4 Lateral Border

The lateral border is less adherent and more dynamic. It is visible in an upright position but becomes more evident in a supine position. The lateral border can be widened or narrowed.

2.1.5 Breast Midline

The midline halves the breast usually at the medio-clavicular line. Ideally the line goes through the NAC and is necessary to determine the new position of the NAC in reduction or mastopexy.

Conclusion

The breast footprint is determined by the upper border, the IMF and the medial and the lateral border. These borders are individual leading to interindividual differences in vertical and horizontal breast shapes.

2.2 Breast Shape

Breast shape is determined by the footprint and the thorax. The third dimension is the volume that projects from the thoracic wall. Projection is measured as distance from thoracic wall to NAC. Ideally the shape is conical that is determined by the position of the breast on the thorax and the NAC in relation to breast volume. The NAC is located centrally on the breast, and the breast does not drop under the IMF. Some studies describe the ideal volume distribution by 45% in the upper pole and 55% in the lower pole resulting in a lightly caudal sagging conus. However the “ideal” shape depends on cultural and social influences.

Breast shape is genetically determined and changes with weight fluctuation, pregnancies, lactation and menopause. In addition, elasticity of the skin and subcutaneous tissue is important.

A caudally sagged lower breast pole has to be moved cranially in mastopexy or removed in reduction. Alternatively the lower pole can be used to auto-augment the breast. However leaving sagged tissue in place will never give an aesthetically pleasing result.

> A downward sagging of the breast over the IMF is called ptosis. There are different types of ptosis: (1) in a nipple ptosis, the NAC is not anymore positioned central on the breast; (2) in a ptosis of the gland, the lower breast pole sags below the IMF, and the NAC appears too high; (3) in a combination of nipple ptosis and glandular ptosis; (4) pseudoptosis where the IMF is too high or has lowered.

2.2.1 Nipple Ptosis

In a nipple ptosis, the nipple is not anymore central on the breast. The nipple position has to be seen with regard to the breast and the IMF. In some cases, the nipple is not ptotic, but the IMF is too high, for example, in tuberous breasts. Lifting the NAC or lowering the IMF can correct this.

2.2.2 Glandular Ptosis

In a glandular ptosis, the lower breast pole sags below the IMF. If the NAC remains centrally on the breast, it is not always considered disturbing. However if the NAC appears to high because to much volume sags down the NAC appears to high. A mastopexy or reduction can solve this problem.

2.2.3 Glandular and Nipple Ptosis

A lowering of breast and NAC together is very common. A mastopexy or reduction can solve this problem.

2.2.4 Pseudoptosis

A pseudoptosis is found if the IMF position has changed or is malformed. A high IMF makes the NAC appear too caudally. A caudally displaced IMF enlarges the vertical base leading to a bottoming out. The NAC appears too cranially.

In most cases, the latter is caused iatrogenically by placing the implant too low. Additionally a lowering can be seen after reduction surgery. The NAC appears too high, and the IMF scar slides up onto the breast.

2.3 Breast Size and Symmetry

Breast size is also individual. There are regional differences. Hypotrophy and hypertrophy have to be assessed together with the patients' build and their evaluation. In most countries the breast size is graded in cup sizes. The cup size depends in the size of the breast and the under bust and the manufacturer. Therefore the surgeon should avoid describing the postoperative size as cup size. The patients should always be informed on possible deviations.

Besides the breast size symmetry is important. Symmetry can differ in size or shape. Symmetry should always be a significant goal in breast surgery.

2.4 Measurement and Planning

The individual breast shape, size and postoperative result have always to be assessed with regard to the patients' build and the desired result. Therefore it is difficult to determine normal measurements. Many books determine standard measurements. However the result after an operation should suit the patient not the measurement. Nevertheless it is important to document breast footprint, shape, size and measurements prior to surgery (◘ Table 2.1).

◘ **Table 2.1** "Ideal measurements" for planning

"Ideal measurements" depend on the patients' build and the desired breast size	
Nipple – jugular notch distance	18–24 cm
Nipple – IMF distance	7–11 cm
Nipple – upper breast border distance	7–10 cm
Nipple – midline distance	9–14 cm
NAC - diameter	3, 5–6 cm

2.5 Markings

Measurements and markings should be made preoperatively with the patient in an upright position with hanging arms. Patients should not moisturize before. The marking pen should be water-resistant and also resist disinfection. Preoperative planning is of importance and should be done unhurriedly and accurately. A perfect marking allows a fast and precise operation. Planning on the operation table should be reserved to revision operations that require a reaction to intraoperative situations. In these cases the patient can be put in a sitting position on the operation table to simulate the upright position as good as possible.

In reduction, mastopexy or reconstructive surgery, the midline should also be marked to position the volume right. The midpoint of the IMF should also be marked as the medial and lateral flap in Wise pattern meet here. If possible all incision should also be marked.

> Measurements and markings should be made preoperatively with the patient in an upright position with hanging arms. Preoperative planning is of importance and should be done unhurriedly and accurately.

2.6 Incisions and Drains

The incisions follow the surgical requirements but should be placed in the relaxed skin tension lines wherever possible to reduce visible scarring.

2.6.1 "Classic" Incisions

"Classic" incisions are (1) around the NAC, periareolar, and this incision can also be semilunar or crescent, and if closed tension free, this usually results in a good scar; (2) the vertical scar from the areolar border down to the IMF, if used as only incision in breast reduction, the scar can be visible, and a dog ear can result in the lower part; and (3) the IMF incision. Usually it is not very conspicuous, but can slide up on the breast if the IMF is not fixed.

> The "classic" incisions are periareolar and vertical and in the IMF.

2.6.2 BCT, Oncoplastic Surgery and Mastectomy

The above-mentioned incisions can be used in breast-conserving therapy (BCT). Tumours in the upper inner pole should be resected via a periareolar approach. The skin should only be resected if there is an oncological need. Tumours in the lateral breast parts can be resected via a direct incision. In the upper part, a curved incision can be used. If the skin has to be resected, this kind of incision can result in the displacement of the NAC. In these cases a rhomboid or radial incision can be better. In the lower pole, the radial incision or the IMF incision can be used.

Mastectomies have to follow oncological needs. In skin-sparing mastectomies (SSM), the NAC is removed. The simplest way is the periareolar incision. If more skin has to be removed, a transverse fusiform incision can be applied. Nipple sparing or subcutaneous mastectomies (NSM) can use vertical or IMF incisions. Lateral IMF incisions have less NAC necrosis. Mastectomies of large or ptotic breasts can be accessed with a Wise pattern (inverted T) incision if a reconstruction with less volume is planned.

In a mastectomy without reconstruction, the incision should be based on oncologic criteria; in most cases it is a transverse incision which should take into account that the scar is not visible in the décolleté.

Tip

In BCT or oncoplastic surgery, the incisions should be placed periareolar or curved on the lateral aspect of the breast. In the lower poles, a radial incision is better. If the skin has to be removed, care should be taken not to misplace the NAC.

2.6.3 Axilla

Axillary incisions for sentinel lymph node (SLN) excisions should be placed over the marked lymph node. Usually the incision should be perpendicular to the course of the pectoralis muscle. A 3–4 cm incision is sufficient in most cases. Complete lymph node dissections can be made via the same widened incision.

2.6.4 Drains

If necessary we prefer a soft Jackson-Pratt drain. They can be diverted in the axilla, the IMF or at the end of the incision.

2.7 Positioning on the Operating Table

General anaesthesia is commonly used. The patient is placed in a supine position. The arms can be abducted to 90° if only one breast is accessed or the patient stays in the supine position. This allows good access to the breast and axilla. If symmetry should be assessed intraoperatively and the patient should be changed to a sitting position, the arms can be positioned with adduction in the shoulder of 30–45° (◘ Fig. 2.1). The elbows are placed on little arm pads, and the hands are placed under the lumbar region (◘ Fig. 2.2). In a two-team approach when both breasts are operated simultaneously, two electrosurgery devices with two electrodes are required. The patients' body temperature can be managed with a convective warming device (e.g. Bair Hugger).

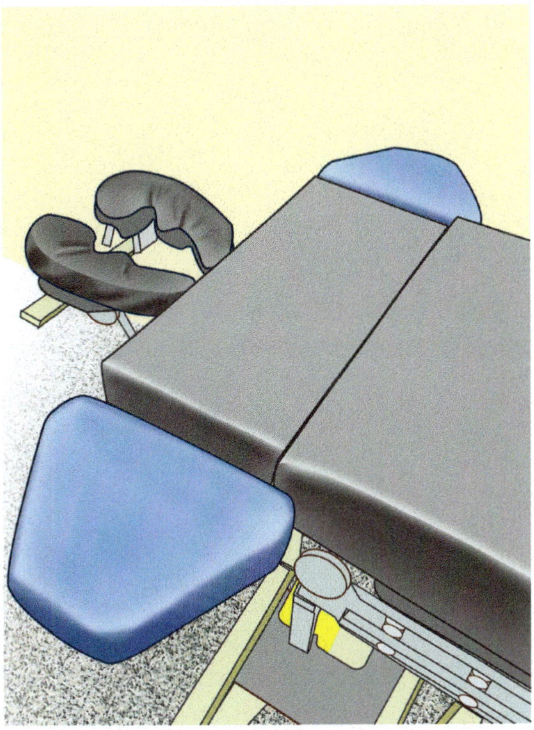

◘ **Fig. 2.1** Operating table for adducted arm position with elbow pads

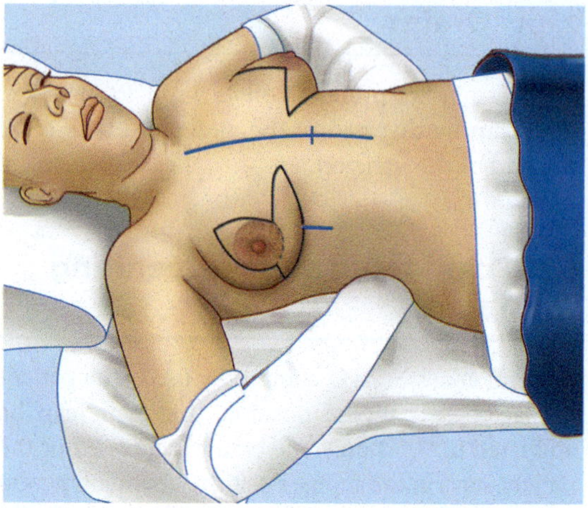

Fig. 2.2 Positioning of a patient for breast reduction. This positioning can be used for almost all breast operations, especially if the patients have to be put intraoperatively in a sitting position. Reconstructive procedures are also positioned this way. The elbows are placed on the pads; the hands are padded and placed under the lumbar region. Pressure sores from venous catheters in the hand should be avoided by adequate padding

2.8 Sutures

Resorbable sutures can be used for deep tissues. Standard is polyglactin (e.g. Vicryl, Ethicon) and poliglecaprone (e.g. Monocryl, Ethicon). The sizes follow the requirements from 3-0 to 2. Buried subcutaneous stitches can be done with Vicryl or Monocryl. The skin should be closed with a running intracutaneous suture. A Monocryl 3-0 or 4-0 can be used if the patients do not report wound-healing problems. Otherwise a polyamide (Ethilon, Ethicon) or polypropylene (Prolene, Ethicon) 3-0 to 0 can be used but must be removed later on. Only little incisions or nipple reconstructions should be closed with simple interrupted sutures (e.g. Ethilon 5-0).

2.9 Photography

All patients should be photographed pre- and postoperatively. Besides proper archiving software, the photographs should be standardized with the same views and light situation. Frontal, oblique and lateral views are necessary. The arms should be adducted. In special cases the arms can be elevated to 90°. This usually elevates the NAC and the IMF. Individual situations should be addressed specially.

The photographs in this book do not show all perspectives due to the limited space.

General

H. Fansa, C. Heitmann, *Breast Reconstruction with Autologous Tissue*,
https://doi.org/10.1007/978-3-319-95468-4_3

According to the German Robert Koch Institute, breast cancer is the most frequent malignant disease in women. They predict 72,000 newly diagnosed patients in 2018. In 2015 mortality was almost 18,000. One of eight women will get breast cancer during her lifetime; 3 out of 10 are younger than 55 when diagnosed. The relative (cancer-related) 5-year survival rate in 2013/2014 was 88%; the 10-year survival rate was 82%. The data is comparable for most developed nations. Although the treatment of breast cancer is very similar in all developed nations, in this chapter we describe the way according to the German guidelines.

3.1 Breast Centre

Cancer treatment follows clinical guidelines. In Germany the treatment is concentrated in the so-called breast centres. The core members of a breast centre are gynaecologists (in Germany they usually perform the breast surgery), plastic surgeons, oncologists, radiologists, radiation therapists and pathologists. Psycho-oncologists are also available. Special fields are consulted (e.g. orthopaedics or complementary medicine) if necessary.

The diagnosis and therapy are discussed pre- and postoperatively in the board. A case manager leads the patient through the treatment. The breast centres are regularly audited and certified according to quality management processes.

3.2 Breast Cancer

Biology of breast cancer is different. This leads to patient-adapted treatment. Invasive cancer and in situ cancer, for example, have different treatment approaches.

Every patient is reviewed in the tumour board. History and family history are registered as well as the tumour biology:

- Tumour size and its relation to the breast size
- Location within the breast (solitary, multifocal, multicentric)
- Type of cancer (histopathology)
- Receptor status for oestrogen and progesterone
- Her2/Neu-status (human epidermal growth factor receptor 2; synonymous erb-B2, c-erbB2)
- Grading and KI-67 (sometimes called MIB1)
- Regional lymph node status
- Individual parameters

The treatment is planned according to the guidelines. First decision is whether surgery or neoadjuvant chemotherapy is the treatment to start with. The board decides which kind of chemotherapy or which kind of surgery is necessary. The surgery is determined:

- Breast-conserving therapy (BCT)
- Oncoplastic surgery
- Mastectomy: skin sparing (SSM) or nipple sparing (NSM)
  - Without immediate reconstruction
  - With immediate reconstruction
    - Reconstruction with autologous tissue
    - Reconstruction with expander/implant
  - Unilateral or bilateral (e.g. with positive genetics or bilateral cancer)
- Sentinel lymph node or axillary dissection (levels 1 and 2)

Thus, treatment follows a complex decision-making. There is always enough time to discuss the findings and put together an accurate treatment plan.

3.3 Time Schedule

Patients should also be informed on the time line. In case the patient will undergo all parts of therapy, surgery, chemotherapy and radiation therapy, the treatment period is 8–9 months. The planned schedule should be respected.

3.3.1 Surgery

In a BCT the patient stays 1–2 days in the hospital; in a mastectomy the patient stays about 5–7 days in hospital if no complication occurs. Bilateral surgery can prolong the stay. Patients who have received prior chemotherapy need a longer convalescence after surgery.

Surgery after neoadjuvant chemotherapy can take place after 4–6 weeks, with respect to the general state, laboratory results or possible study inclusion.

3.3.2 Chemotherapy and Hormone-Blocking Therapy

Chemotherapy takes approximately 4–5 months. It can be administered before or after surgery, depending on the tumour biology. If the chemotherapy follows after surgery, it is administered before radiation therapy. Hormone-blocking therapy is recommended for 10 years.

3.3.3 Radiation Therapy

Adjuvant radiation takes about 5–6 weeks. The dose is fractioned and administered in a daily protocol (e.g. 1.4 Gray per day for 25 days). Interruptions are not reasonable. Radiation should start 4–6 weeks after surgery if no chemotherapy is planned.

3.4 Family History and Genetics

Breast cancer can have genetic cause. Besides BRCA there are other mutations that can cause cancer, such as CHEK2, PALB2 and RAD51C. CHEK2 is supposed to increase the risk moderately, while PALB2 seems to have a similar risk like BRCA. RAD51C is associated with a higher risk for ovarian cancer. The type of cancer depends on the altered gene. While BRCA2-associated cancer resembles sporadic cancer, BRCA1 often shows a triple-negative phenotype with grade 3 cancer. If age of onset, family history or tumour biology are suspicious for a genetic cause, a medical genetic counselling and testing are recommended not only with regard to breast cancer but also to other cancer types.

Criteria for counselling according the German guidelines (cited after S3-Leitlinie Brustkrebs, Diagnostik, Therapie und Nachsorge 2017):

Counselling and genetic testing should be offered if the family history shows the following:

- At least three women with breast cancer
- At least two women with breast cancer, one with onset before the age of 51
- At least one woman with breast cancer and one with ovarian cancer
- At least two with ovarian cancer
- At least one with breast and ovarian cancer
- At least one woman with breast cancer and onset before the age of 35
- At least one woman with bilateral cancer with onset before the age of 50
- At least one man with breast cancer and one woman with breast or ovarian cancer

3.4.1 Intensive Screening

In Germany patients with proven genetic mutations can undergo an intensified screening program. They receive an MRI every year and a sonography every 6 months beginning with their 25th year. Mammography is added every year or second year. This program also depends on the family history (onset of cancer in the diseased family member). Patients who were radiated at the thorax due to Hodgkin's lymphoma and thus have a high risk of developing breast cancer are also enrolled to this program.

3.4.2 Prophylactic/Preventive Mastectomy

Patients who carry genetic mutations can undergo prophylactic or preventive mastectomies if they do not have breast cancer. A bilateral salpingo-oophorectomy should also be discussed. According to the German guidelines, the mastectomy reduces the risk of breast cancer about 95%. Breast cancer-related lethality is reduced by 95%. The prophylactic ovarectomy reduces the risk for ovarian cancer by 97%; it also reduces the overall mortality by 75%. Ovarectomy should take place at the age of 40, after completed family planning. However data on this topic is in a constant state of flux.

Once diseased the rate of secondary cancer on the same side is not significantly increased in patients with genetic mutations. Therefore BCT can be an option for these patients. However these patients have an increased risk for contralateral carcinoma of 25–45% in 15 years. The bilateral or contralateral mastectomy thus reduces the incidence of a second cancer. The risk depends on the type of genetic mutation and the age of the patient at onset of disease. Overall survival seems also to be reduced by contralateral mastectomy. The prognosis of the first cancer however should be taken into account. Currently there is no data available on preventive mastectomy in non-genetically affected women. The indications should be made carefully after meticulous counselling.

Literature

Epidemiological Data (in German)

1. https://www.krebsdaten.de/Krebs/DE/Content/Publikationen/Krebs_in_Deutschland/kid_2017/kid_2017_c50_brust.pdf?__blob=publicationFile

German Guidelines on Diagnosis, Therapy and After Care (in German)

2. http://www.awmf.org/uploads/tx_szleitlinien/032-045OLl_S3_Mammakarzinom_2017-12.pdf
3. Cochrane:Lostumbo L, Carbine NE, Wallace J. Prophylactic mastectomy for the prevention of breast cancer. Cochrane Database Syst Rev. 2010;11:CD002748.
4. Graeser MK, Engel C, Rhiem K, Gadzicki D, Bick U, Kast K, Froster UG, Schlehe B, Bechtold A, Arnold N, Preisler-Adams S, Nestle-Kraemling C, Zaino M, Loeffler M, Kiechle M, Meindl A, Varga D, Schmutzler RK. Contralateral breast cancer risk in BRCA1 and BRCA2 mutation carriers. J Clin Oncol. 2009;27:5887–92.
5. Kuchenbaecker KB, Hopper JL, Barnes DR, Phillips KA, Mooij TM, Roos-Blom MJ, Jervis S, van Leeuwen FE, Milne RL, Andrieu N, Goldgar DE, Terry MB, Rookus MA, Easton DF, Antoniou AC, BRCA1 and BRCA2 Cohort Consortium, McGuffog L, Evans DG, Barrowdale D, Frost D, Adlard J, Ong KR, Izatt L, Tischkowitz M, Eeles R, Davidson R, Hodgson S, Ellis S, Nogues C, Lasset C, Stoppa-Lyonnet D, Fricker JP, Faivre L, Berthet P, Hooning MJ, van der Kolk LE, Kets CM, Adank MA, John EM, Chung WK, Andrulis IL, Southey M, Daly MB, Buys SS, Osorio A, Engel C, Kast K, Schmutzler RK, Caldes T, Jakubowska A, Simard J, Friedlander ML, SA ML, Machackova E, Foretova L, Tan YY, Singer CF, Olah E, Gerdes AM, Arver B, Olsson H. Risks of breast, ovarian, and contralateral breast cancer for BRCA1 and BRCA2 mutation carriers. JAMA. 2017;317(23):2402–16.

Tumour Resection and Breast-Conserving Therapy (BCT)

H. Fansa, C. Heitmann, *Breast Reconstruction with Autologous Tissue*,
https://doi.org/10.1007/978-3-319-95468-4_4

There are benign and malignant tumours. If a malignant tumour is not properly recognized prior to the operation, the therapy is impeded.

4.1 Diagnosis

To treat a possible carcinoma right, it is necessary to operate with a secured diagnosis. Every tumour should be diagnosed earlier to surgery by radiologic imaging and histology. Sonography, mammography and MRI are the common tools for examination. Punch biopsies or vacuum-assisted biopsies to identify the type of tumour are routinely used.

In malignant tumours a preoperative staging (evaluation of distant metastasis) is only recommended in aggressive or locally advanced tumours or if a metastasis is suspected. In early stages a general staging is not indicated according to the German guidelines. Staging consists of a CT scan of the thorax and abdomen and a bone scintigraphy. A PET-CT scan is only recommended in unclear findings.

4.2 Indications

Palpable tumours that were diagnosed as benign can be resected in an excisional biopsy. The indications for a BCT in malignant and premalignant tumours are locally limited in situ carcinomas (DCIS/LCIS) and invasive carcinomas with a favourable relation of tumour size and breast size. Resection margins should be tumour free (R0 resection).

In Germany about 70% of all surgical cancer treatments are done as BCT and only 30% as mastectomy. The BCT is considered oncologically safe. Inflammatory carcinomas should not be treated by BCT. A relative contraindication is seen for multicentric carcinomas and unfavourable relation of tumour size to breast size. A sub-group of patients under the age of 40, with a poorly differentiated carcinoma and insufficient adjuvant therapy, have a higher risk for a local recurrence after BCT compared to a mastectomy. To control local recurrences, a postoperative radiation therapy is always recommended. If the patient does not want to undergo radiation therapy, a mastectomy should be recommended.

BCT is an often underestimated operation. Ten to thirty percent of all patients after BCT and radiation are not pleased with the aesthetic result.

The BCT is considered oncologically safe. The indications for a BCT in malignant and premalignant tumours are locally limited in situ carcinomas (DCIS/LCIS) and invasive carcinomas with a favourable relation of tumour size and breast size. Resection margins should be tumour free (R0 resection). To control local recurrences, a postoperative radiation therapy is always recommended. If the patient does not want to undergo radiation therapy, a mastectomy should be recommended.

4.3 Surgery of a Palpable Tumour

Resection of a palpable tumour resembles an open diagnostic excision biopsy. Small subcutaneous tumours diagnosed as benign can be removed this way. Most benign tumours are fibroadenomas. Only in exceptional cases, a tumour should be removed without prior image-guided needle biopsy.

4.4 Surgery after Localization Wire and Specimen Radiography

Non-palpable tumours or tumours which are difficult to confine should be preoperatively marked with a localization wire. Some tumours may require more than one wire. Even in palpable masses, a localization wire should be considered if a haematoma from the needle biopsy is evident. The wire should be documented after the placement, and the surgeon should control the position prior to surgery (Figs. 4.1 and 4.2) to plan the incision and resection. The tumour and the localization wire should be removed en bloc. A specimen radiography with topographic marking should be done after resection (Figs. 4.3 and 4.4).

In many cases the findings are marked with a clip when needle biopsy takes place. This allows an easy localization of the lesion. After surgical resection the specimen radiography should document the clip. This is also necessary in a mastectomy.

4.5 Histopathology and Margins

All resected specimens should be examined histologically. The specimen has to be marked topographically. We mark the specimen laterally, cranially and pectorally. Frozen sections can be applied if immediate surgical consequences result from the examination. Frozen sections can, for example, evaluate an unclear lesion or sentinel examination. Frozen sections after neoadjuvant chemotherapy or with a present DCIS are prone to false results. A regular histology should be intended.

The resection margins should be free to reduce the risk of a local recurrence. The guideline determines that "no ink on tumour" should be achieved in invasive cancer. Adjuvant treatment like chemotherapy and radiation therapy should be included in this resection concept. DCIS should also be resected with free margins; however a 2 mm margin is recommended if a radiation therapy follows the surgery. Wider margins should be applied if a radiation is abdicated. If a complete resection is not possible by BCT or in an oncoplastic surgery, a mastectomy should be considered.

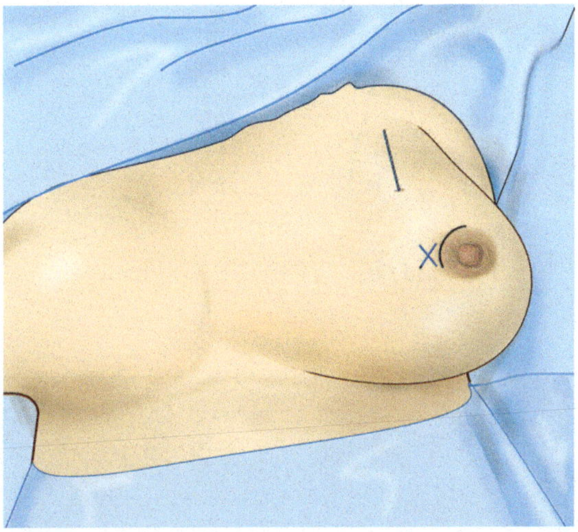

Fig. 4.1 Percutaneous wire localization for BCT. The wire marks the tumour. The X marks the localization in the skin. The tumour is removed from a periareolar incision

4.6 Informed Consent

The disclosure of general and special risks should be documented with standardized and evaluated forms. Infection, haematoma and wound-healing complications can occur in rare cases. Seroma formation, visible scars and asymmetries can occur. Skin irregularities and dents are possible. The resection of the tumour can reduce breast size, and scarring can distort the NAC. A loss of sensitivity can disturb the patient if evident at the NAC. In rare cases a NAC necrosis can appear. A NAC resection may be necessary due to oncologic reasons. If surgery is performed properly, complications are rare.

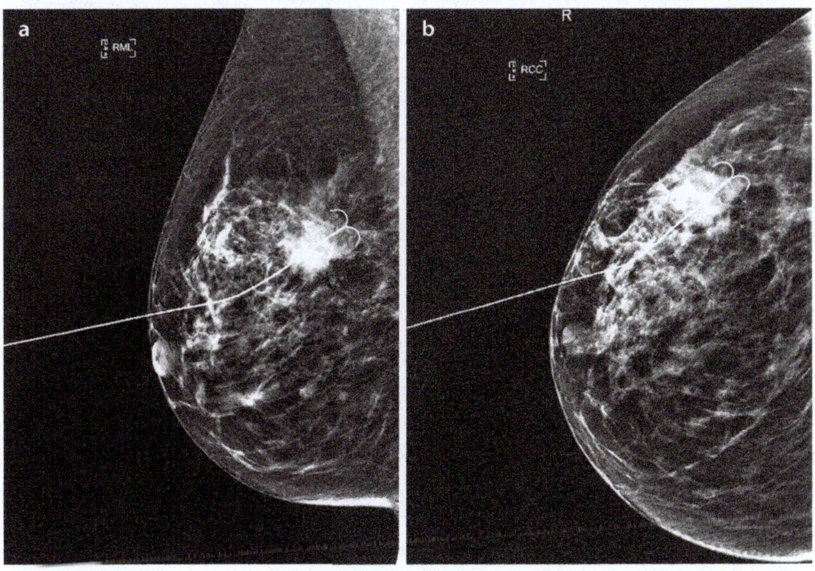

Fig. 4.2 Preoperative control of a wire localization in a mammography. The tumour is located in the right upper lateral breast pole. The wire penetrated the tumour. **a** medial-lateral; **b** craniocaudal. (By courtesy of Dr. B. Uphus, Die Radiologie, Munich)

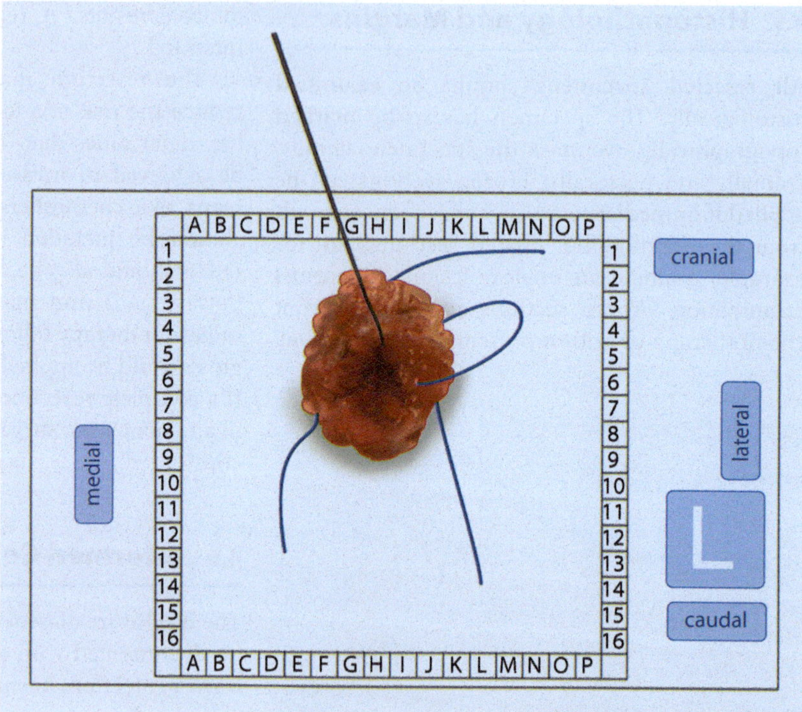

Fig. 4.3 Placement of topographically marked specimen for radiography

Second operations should be mentioned if histopathology is unclear. A drawing, e.g. of the incision, can make the disclosure more comprehendible. If tumour and sentinel lymph node/axillary dissection are performed in one operation, the risks can be discussed in one informed consent.

4.7 Surgery

4.7.1 Preoperative Markings and Incisions

Palpable tumours, the IMF and the planned incision should be marked on the upright patient. There are many possible incisions (Fig. 4.5). In the upper part of the breast, incisions should be rather curved or periareolar. In the lower pole, the incision should be radial. As the scar can shrink, incisions beginning from the areola to the periphery can distort the NAC. This is disturbing and is difficult to correct especially after radiation therapy. If skin resection is necessary, a deformation of the breast and NAC malposition should be avoided. Tumours in the upper inner pole of the breast should be rather treated with oncoplastic techniques. If the tumour is located in the upper lateral pole, the sentinel or axillary dissection

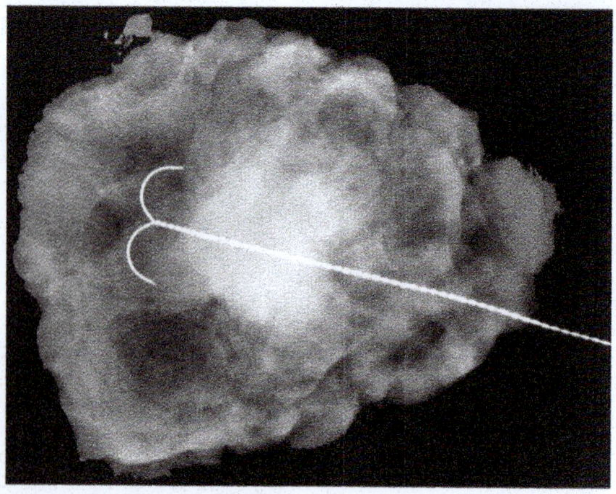

Fig. 4.4 Radiography after resection. Wire and tumour are located within the resected tissue. The margin can be assessed in the projected plane

can be tried from the same incision. Otherwise a separate incision is necessary.

4.7.2 Position

Before the patient is transferred to the OR, the team should examine if a planned marking (sentinel or wire marking) has taken place sufficiently and all findings are available.

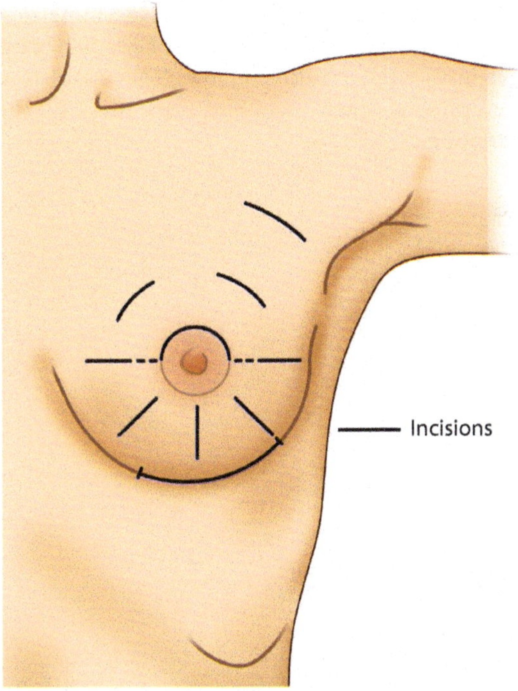

Fig. 4.5 Possible incisions for BCT. The periareolar incision can be altered according to the tumour localization. A combined horizontal radial and periareolar incision can distort the NAC due to the later shrinkage. An incision in the upper inner pole should only be used if oncologically necessary

General anaesthesia is recommended. Only small palpable tumours which are easy accessible should be resected under local anaesthesia. The patient is placed supine; arms are abducted by 90° in the shoulder, allowing access to the breast and axilla. If an intraoperative change to a sitting position is mandatory, then the arms should be adducted by 45–30° in the shoulder. The elbows are placed on little arm pads, and the hands are placed under the lumbar region. In a two-team approach when both breasts are operated simultaneously, two electrosurgery devices with two electrodes are required. The patients' body temperature can be managed with a convective warming device (e.g. Bair Hugger).

4.7.3 Tumour Resection

After incision the tumour is dissected. If wires are used, the tumour and the wires should be removed en bloc. The specimen is marked to allow topographic orientation and is then radiographed. Preoperatively placed clips to mark the tumour should be removed with the tumour. Histopathology should follow. If a clinical suspicion demands a wider resection, this can be done at this point. Careful haemostasis and if necessary a clip marking for the later radiation therapy can be applied. If a sentinel lymph node or the axillary dissection is done forming the same incision, it can be done now. If necessary a drain is placed. Smaller tumours do not require a reconstruction. The wound layers are closed.

4.7.4 Further Resections

If a frozen section is performed, a wider resection can be done in the same surgery if the margins are not free. Otherwise the resection has to take place in a second surgery.

4.7.5 Aftercare

The patients are mobile. Thromboprophylaxis is recommended. Drains should be removed with regard to the fluid amount. A bra can be used if necessary.

Sporting, work and daily activities should not exceed the standard. Sauna and sun tanning should be avoided for about 6 weeks. Radiation therapy can start after 4–6 weeks post-surgery.

4.7.6 Complications

Complications are rare if surgery is properly performed. Little haematomas can be tolerated; larger haematomas that cause pain, impair the aesthetic outcome or cause severe blood loss require revision.

Acute infections are evident after 2–3 days. The incision is red; the axilla swells up. Lab work shows increased leucocytes and CRP. A wound swab and a surgical revision are necessary.

Chronic infection and seroma cause redness and delayed wound healing and lead to seroma or lymphatic discharge from the wound. In many cases local antiseptic treatment, wound punctures and systemic antibiotic treatment can support healing.

A complication that is more evident lately is an *oedema* of the thoracic wall. This oedema is only present if a BCT, lymph node surgery and radiation therapy are applied together. If a complex decongestive therapy (CDT) does not improve the situation, reconstructive procedures can help to relieve the symptoms.

Aesthetic complications include asymmetries, dents and skin irregularities. Shrinkage of the scar can distort the position of the NAC. Radiation therapy and their sequelae can amplify the symptoms.

Oncoplastic Surgery

H. Fansa, C. Heitmann, *Breast Reconstruction with Autologous Tissue*,
https://doi.org/10.1007/978-3-319-95468-4_5

In a BCT, the focus is on an oncologically safe local resection following radiation therapy. Oncoplastic surgery includes wider margins and a partial mastectomy to (1) allow better local oncologic control. (2) The breast is shaped to improve the aesthetic outcome, which includes (3) the contralateral side, as symmetry is an essential part of breast aesthetics. (4) Some studies advocate a primary reconstruction of the breast avoiding cavities which in turn lead to better results after radiation therapy.

Oncoplastic surgery underlines the paradigm shift that primary resection and reconstruction are safely performed in a single-stage operation. Furthermore, it is more difficult to correct an aesthetically less pleasing result after radiation therapy.

Like in a BCT, radiation therapy is a crucial part of the oncoplastic concept. Most available studies underline the safety of this concept if wide margins are met. The studies have collected retrospective data. In the USA oncoplastic surgery is more popular than in Germany. The technique is convincing, and following the right indication, it improves oncologic and aesthetic outcome.

Oncoplastic surgery focuses on wide margins, new breast shape, inclusion of the contralateral side and the improved outcome after radiation therapy. Thus patients' quality of life can be enhanced.

5.1 Indications for Oncoplastic Techniques

Wide margins are essential. The indication depends on the diagnosis, tumour size and position, tumour biology, patients' request and breast size and shape. If a skin resection is oncologically necessary, a careful planning is mandatory. A skin resection in the upper breast poles is difficult to combine with reduction/mastopexy incision patterns. If on the other hand a resection is necessary in the lower part, it can often be combined with skin resections from reduction patterns.

If oncologically possible skin resections in the upper inner and medial pole of the breast should be avoided. The desired NAC position should also be planned. Some resection patterns lead to distortion of the NAC laterally or caudally. This malposition should be avoided and corrected. A correction after the radiation therapy took place is difficult in most cases. Additionally malpositions cranially or within the décolleté are difficult to improve.

The defect that results from resection can be filled with local transposition of breast tissue and local flaps (*volume displacement*) and by free flaps (*volume replacement*). Local transposition requires the knowledge of the vascular patterns. The dissection plane is above the gland like in central pedicles or for larger mobilization within the gland. Closure without tension is mandatory.

Shaping a breast after BCT and radiation therapy is difficult. Including the primary aesthetic concept leads to better results. Especially in large or ptotic breasts, a valuable oncoplastic concept even with mastectomy and free autologous flaps is the better way than a local aesthetically insufficient shaping.

5.2 Resection and Reconstruction

Oncoplastic resection does not only hollow out the tumour but resembles a partial mastectomy. The tumour should be located with a wire preoperatively if it is not palpable. Some tumours require more than one wire. Especially in DCIS wide margins are beneficial. Some studies demand to remove the pectoral fascia. The resulting defect is closed by local volume displacement. Cavities within the breast should be avoided.

5.2.1 Incisions and Local Tissue Transposition

Many kinds of incisions are used. Some were presented in ▶ Chap. 4. Additional incisions are shown here.

Radial/elliptic incisions are possible *in all parts* of the breast. Central tumours are best accessed from periareolar incisions. If a skin resection in the upper or central pole is not necessary, a reduction/mastopexy incision pattern (like Wise pattern) is possible.

Tumours in the upper breast pole are removed from a crescent periareolar incision or a batwing incision (◘ Fig. 5.1). The batwing incision com-

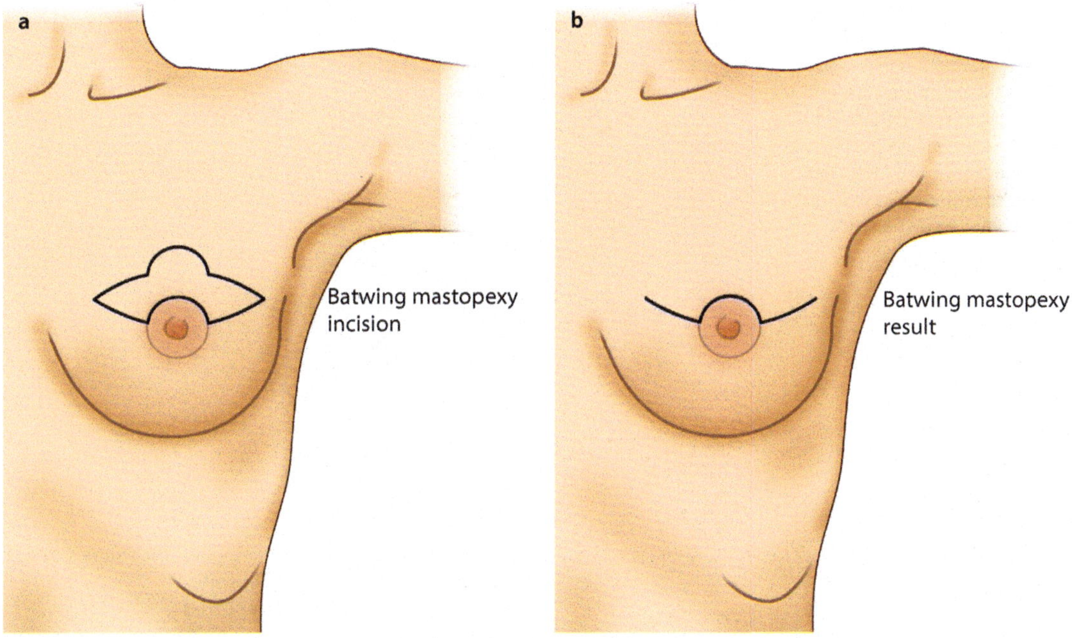

Fig. 5.1 **a** The batwing incision combines the cranial periareolar incision with a lateral and medial ellipse. The lateral incision should avoid a dog ear. In some cases a single-sided batwing incision can be sufficient. **b** However the mastopexy effect is only moderate. Incisions that alter the NAC position should always include the contralateral side for symmetry purposes. The lower breast parts can be accessed from the IMF. Triangular incisions (narrow side pointing to IMF) are also possible. They are usually combined with an IMF incision to approximate the skin. Larger resection can be performed by a trapezoid-shaped incision, usually combined with a periareolar incision to distribute the skin

bines the cranial periareolar incision with a lateral and medial ellipse. In some cases, a single-sided batwing incision can be sufficient. However the mastopexy effect is only moderate. It is important to close all layers of the wound in this incision to avoid dents above the NAC or widening of the scar. Incisions that alter the NAC position should always include the contralateral side.

The lower breast parts can be accessed from the IMF. Triangular incisions (narrow side pointing to IMF) are also possible. They are usually combined with an IMF incision to approximate the skin. Larger resection can be performed by a trapezoid-shaped incision, usually combined with a periareolar incision to distribute the skin (Fig. 5.2).

5.2.2 Local Tissue Transposition in Large or Ptotic Breasts with Reduction/Mastopexy

Oncoplastic techniques are best executed in large or ptotic breasts. Local volume resection and volume redistribution allow a safe oncologic therapy and aesthetic outcome. After resection the breast skin and volume are completely reshaped allowing wide margins and avoiding cavities. Tumours that are not located in the skin resection pattern can also be accessed if no additional skin resection is necessary.

The contralateral side can and should be included into this concept. Using these techniques, the breasts are reduced by the amount of resection, but an aesthetic result can be achieved. We prefer the inverted T-pattern (Wise) for reduction or mastopexy. The pure periareolar techniques have failed in our hands to achieve long lasting aesthetic results. Additionally the pure vertical mastopexy/reduction patterns are difficult, because the breast shape undergoes postoperative changes that can interfere with the radiation therapy, resulting in a not predictable result.

5.2.2.1 Oncoplastic Mastopexy with the Ptotic Breast

Oncoplastic surgery in a ptotic breast includes the oncologic resection and reshaping of the breast with local tissue transposition and excess skin resection. Planning is essential. The following

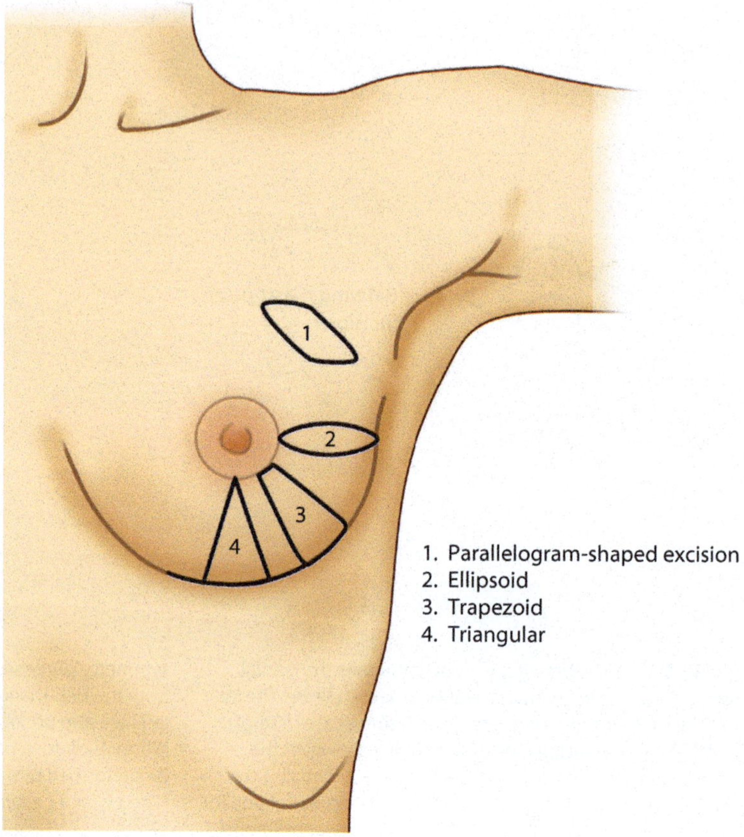

Fig. 5.2 Possible incisions for BCT or oncoplastic surgery. The parallelogram-shaped excision reduces distortions of the NAC with a longer scar. Other excisions are elliptical, trapezoid or triangular shaped, if necessary combined with periareolar and IMF incisions to reshape the skin

questions have to be answered prior to surgery: Where is the tumour located? How much tissue has to be removed? Is a local transposition sufficient or is a flap needed? If a local transposition is sufficient, the tumour resection and the resection pattern should be marked. The pedicles for the NAC and the breast as well as the pedicle for the local transposition to fill the defect are also marked. Although the mastopexy should lead to an aesthetic outcome, new NAC position and nipple-IMF distance should allow a tension-free closure. A moderate ptosis is better tolerated than a wound breakdown that prolongs further oncologic treatment.

In many cases it is better to separate the pedicles in oncoplastic surgery: one pedicle for the breast and the NAC and one pedicle for the volume that fills the defect. This allows more flexible shaping. In some cases a common pedicle for both purposes is used. An extended superomedial pedicle can, for example, fill lateral defects.

The superior-medial or superior-central pedicle is a standard technique for a tumour resection in the lateral upper breast pole. The tissue that fills a defect in the upper lateral pole can be pedicled inferiorly (e.g. Ribeiro technique) or centrally (Fig. 5.3 and 5.4, Table 5.1).

5.2.2.2 Oncoplastic Reduction in Large Breasts

In large and ptotic breasts, the same transposition can take place. However if the breast is large and a reduction is planned, it is easier to perform the tumour resection with wide margins and then reshape the breast with a reduction (Figs. 5.5, 5.6 and 5.7). This works with almost all tumour locations within the breast.

Especially after resection in the upper lateral pole where most carcinomas are encountered, reduction is best performed with a superior-medial or central pedicle. If a dent or defect develops, it can be filled with an inferior flap according to Ribeiro. The flap is perfused from the inferior part of the breast, which is normally resected in a reduction. The inferior and intercostal vessels

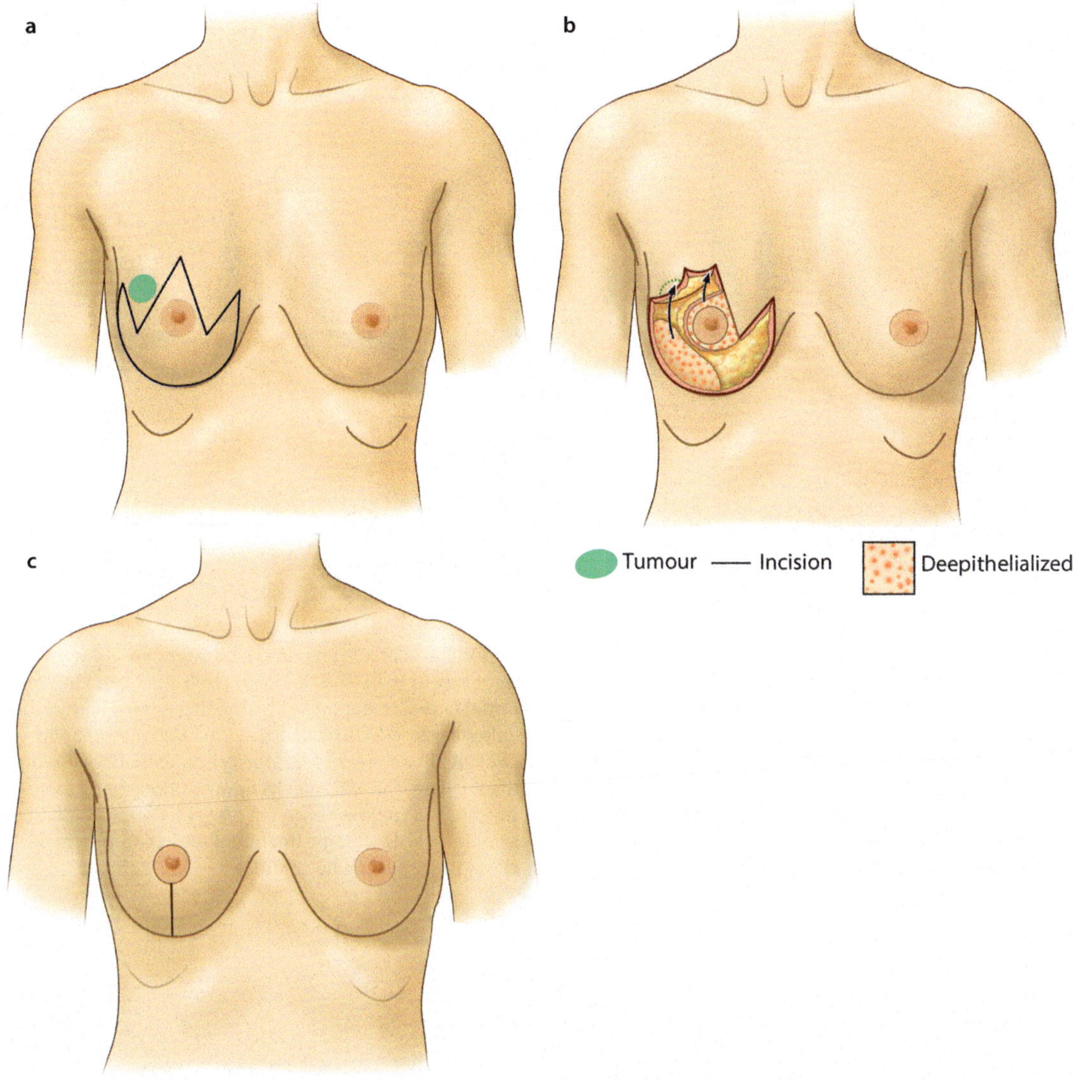

Fig. 5.3 **a–c** Besides oncologic safe resection volume displacement and resection of excess skin are the techniques of choice in ptotic breasts. This example shows an upper lateral tumour. **a** No skin resection above the tumour is necessary. The NAC is pedicled centrally/superiomedially. The volume to fill the defect comes from an inferior pedicle (e.g. Ribeiro flap, **b**) or from an extended central pedicle. This results in a mastopexy figure of an inverse T(C). Cavities or distortions of the NAC are avoided; the scars are usually good

usually safely perfuse the transposition flap. If the skin has to be resected, alternative incision patterns have to be used (Fig. 5.8). For symmetry the contralateral side has to be included.

5.2.3 Local and Free Flaps

Partial mastectomy defects can be filled with local transposition from the breast itself, local flaps or free flaps. These techniques are the same like in complete or partial mastectomy defects (see ▶ Chaps. 10 and 11.). Especially in small breast with a larger tumour, local transposition might be insufficient to create an aesthetic breast shape. One should discuss if from an oncological or aesthetic point of view a complete mastectomy is to be preferred over a partial resection, which requires a radiation therapy. Complete mastectomies are best treated with free flaps or if applicable implant reconstruction.

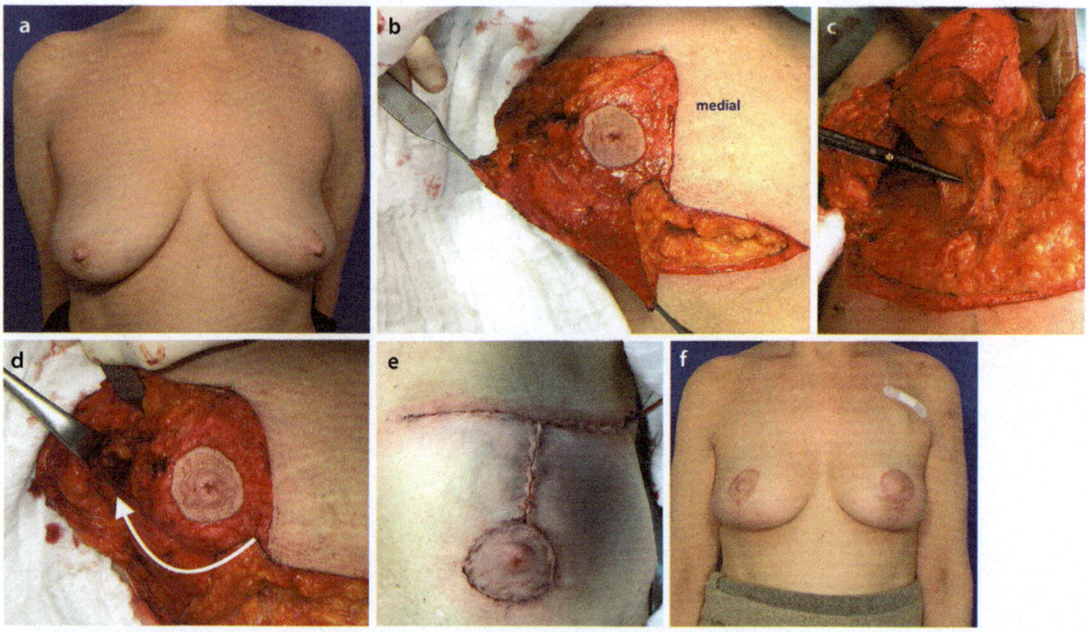

Fig. 5.4 **a** 2.4 cm invasive carcinoma, the right upper lateral breast pole; slight asymmetry and nipple-jugular notch distance of 27 cm. Planned oncoplastic resection with a bilateral inverse T-resection and mastopexy. **b** The tumour is resected with wide margins. Reduction and mastopexy are planned. The NAC is pedicled superiorly and centrally. The caudal parts are deepithelialized. **c** The central pedicle from the Würinger septum is demonstrated and left intact (scissors). The cavity from tumour resection is seen in the background. **d** The breast is rotated (arrow). The caudal part fills the defect in the upper lateral resection cavity. The flap is fixed with resorbable sutures. **e** Closure like in a reduction mammaplasty. **f** Result after 4 weeks. Mastopexy and reduction also on the left side. The NAC is in its new position; no distortion and no volume deficit are present. Breast shape is symmetrical. Oncologic treatment (radiation treatment, chemotherapy) can be continued

Table 5.1 Possible pedicles in oncologic reductions and mastopexies

Tumour location	Pedicle for NAC and breast	Pedicle to fill the defect
Upper lateral	Superior/medial or central	Inferior
Lower lateral	Superior/medial or central	Central or extended superior-medial pedicle
Central	Superior or inferior, NAC resection when indicated	Superior or inferior
Upper medial	Central, superior, inferior	Inferior, central
Lower medial	Superior, central	Inferior/lateral, central

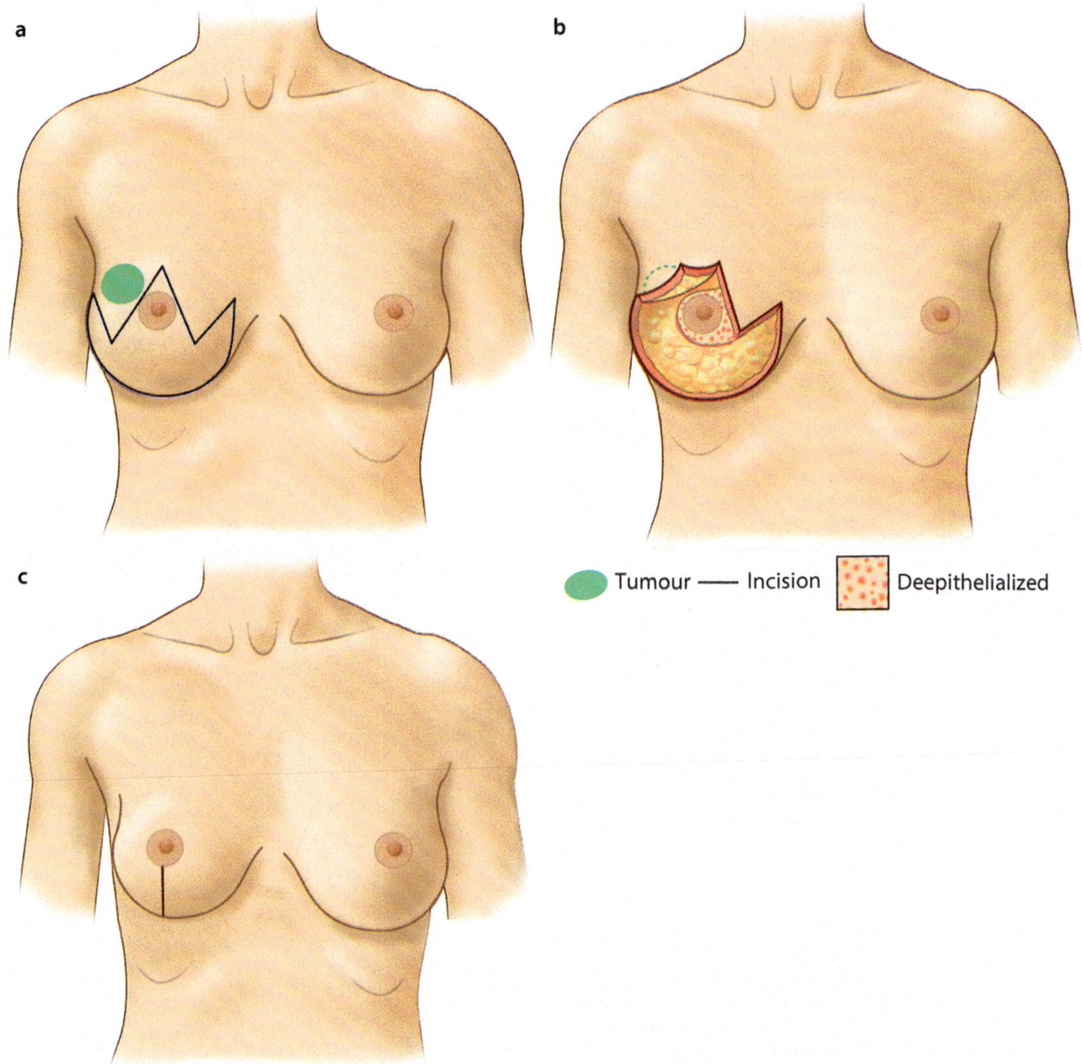

Fig. 5.5 In a large breast, the same principles like in ptotic breast can be applied. This example shows a tumour in the upper lateral pole. **a** No skin resection above the tumour. The NAC is pedicled centrally/superiomedially. As the breast is reduced, the upper lateral pole is completely resected, and no volume displacement is necessary. **b** Additional resections follow the patient's desire. This results in a mastopexy figure of an inverse T(C). Cavities or distortions of the NAC are avoided; the scars are usually good

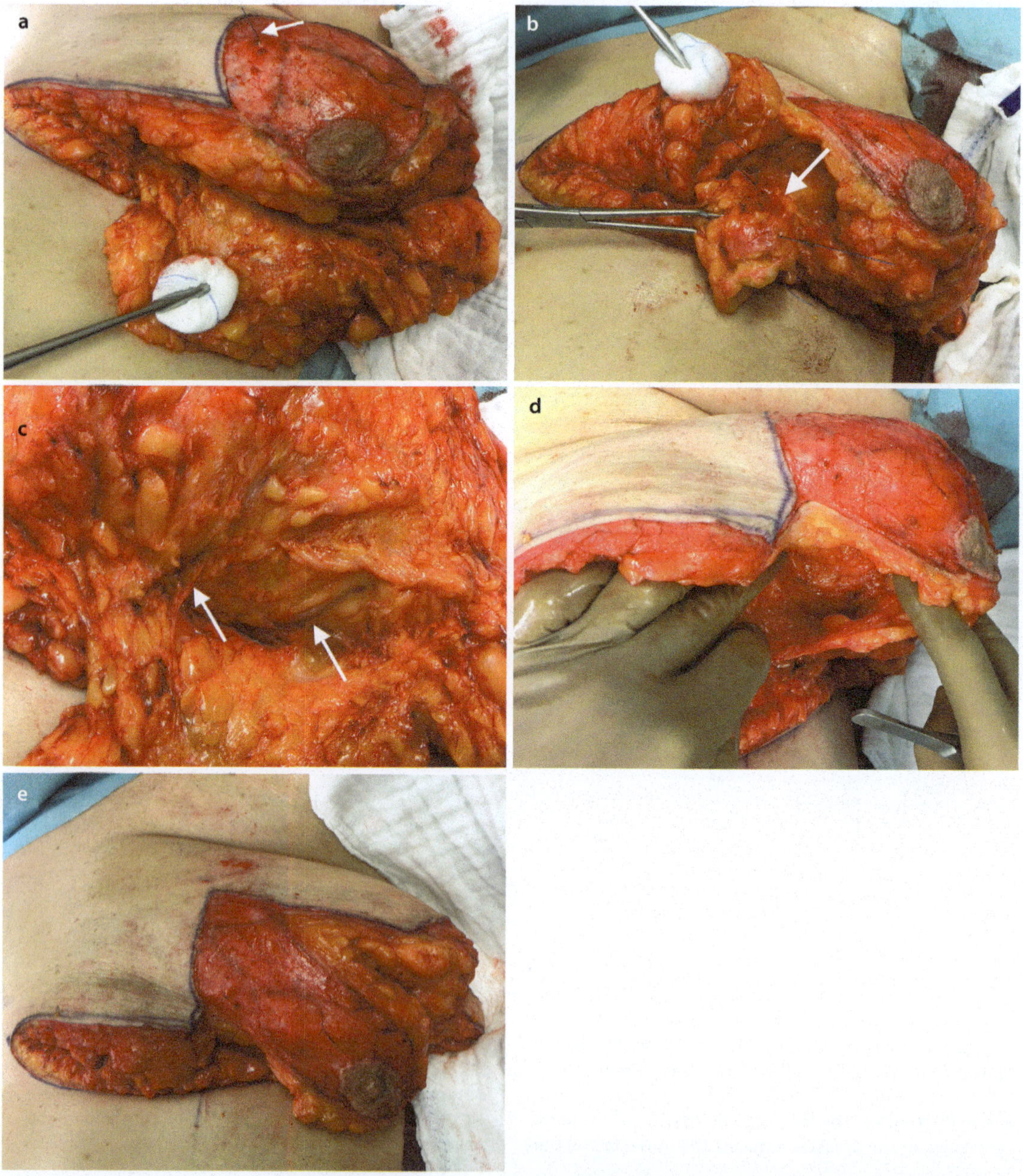

Fig. 5.6 **a** Intraoperative example of an oncoplastic resection left. A reduction and mastopexy are planned. The tumour is centrally located and marked with a wire (arrow). The NAC is pedicled centrally and superiomedially. The caudal parts are not used and just resected. **b** Resection with wire and topographic marking. **c** The arrows show the vessels of the Würinger septum, which was left intact. **d** The resection results in a central defect. The septum is seen in the hand of the surgeon. **e** Before closure, the NAC is safely perfused and placed cranially

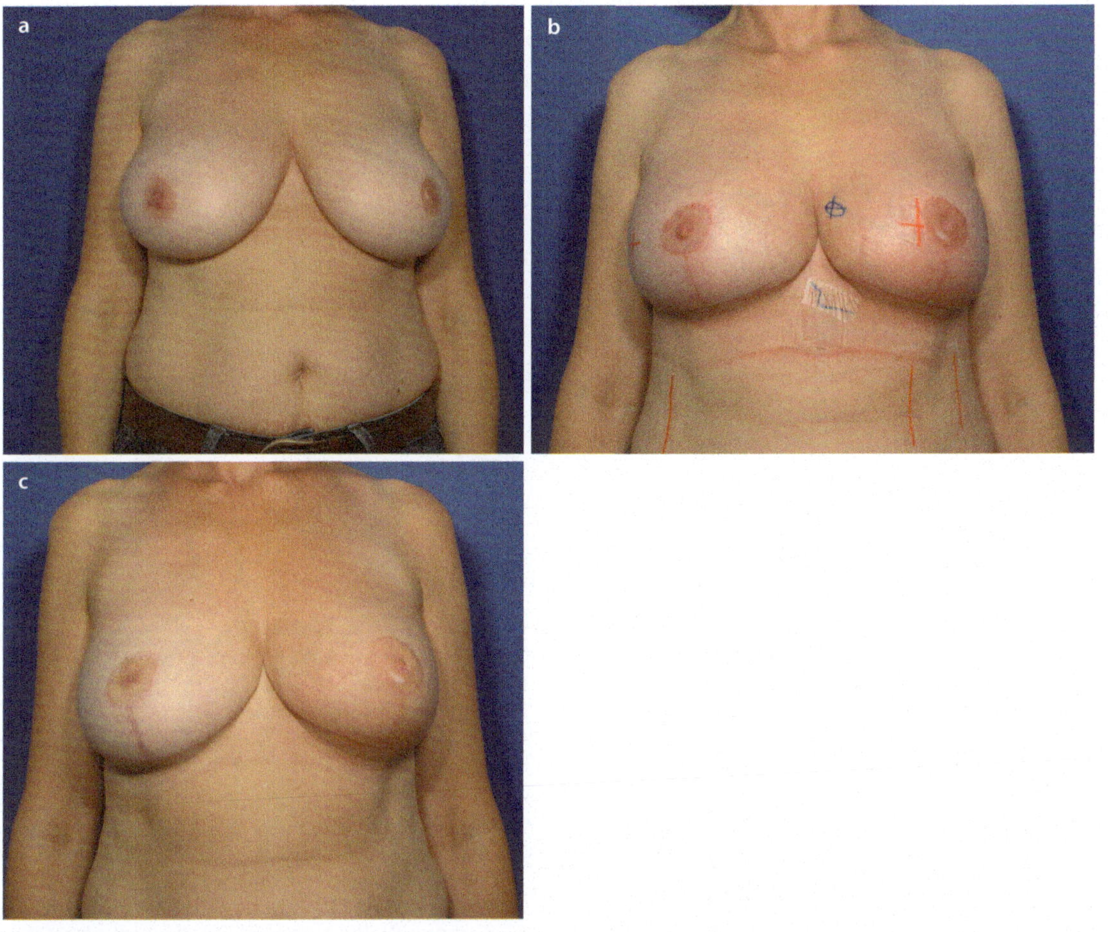

Fig. 5.7 **a** Patient with breast cancer, left side. Oncoplastic resection. **b** Radiation therapy; **c** immediately after radiation has finished

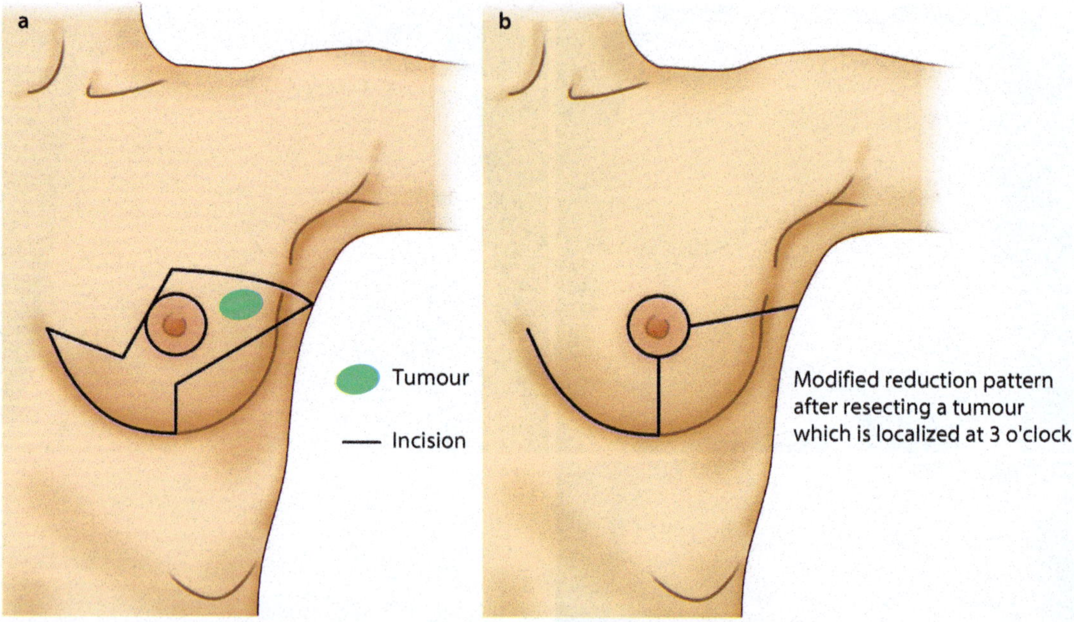

Fig. 5.8 **a** Modified reduction according to Silverstein (2014). If the skin has to be resected above the lateral pole, the reduction is not possible with an inverted T-pattern. **b** The lateral IMF incision is therefore transferred in transverse horizontal scar. The pedicle for the NAC is central or superiomedial

5

Defects after resection of a tumour can be filled with local tissue from the breast (*volume displacement*) or local/free flaps (*volume replacement*). Oncoplastic surgery is well applied in large and/or ptotic breasts where a reduction or mastopexy pattern can be used to reshape the breast. The contralateral side should always be included in this concept of symmetry.

Literature

1. Anderson BO, Masetti R, Silverstein MJ. Oncoplastic approaches to partial mastectomy: an overview of volume-displacement techniques. Lancet Oncol. 2005;6:145–57.
2. Hamdi M. Oncoplastic and reconstructive surgery of the breast. Breast. 2013;22(Suppl 2):S100–5.
3. Losken A, Hart AM, Broecker JS, Styblo TM, Carlson GW. Oncoplastic breast reduction technique and outcomes: an evolution over 20 years. Plast Reconstr Surg. 2017a;139:824e–33e.
4. Losken A, Hart AM, Chatterjee A. Updated evidence on the Oncoplastic approach to breast conservation therapy. Plast Reconstr Surg. 2017b;140(5S Advances in Breast Reconstruction):14S–22S.
5. Losken A, Hart AM, Dutton JW, Broecker JS, Styblo TM, Carlson GW. The expanded use of autoaugmentation techniques in Oncoplastic breast surgery. Plast Reconstr Surg. 2018;141:10–9.
6. Nahabedian M. Oncoplastic surgery of the breast. Philadelphia: Saunders; 2009.
7. Ribeiro L, Accorsi A Jr, Buss A, Marcal-Pessoa M. Creation and evolution of 30 years of the inferior pedicle in reduction mammaplasties. Plast Reconstr Surg. 2002;110:960–70.
8. Silverstein MJ, Mai T, Savalia N, Vaince F, Guerra L. Oncoplastic breast conservation surgery: the new paradigm. J Surg Oncol. 2014;110:82–9.
9. Tong WM, Baumann DP, Villa MT, Mittendorf EA, Liu J, Robb GL, Kronowitz SJ, Garvey PB. Obese women experience fewer complications after Oncoplastic breast repair following partial mastectomy than after immediate total breast reconstruction. Plast Reconstr Surg. 2016;137:777–91.

Sentinel Lymph Node and Axillary Dissection

H. Fansa, C. Heitmann, *Breast Reconstruction with Autologous Tissue*,
https://doi.org/10.1007/978-3-319-95468-4_6

The removal of axillary lymph nodes is nowadays used more for the diagnosis and initiation of adjuvant measures. Surgical therapy can only be one of many approaches to lymph node infiltration caused by cancer. Since the removal of axillary lymph nodes can lead to high morbidity and ultimately the survival rate is not improved by an aggressive lymph node dissection, the removal of sentinel lymph nodes has become popular. The sentinel lymph node (SLN) is the lymph node that is the first filter station in the drainage of the breast. If the lymph node is tumour-free, no further measures are necessary. If the lymph node is affected by macrometastasis, axillary dissection should take place as a follow-up intervention. The frozen section test has proven to be sufficiently safe in our hands. After frozen section examination, the axillary dissection can be performed in the same procedure in case of infiltration. If a frozen section examination is not possible or if a metastasis appears later in the workup, the axillary dissection must be carried out in a second operation. Isolated tumour cells and micrometastases in the SLN are not an indication for axillary lymphadenectomy.

6.1 Anatomy

The breast lymphatic fluid drains significantly into the axillary lymph nodes. Only a few paths lead primarily to the internal mammary station. The axilla is bounded at the anterior margin by the pectoral muscle and dorsally by the latissimus muscle. In the depth lie the rib cage and the anterior serratus muscle. The cranial boundary is the axillary vein. This makes the axilla a three-sided pyramid. The lymph node pad is divided by the minor pectoral muscle into its levels (see ▶ Chap. 1.4).

The sentinel concept is based on the fact that the lymph drainage of a region is usually filtered at one first lymph node or a smaller group. If cancer cells migrate through the lymphatics, they are likely to travel this way. In recent years, this concept has successfully established itself for a number of carcinomas. If the lymph node is affected, it can no longer perform its filtering function after a certain tumour size. In these cases, a bypass circuit is formed for the lymph. If an SLN is then removed, it can be false negative.

6.2 Indication

If the clinical and radiological examination of the axilla is inconspicuous in a malignant tumour of the breast, the indication for SLN removal is given. In the case of a suspicious lymph node, a punch biopsy can also be performed primarily for histological clarification, if this is anatomically possible. The current German guidelines provide for SLN removal in DCIS only if subsequent SLN removal is no longer possible, e.g. in the case of mastectomy or in the outer upper quadrant. There is an increased risk aft lymph node infiltration in palpable lesions or tumours larger than 4 cm. If an invasive lesion is found in the breast preparation during histological processing, SLN can be removed later. In small carcinomas with a good prognosis and subsequent percutaneous irradiation via tangential opposing fields (tangential irradiation), it is discussed not to perform axillary dissection if one or two sentinel lymph nodes are affected.

In the case of radiologically or clinically visible infestation, SLN removal is currently contraindicated. Axillary lymphadenectomy is required here. In the case of unclear tumours for which a histological diagnosis has not yet been made but which are classified as suspected malignant, SLN marking can be performed preoperatively. If the tumour is then classified as malignant, SLN can be removed in the same operation.

Patients with distant metastasis do not require axillary lymph node removal as a staging measure.

6.2.1 Sentinel and Neoadjuvant Chemotherapy

If the patient receives primary chemotherapy due to tumour biology before surgery and if the axilla is clinically and radiologically unremarkable, SLN removal after chemotherapy should be performed according to the current guideline. Patients with a clinically positive nodal status after chemotherapy should undergo axillary dissection. The same applies to patients who still have positive nodal status even after primary chemotherapy.

6.3 Marking of the Sentinel

Currently, the SLN is labelled with a blue dye or with metastable technetium-99 (99mTc) in nuclear medicine. The 99mTc has proven itself in our setting. The technetium has a half-life of 6 h and emits gamma radiation. It is applied to the skin near the tumour on the evening before or on the day of the operation. The SLN or possible accompanying lymph nodes are marked after finding them in the axilla with a pen. In the operating room, a gamma probe can be used to locate and mark the lymph nodes. It is important to measure its activity and the residual activity of the axilla after the removal of the SLN to ensure that it is the correct lymph node. If no lymph node is detected in the axilla after sentinel marking, axial dissection is usually necessary. A different therapy should be discussed with the patient in any case.

A newer technique is the visualization of the SLN with indocyanine green. However, this form is not yet widely used.

6.4 Informed Consent

The disclosure of general and special risks should be documented with standardized and evaluated forms. Infection, haematoma and wound-healing complications can occur in rare cases. In most cases, SLN is removed together with the tumour or a mastectomy, so that everything can be clarified together. If an axillary dissection is performed in the same operation, this can also be clarified. It is advisable to determine the incision in advance with the patient and, if necessary, to point out oncological necessities. SLN removal can also produce lymphatic fluid/seroma that may need to be punctured. Scarring in the axilla can lead to later pain. Newly formed lymph channels can also cause palpable and visible strands. These usually heal without consequences after physiotherapeutic treatment but irritate the patients. Numbness is possible after injury or scarring of the intercostobrachial nerves on the upper arm and the axilla. Lymph congestion and later oedema in the arm, chest and thoracic wall can also occur in rare cases during SLN removal. In axillary lymphadenectomy the rate is higher than in sentinel.

If an axillary dissection is planned later in the case of infiltration of the SLN, this should also be fixed. According to the German guidelines, in the case of small carcinomas with a good prognosis and subsequent percutaneous irradiation via tangential opposing fields (tangential irradiation), axillary dissection should be dispensed with if one or two sentinel lymph nodes are affected. The advantages and disadvantages of this approach should be discussed based on guidelines and recorded in writing. It is also important to document that any recommended interventions are not desired.

6.5 Surgery

6.5.1 Preoperative Markings

If a separate incision is planned, the marking should be made on the patient with a 90° abducted arm. The incision should be above the marked SLN, following the axillary relaxed skin tension lines. Thus, the incision is usually perpendicular to the pectoralis muscle between pectoralis and latissimus in the caudal axilla. Usually an incision of 3–4 cm is sufficient. In obese patients, a longer incision must be made. The incision can be extended for the axillary dissection, lengthwise, or at a 90° angle to the incision at the anterior edge of the axilla.

6.5.2 Position

Before the patient is transferred to the OR, the team should examine if a planned marking (sentinel or wire marking) has taken place sufficiently and all findings are available.

General anaesthesia is recommended. The patient is placed supine; arms are abducted by 90° in the shoulder, allowing access to the breast and axilla. If an intraoperative change to a sitting position is mandatory, then the arms should be adducted by 45–30° in the shoulder. The elbows are placed on little arm pads, and the hands are placed under the lumbar region. In a two-team approach when both breasts are operated simultaneously, two electrosurgery devices with two electrodes are required. The patients' body temperature can be managed with a convective warming device (e.g. Bair Hugger).

6.5.3 Sentinel Surgery

In the case of BCT or mastectomies of tumours located in the upper outer pole of the breast, SLN removal can usually be performed using the same incision. An assistant can allow the way to the axilla using longer Langenbeck hooks. Longer instruments are important here. In the axilla, the dissection should be done with scissors (Metzenbaum) and bipolar forceps.

A separate incision should follow the SLN mark on the skin. Usually the SLN are in level 1 or 2 of the axilla, near the breast, rarely in the direction of the axillary vein. First, the axillary fascia must be opened sharply. Then you immediately notice the different, i.e. softer tissue consistency. As soon as you are in the axilla, the structures should be exposed and wound margins lifted up with a hook or a retractor. With the gamma probe, you can now search the axilla and find the direction of the SLN. This is naturally easier with thinner patients than with obese patients. Frequently, even if no tumour is found in the SLN, swelling of the SLN occurs due to the preceding punch, marking, etc., so that it is usually also palpable and visible. If the SLN is more likely to be found in the depth of the axilla, it is best to dissect by spreading with the branches of the scissors. Visible vessels that can tear or obstruct the path should always be bipolar coagulated. If possible, the lateral thoracic arteries and the thoracodorsal vessels should be protected. The accompanying thoracodorsal nerve should also be preserved. At the "bottom" of the axilla, the long thoracic nerve runs on the anterior serratus muscle, where it innervates. This nerve is also to be spared. Small nerves, the so-called intercostobrachial nerves, run transversely. These provide sensitivity to the axilla and the inner upper arm. If possible, these nerves should be preserved, as the loss of sensitivity is perceived as disturbing by many patients. Visible lymph vessels that do not obstruct the preparation should be protected.

Once the SLN has been found and identified with the probe, it can be removed bluntly, with scissors and bipolar forceps. The SLN should be grasped with one hand with an instrument that does not squeeze it (e.g. with a Museux forceps, or an Overholt forceps placed below the SLN), and with the other hand, the node is resected with the scissors and a proactive coagulation. If further lymph nodes stick to the SLN, they should also be removed if there is a suspicion. It is important to control the SLN and the dissected axilla with the probe so that the SLN can be clearly identified. The probe counts should be documented. The SLN can then be sent to histopathological examination. If additional lymph nodes are removed, they should be sent in separately.

A Redon drain can be inserted but is usually not necessary for SLN removal. The fascia of the axilla can be closed with an absorbable suture. The skin is closed in several layers as usual.

6.5.4 Axillary Lymph Node Dissection

If axillary lymphadenectomy is indicated, it can be performed directly. If possible, it is done through the incision of the breast. Otherwise, the pre-existing incision is used and extended if necessary. The measures to protect the axillary structures as with SNL removal must be observed. The German guidelines currently recommend the removal of ten lymph nodes from level 1 and level 2, whereby the lymph nodes can also be removed according to size and palpation. If an invasive procedure has taken place in advance, e.g. a punch biopsy, the lymph nodes may already have been reactively enlarged. It is important to preserve existing lymph collectors in the axilla and especially towards the axillary vein if possible in order to reduce the risk of arm oedema.

In the normal procedure, the lateral margin of the pectoral muscle is exposed. After the nerve bundle of the lateral pectoral nerve has been protected, the axillary vein is identified. The thoracodorsal bundle is also spared. The preparation of the axillary fat body is performed craniomedially (from medial border of the pectoralis minor – level 2) to caudal and lateral. The fatty tissue between the major and minor pectoral muscles is also resected, as is the fatty tissue up to the latissimus dorsi and subscapular muscles. The intercostobrachial nerves should be spared. If axillary dissection is limited to level 1 and 2 lymph nodes, consequences of axillary dissection such as pain, loss of sensitivity and upper limb lymphedema can be greatly reduced. Drainage is often necessary.

6.5.5 Isolated Metastases

Isolated metastases in the axilla can also occur after years, depending on the tumour biology. Imaging diagnostics are necessary in advance. From a surgical point of view, a CT-scan is usually more informative, as it can evaluate the involvement of the arm vessels and nerves. If there is an indication to remove isolated metastases in the axilla, the same incisions can be used. As a rule, these metastases continue on lymphatic routes to cranial. This surgical therapy can only be curative in rare cases and always requires accompanying therapies, such as anti-hormonal, chemotherapeutic and radiation measures, depending on the type and extent of the tumour.

With axillary metastases there is always the danger of injury to the vessels and nerves in the axilla, which can also be infiltrated. An injury of the axillary vein is always difficult to manage and requires vascular surgery. Resection of the axillary vein is only possible in emergencies and with sufficient collateralization. Resection of nerves of the arm plexus is usually associated with a high morbidity and often not curative. It can only make sense if other measures are not appropriate.

6.5.6 After-Treatment

Patients can get up immediately and are mobile. The arm can also be moved normally, but should not be subjected to excessive strain. If SLN is removed together with BCT or mastectomy, thromboprophylaxis is recommended. Drains can be removed according to the amount of drainage. A bra may be necessary depending on the extent of the procedure.

Sports activities, professional and everyday efforts beyond the normal extent as well as sauna and solarium visits depend on the main intervention.

6.5.7 Complications

The surgical complication rate is low if the procedure is carried out properly. Acute smaller hematomas can be tolerated; larger hematomas that cause pain, impair the aesthetic outcome or cause severe blood loss require revision.

Acute infections usually manifest after 2–3 days with the classic indicators. The incision is red; the axilla swells up. Lab work shows increased leucocytes and CRP. A wound swab and a surgical revision are necessary.

Chronic infection and seroma cause redness and delayed wound healing. Lymphorrhea caused by the procedure can maintain such a situation. In many cases local antiseptic treatment, punctures and systemic antibiotic treatment can support healing. A protein-rich diet and immobilization of the arm may reduce lymphorrhea. It becomes difficult when the chemotherapy has already started. Usually the healing process is then slowed down and protracted.

Injuries or *scarring* of the intercostobrachial nerves can cause numbness in the axilla and upper arm. Injuries to the thoracodorsal nerve paralyse the latissimus dorsi muscle; injuries to the long thoracic nerve lead to a winged scapula. If the axillary vein is injured, severe bleeding occurs. Vascular surgery is necessary here.

Lymph congestion/oedema in the arm can rarely occur after SLN removal and somewhat more frequently after axillary dissection. The rates vary between 9% and 37% and are probably also dependent on the respective accompanying therapies, such as chemotherapy and radiation, which can contribute to congestion through scarring and healing impairment of lymphangioneogenesis. Most lymphatic congestions can be treated well with lymph drainage. If chronic lymphedema develops, the possibility of surgery (lymph node transplantation or lymphovenous anastomosis) should be discussed in addition to classical decompression and physical decongestion therapy.

6.5.8 Re-sentinel

After BCT, a recurrence or a new disease, a new SLN removal may be necessary. A success rate of more than 90% was reported here.

Literature

1. Bromham N, Schmidt-Hansen M, Astin M, Hasler E, Reed MW. Axillary treatment for operable primary breast cancer. Cochrane Database Syst Rev. 2017;1: CD004561. https://doi.org/10.1002/14651858.

2. Crane-Okada R, Wascher RA, Elashoff D, Giuliano AE. Long-term morbidity of sentinel node biopsy versus complete axillary dissection for unilateral breast cancer. Ann Surg Oncol. 2008;15:1996–2005.
3. Del Bianco P, Zavagno G, Burelli P, Scalco G, Barutta L, Carraro P, Pietrarota P, Meneghini G, Morbin T, Tacchetti G, Pecoraro P, Belardinelli V, De Salvo GL. GIVOM Morbidity comparison of sentinel lymph node biopsy versus conventional axillary lymph node dissection for Breast cancer patients: results of the sentinella-GIVOM Italian randomised clinical trial. Eur J Surg Oncol. 2008;34:508–13.
4. Fleissig A, Fallowfield LJ, Langridge CI, Johnson L, Newcombe RG, Dixon JM, Kissin M, Mansel RE. Post-operative arm morbidity and quality of life. Results of the ALMANAC randomised trial comparing sentinel node biopsy with standard axillary treatment in the management of patients with early breast cancer. Breast Cancer Res Treat. 2006;95:279–93.
5. Giuliano AE, McCall L, Beitsch P, Whitworth PW, Blumencranz P, Leitch AM, Saha S, Hunt KK, Morrow M, Ballman K. Locoregional recurrence after sentinel lymph node dissection with or without axillary dissection in patients with sentinel lymph node metastases: the American College of Surgeons Oncology Group Z0011 randomized trial. Ann Surg. 2010;252:426–32.
6. Giuliano AE, Ballman KV, McCall L, Beitsch PD, Brennan MB, Kelemen PR, Ollila DW, Hansen NM, Whitworth PW, Blumencranz PW, Leitch AM, Saha S, Hunt KK, Morrow M. Effect of axillary dissection vs no axillary dissection on 10-year overall survival among women with invasive breast cancer and sentinel node metastasis: the ACOSOG Z0011 (alliance) randomized clinical trial. JAMA. 2017;318:918–26.
7. Intra M, Viale G, Vila J, Grana CM, Toesca A, Gentilini O, Galimberti V, Veronesi P, Luini A, Rotmensz N, Bagnardi V, Mattar D, Colleoni M. Second axillary sentinel lymph node biopsy for breast tumour recurrence: experience of the European Institute of Oncology. Ann Surg Oncol. 2015;22:2372–7.
8. Janni W, Kühn T, Schwentner L, Kreienberg R, Fehm T, Wöckel A. Sentinel node biopsy and axillary dissection in breast cancer: the evidence and its limits. Dtsch Arztebl Int. 2014;111:244–9.
9. Kuehn T, Bauerfeind I, Fehm T, Fleige B, Hausschild M, Helms G, Lebeau A, Liedtke C, von Minckwitz G, Nekljudova V, Schmatloch S, Schrenk P, Staebler A, Untch M. Sentinel-lymph-node biopsy in patients with breast cancer before and after neoadjuvant chemotherapy (SENTINA): a prospective, multicentre cohort study. Lancet Oncol. 2013;14:609–18.
10. Krag DN, Anderson SJ, Julian TB, Brown AM, Harlow SP, Costantino JP, Ashikaga T, Weaver DL, Mamounas EP, Jalovec LM, Frazier TG, Noyes RD, Robidoux A, Scarth HM, Wolmark N. Sentinel-lymph-node resection compared with conventional axillary-lymph-node dissection in clinically node-negative patients with breast cancer: overall survival findings from the NSABP B-32 randomised phase 3 trial. Lancet Oncol. 2010;11:927–33.
11. Russo L, Betancourt L, Romero G, Godoy A, Bergamo L, Delgado R, Ruiz Á, Gutiérrez M, Salas E, Puzzi M. Frozen section evaluation of sentinel lymph nodes in breast carcinoma: a retrospective analysis. Ecancermedicalscience. 2017;11:774. https://doi.org/10.3332/ecancer.2017.774.
12. Tucker NS, Cyr AE, Ademuyiwa FO, Tabchy A, George K, Sharma PK, Jin LX, Sanati S, Aft R, Gao F, Margenthaler JA, Gillanders WE. Axillary ultrasound accurately excludes clinically significant lymph node disease in patients with early stage breast cancer. Ann Surg. 2016;264:1098–102.
13. Zuber M, Oertli D, Marti WR, Kocher T, Wildisen A, Berclaz G, Köchli OR, Harder F. Für die Arbeitsgruppe FMH Guideline Mammakarzinom. FMH Guideline. Axillachirurgie beim Mammakarzinom Schweiz Ärztezeitung. 2003;84:1967–73.

Mastectomy

H. Fansa, C. Heitmann, *Breast Reconstruction with Autologous Tissue*,
https://doi.org/10.1007/978-3-319-95468-4_7

Mastectomy has become less invasive. The radical mastectomy published by William Halsted in1894 included resection of skin, gland, the pectoral muscles and axillary lymph nodes en bloc. This approach was partially due to the late and extensive stages of the disease. Nowadays most mastectomies are performed as nipple-sparing mastectomies (NSM), leaving the skin and the nipple intact. It was shown that the risk for recurrence is not much increased in the right indications. Skin- and nipple-sparing mastectomies (SSM and NSM) have shifted the paradigm in breast reconstruction. Leaving the skin intact requires a primary reconstruction and involves the plastic surgeon early in the surgical and oncological concept.

7.1 Indication

The indication is given if a BCT is not possible or not wanted, for example, in small breasts with a large tumour, a more aggressive cancer biology or a multicentric localization. Some patients demand a mastectomy because they are afraid of a recurrence or do not want a radiation therapy.

7.2 Informed Consent

The disclosure of general and special risks should be documented with standardized and evaluated forms. Infection, hematoma and wound healing complications can occur. Seroma formation and visible scars can result. Loss of sensitivity to the breast skin and the NAC is often. A skin necrosis and NAC necrosis can occur and may require a reoperation. Smaller wound healing problems can remain conservatively treated if an autologous reconstruction is applied. A lymph oedema of the breast and thoracic wall is possible in rare cases. In most cases a reconstruction is planned too. Therefore the risks of the reconstructive procedure should also be included, as well as risks from a possible lymph node dissection (◘ Fig. 7.1). The patient should be aware that breast shape, colour and symmetry are altered. Aesthetic change can

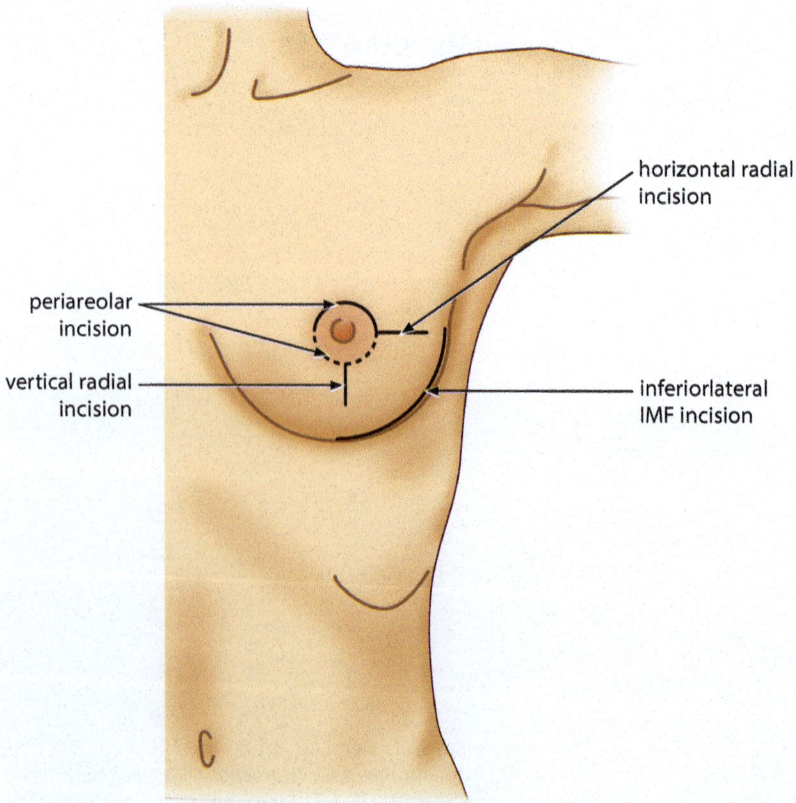

◘ **Fig. 7.1** SSM and NSM incisions can be periareolar, radial, elliptical or as an inverted T. Studies have shown that a vertical incision more often leads to nipple necrosis. Incisions in the mediolateral IMF, caudal periareolar or periareolar with extensions laterally or vertically caudal (Y-shaped) have induced less necrosis. Lateral incisions that connect to the periareolar incision can result in scarring that distorts the NAC. The breast skin should only be resected if oncologically necessary. Mastopexy techniques should always be considered in an immediate setting result in psychological problems which may require psycho-oncologic consultation.

The incisions should be visualized in a drawing. The indication for a SSM or NSM should be discussed carefully. Scarring can distort the NAC in an NSM.

Second operations should be mentioned if histopathology is unclear or wound healing problems occur. If the patient does not want recommended surgery or parts, this should also be documented.

7.3 General Information for Mastectomies

7.3.1 Preoperative Markings

The markings follow the kind of mastectomy and are made in accordance to oncologic and aesthetic aspects.

7.3.2 Position

Before the patient is transferred to the OR, the team should examine if a planned marking (sentinel or wire marking) has taken place sufficiently and all findings are available.

General anaesthesia is recommended. Only small palpable tumours which are easy accessible should be resected under local anaesthesia. The patient is placed supine, and the arms are abducted by 90° in the shoulder, allowing access to the breast and axilla. If an intraoperative change to a sitting position is mandatory, then the arms should be adducted by 45–30° in the shoulder. The elbows are placed on little arm pads and the hands are placed under the lumbar region. In a two-team approach when both breasts are operated simultaneously, two electrosurgery devices with two electrodes are required. The patients' body temperature can be managed with a convective warming device (e.g. Bair Hugger).

7.3.3 Surgery

In most cases the border between the subcutaneous and glandular tissue is well defined. The gland is whitish and firm. The fat is yellow and soft. In involutional breasts the differentiation can get difficult. Sometimes the cranial border does not allow to clearly distinguishing between fat, fascia and gland too. Mastectomy should always include the pectoral fascia. It is regarded as a safe border, which allows better histopathologic diagnostic and safer dorsal margins.

It should be taken care that the axillary part of the gland is always also removed. Glandular tissue can also be seen at the level of the IMF. Especially in preventive/prophylactic mastectomies, the safety is improved with a radical glandular resection. Haemostasis follows the anatomy and is more tedious medially, caudally and towards the axilla. Bleeding can also be more severe from the pectoral muscle and from the medial perforators of the IMA. In most cases they can be left intact to improve skin perfusion. If they are sufficient in calibre, they can also be used as recipient vessels for autologous tissue.

> **Tip**
>
> It is easier to start with the dissection between the skin and gland and then between the gland and muscle and the lateral thoracic wall. The specimen has to be marked topographically to allow proper histopathology. If permanent clips were placed during diagnostic procedures, the specimen should be radiographed before it is sent to histopathology. In cases where the tumour is not palpable within the breast, a wire localization before surgery can help the pathologist find the suspect area.

Mastectomy leaves behind a big cavity, and the skin is always impaired in terms of perfusion and sensitivity. A significant complication is skin necrosis due to impaired perfusion. Necrosis cannot always be avoided. However gentle tissue handling can reduce the problems. Avoid (1) aggressive electrocautery that causes too much heat. This leads to local tissue damage with impaired perfusion and necrosis, and it is associated with more seroma development, which in turn can impair the result. Avoid (2) sharp and inappropriate hooks, or do not exert too much tension on the hooks. Inappropriate use of hooks can lead to mastectomy flap necrosis. Avoid (3) haematoma that puts tension on the skin and in turn advance impaired perfusion. Drains are necessary in most cases.

7.3.4 Aftercare

The patients are mobile. Thromboprophylaxis is recommended. Drains should be removed with regard to the fluid amount. A mastectomy without reconstruction can require a compression dressing. A bra can be used if necessary. If a reconstruction is performed, aftercare follows the needs of the reconstruction.

Sporting, work and daily activities should not exceed the standard. Sauna and sun tanning should be avoided for about 6 weeks.

7.3.5 Complications

Complications are rare if surgery is properly performed. Little hematomas can be tolerated; larger hematomas that cause pain, impair the aesthetic outcome or cause severe blood loss require revision.

Acute infections are evident after 2–3 days. The incision is red, the surgical site swells up. Lab work show increased leucocytes and CRP. A wound swab and a surgical revision are necessary.

Chronic infection and seroma cause redness and delayed wound healing and lead to seroma or lymphatic discharge from the wound. In many cases local antiseptic treatment wound punctures and systemic antibiotic treatment can support healing. Protein-rich diet and immobilization of the arm can help to reduce seroma production. If chemotherapy has started, the healing is very slow. A surgical revision might become necessary.

Wound Healing Breakdown and Necrosis

If no reconstruction is performed, a conservative treatment can be tried. Larger defects should be revised. In special cases a local or distant flap has to be used to cover the defect. A negative-pressure wound therapy can be used for temporary treatment.

Aesthetic complications include asymmetries, dents and skin irregularities. Shrinkage of the scar can distort the position of the NAC. Radiation therapy and their sequelae can amplify the symptoms.

7.4 Skin-Sparing Mastectomy, SSM

Skin-sparing mastectomy, SSM, includes the resection of the NAC and if necessary the skin above the tumour. Many studies have shown that in most indications this technique is oncologically safe. A recent alternative therapy is a mastectomy with resection of the nipple, but leaving of the areola. There are no sufficient studies available regarding oncologic and aesthetic results regarding this technique. The SSM incisions can be periareolar, radial, elliptical or as an inverted T (Figs. 7.1 and 7.2).

If an autologous reconstruction is planned in smaller breasts, the mastectomy and NAC removal can be performed from a periareolar incision. Incision should follow the NAC diameter; however, 42 mm is necessary to perform the mastectomy and to later reconstruct the defect. The former NAC can be replaced with tissue from the flap.

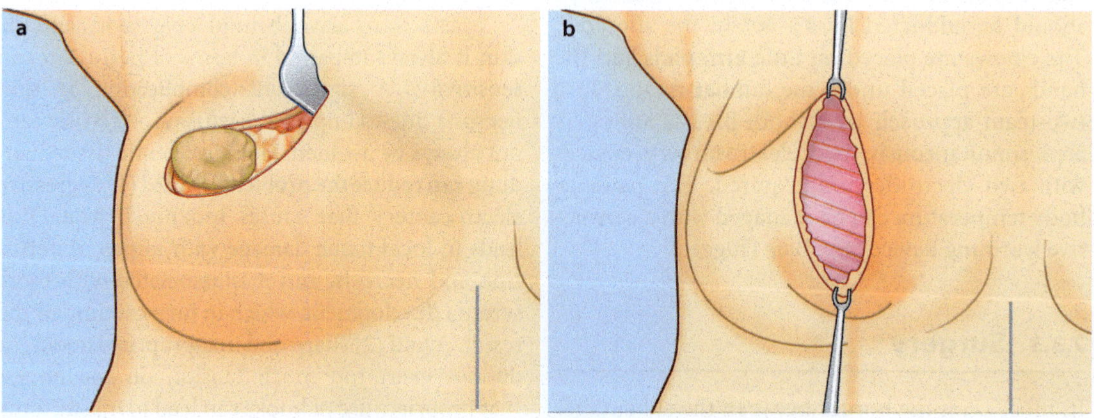

Fig. 7.2 **a** Periareolar SSM. The gland is resected together with the NAC. Gentle tissue handling reduces skin necrosis. This kind of resection is suitable for autologous reconstructions. **b** After the SSM the pectoral muscle is seen dorsally. The fascia should be removed with the gland

In larger or ptotic breasts where a reduction or mastopexy is planned, the SSM can be performed using an inverted T-pattern. The patient is marked prior to surgery in an upright position like a reduction surgery. As the skin is always thinner after mastectomy, a tension-free closure is mandatory. The vertical limbs should be long enough: if the NAC requires about 4 cm, and the areola border to IMF distance is usually 6–7 cm, the vertical limb should measure at least 10–11 cm, in larger breasts even more. The use of autoderm can improve the breast shape and facilitate reconstruction (see ► Sect. 7.6).

7.5 Nipple-Sparing and Prophylactic Mastectomy

▪▪ Oncological Aspects

Recently the NSM has shown to be a valuable technique in invasive carcinomas, DCIS and also with the prophylactic/preventive mastectomies. The entire breast skin remains intact; only the gland is resected. However glandular tissue and ducts remain within the nipple and may cause recurrence. Leaving the nipple on the other hand improves the aesthetic outcome and helps the patients psychologically.

Most studies on the oncological safety are retrospective. The risk for local recurrence is seen at 2.4% with a follow-up of 38 months. Carcinomas that are larger than 5 cm have a distance from the nipple of less than 2 cm, with a negative hormone status and positive HER2-Neu status which show a higher recurrence rate in an NSM. Multicentric or multifocal carcinomas and lympho-vascular invasion have also an unfavourable prognosis.

Regarding the safety of NSM and prophylactic mastectomies, there are only retrospective studies available with a low number of patients and a follow-up of less than 5 years. Although it is regarded safe, a cancer development cannot be excluded. Therefore the decision whether to perform a NSM or SSM should be made together with the patient.

In a NSM the gland facing the nipple should be additionally marked to allow a histopathologic examination. If cancer is evident, the NAC should be resected later on.

▪▪ Surgical Aspects

Besides the risk for a skin necrosis in a NSM, the risk for nipple necrosis is possible. Complication rates on skin necrosis are reported to occur in up to 22%. The rate of NAC necrosis is between 1% and 37.5%. Besides the psychological implications, a full-thickness nipple necrosis is difficult to manage in an implant reconstruction.

Gentle tissue handling (see above) and special incision types are helpful to prevent skin and nipple necrosis. The incision can influence the perfusion. Studies and our own experience have shown that a vertical incision more often leads to nipple necrosis. Incisions in the mediolateral IMF, caudal periareolar or periareolar with extensions laterally or vertically caudal (Y-shaped) have induced less necrosis.

▪▪ Aesthetic Aspects

Leaving the NAC gives a better aesthetic outcome if oncologically possible. Although sensitivity is reduced, patients embrace the preservation of their NAC.

Care has to be taken that mastectomy and following reconstruction does not lead to a malposition of the NAC. A fixed malposition can ruin the result. Reasons for a malposition can be wound healing problems, insufficient reconstruction, or the sequelae after radiation therapy. Capsular contracture in implant reconstruction can place the NAC too cranial (◘ Fig. 7.3). If the skin shrinks, a symmetric positioning can become difficult in a secondary procedure.

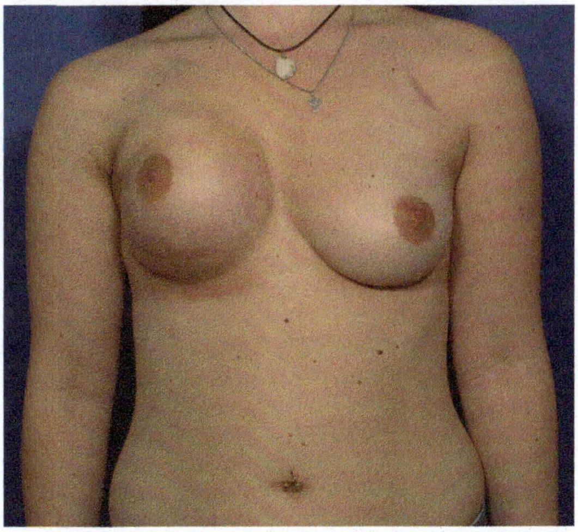

◘ **Fig. 7.3** NSM with immediate implant reconstruction and radiation therapy. Capsular contracture leads to a stone hard breast and malposition of the NAC. An immediate autologous reconstruction is more favourable, even if a radiation therapy has to be applied. A secondary conversion from implant to autologous tissue is possible and indicated, but it is not always successful in terms of lowering the nipple due to rigid skin after radiation

Depending on the incision, a SLN biopsy or axillary dissection can be performed from the same or a second incision.

Radiation Therapy

There is no standard whether after an NSM a radiation should be applied to reduce the risks of recurrence.

Specific Features

In large or ptotic breasts that should be reduced, the NSM can be made with an inverted T incision. Before the operation the patient is marked in an upright position like for a reduction operation. As the skin is always thinner after mastectomy, a tension-free closure is mandatory. The vertical limbs should be long enough: if the NAC requires about 4 cm, and the areola border to IMF distance is usually 6–7 cm, the vertical limb should measure at least 10–11 cm, in larger breasts even more. We prefer a cranial/medial pedicle for the NAC. The de-epithelialized corium should only be incised as necessary to put the NAC in the desired position.

If an impaired NAC perfusion is evident within the surgery, the pedicled NAC can be converted to a free NAC graft. This results in a total loss of sensitivity and may lead to depigmentation of the NAC. This option should be discussed prior to the operation. If the skin is not viable intraoperatively, the reconstruction can be delayed, or if autologous tissue is used, the skin can be replaced by the skin of the flap.

7.6 Mastectomy and Autoderm

In SSM and NSM of large or ptotic breasts where a reduction is planned and an inverted T-pattern is used, the caudal skin, which is resected in regular mammaplasties, is kept and de-epithelialized. The gland is resected and the subcutaneous tissue and the dermis are kept intact. This result in an inferior flap is well perfused from the caudal perforators and the axial vessels from the IMF. Bostwick has published this technique and named it *Autoderm*. Basically it resembles the caudal flap (with glandular tissue) in Ribeiro's technique of reduction mammaplasty (Fig. 7.4).

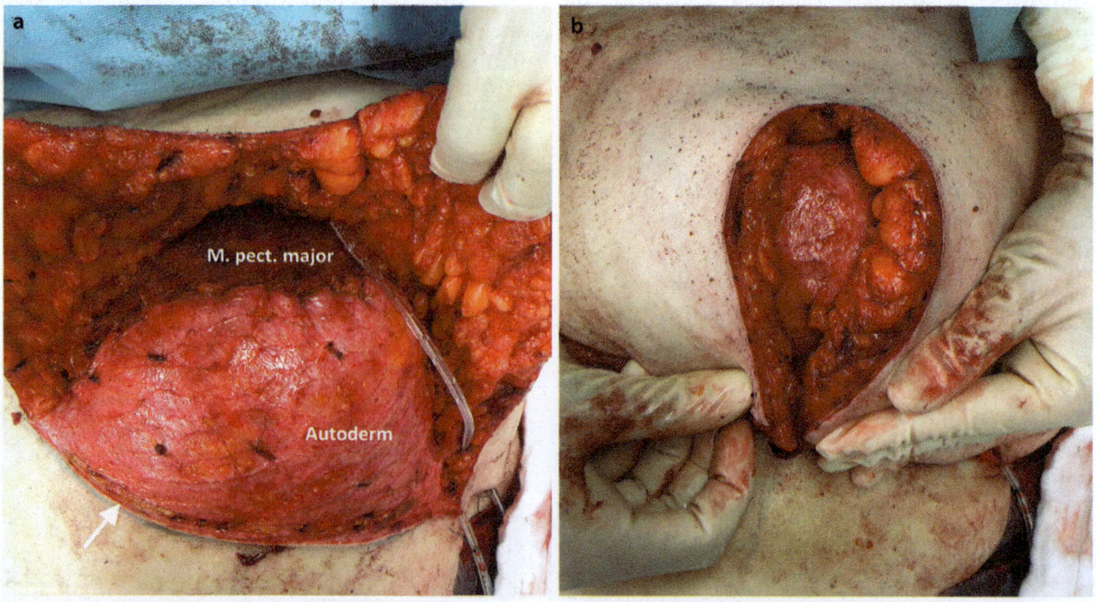

Fig. 7.4 **a** Subpectoral implant reconstruction with a caudal dermis flap (autoderm). After the inverted-T incision is marked, the lower part which is usually removed is de-epithelialized. The mastectomy follows. Here the implant is placed subpectorally, and the dermis flap is sutured against the muscle. The caudal dermis is incised along the IMF (arrow), to avoid a misplacement of the IMF. In some cases the IMF has to be fixed additionally. **b** The medial and lateral legs of the T are closed like in a mammoplasty

The caudal flap can be used to (1) stabilize a subpectoral implant. It is then sutured to the muscle. The implant is completely covered. The shape is pleasing and the closure in all layers prevent wound break down. If a wound healing complication occurs, the caudal dermis flap covers the implant. Revision surgery is reduced. But also in (2) autologous reconstructions, this technique is beneficial. The caudal flap is not sutured against the muscle but to the autologous flap. This results in an aesthetically pleasing lower pole. In case of a flap loss, the dermis flap can be used to cover a replacing implant (■ Figs. 7.5 and 7.6).

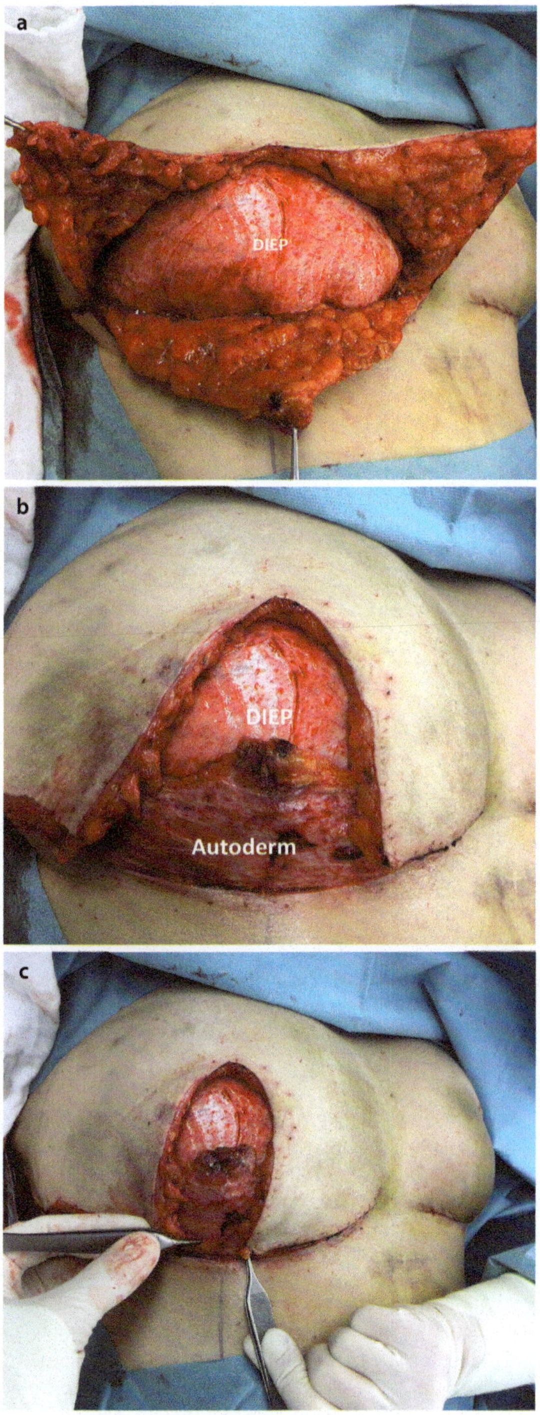

Tip

If the autoderm flap is used the IMF can be unstable. We recommend some fixation sutures to pexy the IMF in its position. Shaping and suture are improved if (only) the dermis is incised in the IMF.

7.7 Complete Mastectomy without Immediate Reconstruction

A complete mastectomy that removes the gland, skin and NAC is indicated in large or special tumours to achieve a free margin or in patients who do not want or are not suitable for a reconstruction.

The incision is usually placed transverse and follows oncologic requirements. The scar should be placed as low as possible. A visible scar in the décolleté should be avoided. The incision line should be marked with the patient in an upright position. The incision allows access to the axilla if necessary.

■ **Fig. 7.5** **a** DIEP reconstruction with a caudal dermis flap. After the inverted-T incision is marked, the lower part which is usually removed is de-epithelialized. The DIEP is placed and anastomosed. The abdominal skin is removed. The DIEP dermis shows a good perfusion. The dermis flap (autoderm) lies caudal and is **b** sutured against the DIEP flap. The lower breast pole is well shaped with that technique. The caudal dermis is incised along the IMF, to avoid a misplacement of the IMF. In some cases the IMF has to be fixed additionally. **c** The medial and lateral legs of the T are closed like in a mammoplasty

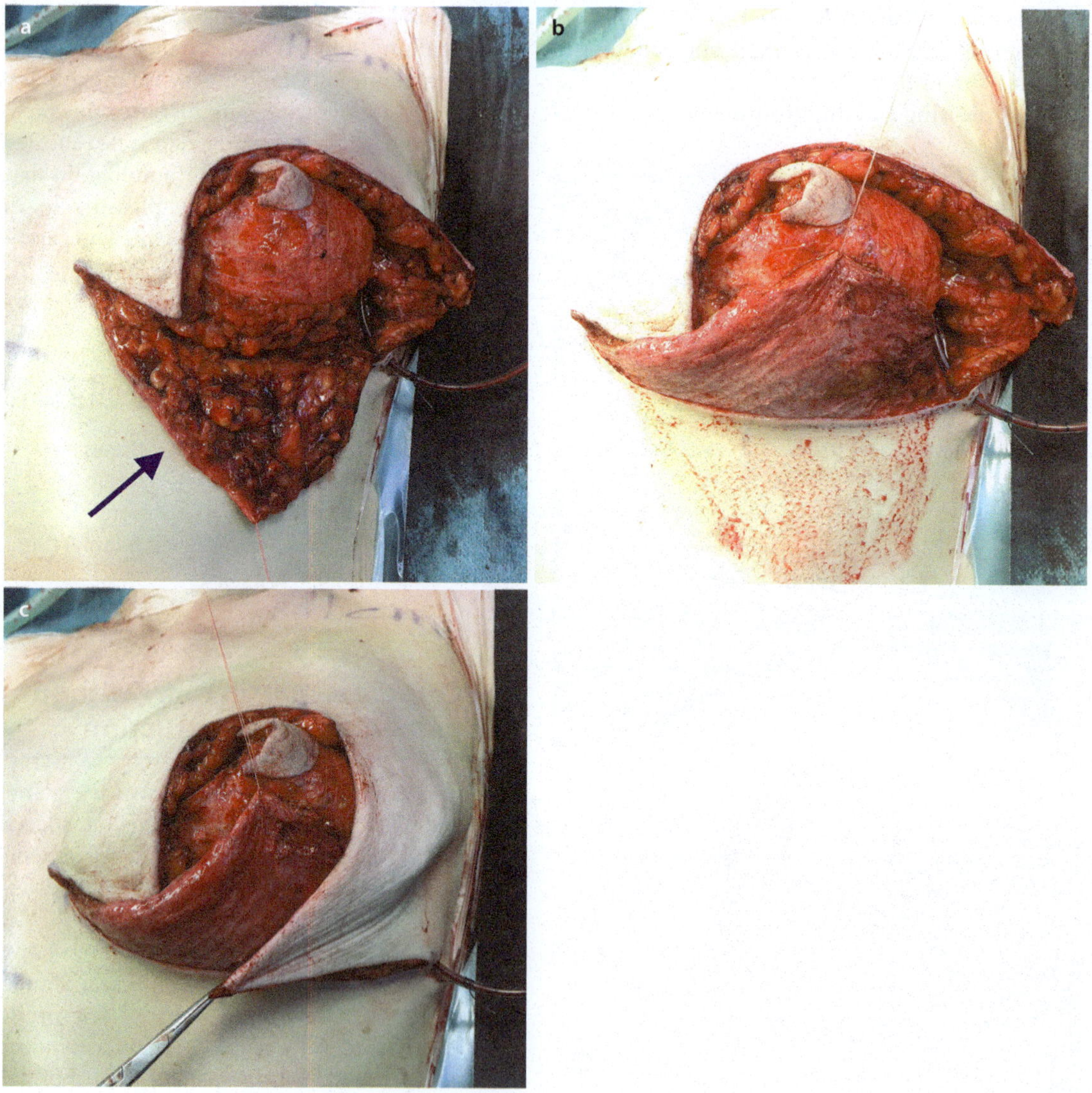

Fig. 7.6 **a** Same procedure like with a DIEP flap (Fig. 7.6), but with an upper thigh flap, also de-epithelialized. Only the skin for the nipple reconstruction is left from the flap skin. **b** The caudal dermis flap (autoderm) is marked with the suture and held upwards. **c** The medial and lateral legs of the T are closed like in a mammoplasty. Especially with the thigh flap the lower pole is better shaped with this procedure

Literature

1. Bostwick J. Prophylactic (risk-reducing) mastectomy and reconstruction. In: Plastic and reconstructive breast surgery, vol. II. St. Louis: Quality Medical Publishing; 1990. p. 1369–73.
2. Colwell AS, Tessler O, Lin AM, Liao E, Winograd J, Cetrulo CL, Tang R, Smith BL, Austen WG Jr. Breast reconstruction following nipple-sparing mastectomy: predictors of complications, reconstruction outcomes, and 5-year trends. Plast Reconstr Surg. 2014;133:496–506.
3. Colwell AS, Christensen JM. Nipple-sparing mastectomy and direct-to-implant breast reconstruction. Plast Reconstr Surg. 2017;140(5S Advances in Breast Reconstruction):44S–50S.
4. Colwell AS, Taylor E, Specht M, Orringer JS. Optimizing nipple position following nipple-sparing mastectomy. Plast Reconstr Surg Glob Open. 2017;5:e1490. https://doi.org/10.1097/GOX.0000000000001490.
5. Headon HL, Kasem A, Mokbel K. The oncological safety of nipple-sparing mastectomy: a systematic review of the literature with a pooled analysis of 12,358 procedures. Arch Plast Surg. 2016;43:328–38.
6. Jakub JW, Peled AW, Gray RJ, Greenup RA, Kiluk JV, Sacchini V, McLaughlin SA, Tchou JC, Vierkant RA, Degnim AC, Willey S. Oncologic safety of prophylactic nipple-sparing mastectomy in a population with BRCA mutations: a multi-institutional study. JAMA Surg. 2017:123. https://doi.org/10.1001/jamasurg.2017.3422.

7. Ladizinsky DA, Sandholm PH, Jewett ST, Shahzad F, Andrews K. Breast reconstruction with the Bostwick autoderm technique. Plast Reconstr Surg. 2013;132:261–70.
8. Manning AT, Wood C, Eaton A, Stempel M, Capko D, Pusic A, Morrow M, Sacchini V. Nipple-sparing mastectomy in patients with BRCA1/2 mutations and variants of uncertain significance. Br J Surg. 2015;102:1354–9.
9. Marta GN, Poortmans P, de Barros AC, Filassi JR, Freitas Junior R, Audisio RA, Mano MS, Meterissian S, DeSnyder SM, Buchholz TA, Hijal T. Multidisciplinary international survey of post-operative radiation therapy practices after nipple-sparing or skin-sparing mastectomy. Eur J Surg Oncol. 2017;S0748-7983(17):30704–7.
10. Meijers-Heijboer H, van Geel B, van Putten WLJ, Henzen-Logmans SC, Seynaeve C, Menke-Pluymers MBE, Bartels CCM, Verhoog LC, van den Ouweland AMW, Niermeijer MF, Brekelmans CTM, Klijn JGM. Breast cancer after prophylactic bilateral mastectomy in women with a BRCA1 or BRCA2 mutation. N Engl J Med. 2001;345:159–64. 2001
11. Mota BS, Riera R, Ricci MD, Barrett J, de Castria TB, Atallah ÁN, Bevilacqua JLB. Nipple- and areola-sparing mastectomy for the treatment of breast cancer. Cochrane Database Syst Rev 2016;11. Art. No.: CD008932. https://doi.org/10.1002/14651858.CD008932.pub3.
12. Smith BL, Tang R, Rai U, Plichta JK, Colwell AS, Gadd MA, Specht MC, Austen WG Jr, Coopey SB. Oncologic safety of nipple-sparing mastectomy in women with breast cancer. J Am Coll Surg. 2017;S1072-7515(17):30595–1. https://doi.org/10.1016/j.jamcollsurg.2017.06.013.
13. van Verschuer VM, Mureau MA, Gopie JP, Vos EL, Verhoef C, Menke-Pluijmers MB, Koppert LB. Patient satisfaction and nipple-areola sensitivity after bilateral prophylactic mastectomy and immediate implant breast reconstruction in a high breast cancer risk population: nipple-sparing mastectomy versus skin-sparing mastectomy. Ann Plast Surg. 2016;77:145–52.

Autologous Reconstruction: Basic Principles for Free Flaps

H. Fansa, C. Heitmann, *Breast Reconstruction with Autologous Tissue*,
https://doi.org/10.1007/978-3-319-95468-4_8

Autologous tissue is the best and long lasting kind of reconstruction. The tissue is warm, soft and feels like breast tissue. Autologous tissue ages naturally. It sags with gravity or gains and loses weight together with the patient's constitution.

The adverse effect is the resulting scar at the donor site. History of autologous tissue shows that surgeons as well as patients have always looked for the ideal donor site, where a surplus of tissue is available and the scar is well hidden.

Breast autologous tissue reconstructions have started with pedicled flaps. However pedicled flaps demonstrate that they either do not have the optimal perfusion (pedicled TRAM-flap) or their volume is not sufficient without adding an implant. With increasing experience in microsurgery, free flaps became routine procedures. Initially free flaps were used in traumatic cases, but soon the indications expanded for reconstructive procedures after tumour defects.

The principle is quite easy. The surgeon can resect the tumour without limitations according to the oncological needs. The surgeon does not need to respect local pedicles, and no trade-offs need to be made regarding oncological needs. After the defect is set, the ideal tissue can be taken from a distant donor site with its artery and vein. The vessels are then anastomosed at the defect site to recipient vessels using a microscope. Usually one artery and vein are sufficient; in rare cases a second vein is needed.

This freedom to resect is oncologically necessary and using the best available tissue leads to safe and more aesthetic results. Nowadays the microsurgical dissection of the recipient vessels, harvest of the free flap and microsurgical anastomoses are routine procedures. Free flaps in breast reconstruction achieve high success rates of up to 98%. The practised hand does not only have high flap survival rates but also aesthetically pleasing results. This is not only due to standard techniques in high-volume breast centres. Additionally the patients are healthy, have only little co-morbidities and do not need intensive care. A standard single-sided free flap breast reconstruction does not take longer than 2.5–4 h in a two-team approach.

In the following we describe the basics of microsurgery and the "workhorse"- flaps in breast reconstruction There are always additional flaps that can be used, however we want to focus on standard flaps that have proven to work in almost all cases. We added some citations on the "niche flaps" at the end of ► Chap. 10.

> Autologous tissue is the best and long lasting kind of reconstruction. The tissue is warm, soft and feels like breast tissue. Autologous tissue ages naturally. The adverse effect is the resulting scar at the donor site. Free flaps in breast reconstruction achieve high success rates of up to 98% and also aesthetically pleasing results.

8.1 Timing

When is the ideal moment for autologous breast reconstruction? If no radiation therapy is planned and the indication for autologous breast reconstruction is given, an immediate reconstruction can take place. If the recipient vessels and the skin were not altered by prior surgeries, the best results are expected.

Even if a radiation therapy is planned, the newest studies demonstrate safe immediate reconstructions with free flaps. The requirement is that the flap is well-perfused. This is underlined by our experience from the last 15 years. All newer studies show that radiation therapy does not alter the aesthetic result of well perfused free flaps for breast reconstruction. Flaps with complications and decreased perfusion can experience problems from radiation. Additionally a pedicled flap with a not ideal perfusion and a high flap volume (e.g. a pedicled TRAM-flap) might develop more post-radiation problems. If a pedicled TRAM is planned, a delayed reconstruction might be considered.

A delayed reconstruction is planned with or without preservation of breast skin. If the skin is preserved, an implant or expander is initially placed. This acts as a placeholder. The oncological therapy can be completed, and at the earliest about 6 months after termination of radiation, the conversion to autologous tissue can follow.

In a complete delayed reconstruction, the mastectomy is done, and no temporary reconstruction takes place. The breast skin is usually removed. At the earliest about 6 months after termination of radiation, the reconstruction can be undertaken. Disadvantage in these delayed techniques are the following: (1) higher numbers of surgeries, (2) scars and tissue changes from radiation and implants make the reconstruction more difficult and (3) fibrosis after radiation and scarring after implants, matrices and meshes can hamper aesthetics.

A delayed autologous reconstruction is almost always possible.

8.2 Perioperative Features

Microsurgical operations require appropriate instruments and an operating microscope (with a 90° tube). Essential, however, is the expertise of the surgeon. Harvesting the flap should cause minimal donor site morbidity and result in a well-perfused flap. The dissection of the recipient vessels and the anastomoses demand high skills. After all the aesthetic shaping of the breast is the goal.

8.2.1 History and Coagulation

Microsurgery is a routine procedure. Dissection of the flap, recipient vessels and the anastomoses are standardized procedures. Especially in breast reconstruction surgery is highly elective and follows specified steps. The patients are usually healthy and have almost no co-morbidities. The surgery can be prepared meticulously. While in the early days fighting microsurgical complications was the focus, nowadays we do care about improving aesthetic results. Microsurgery has become a standard technique and not the goal of reconstruction.

However, a special patient group is affected by microsurgical complications: patients who suffer from thrombophilia/hypercoagulability. They can present a thrombosis caused by the *Virchow triad* of hemodynamic stasis, endothelial injury and hypercoagulability. These patients can be identified by careful history and then diagnosed with the corresponding laboratory. However, many patients indicate a history of thrombosis/embolism themselves. A thorough history is necessary not only to prevent flap loss but also to avoid possible lethal complications such as pulmonary embolism or strokes.

Unclear findings and positive history should demand a meticulous lab work. The usual global testing such as PT/INR, PTT and TT do not catch thrombophilia. The common causes in Europe are:

- Factor V Leiden mutation
- ATIII-, Protein S- and C-deficiency
- Hyperhomocysteinaemia (due to drugs, diet or genetic causes (e.g. MTHFR))
- Prothrombin mutation (20210A mutation)
- Antiphospholipid syndrome (APS)
- Increased factor-VIII activity

History of a possible thrombophilia according to the criteria of Sapporo:

- Arterial/venous thrombosis and/or pulmonary embolism
- Pregnancies with:
  - One or more unexplained deaths of a foetus at or beyond the 10th week of gestation and/or three or more unexplained abortions before the 10th week of gestation
  - One or more premature birth before 34th week of gestation

In addition there is some evidence that thrombocytosis and tamoxifen can increase flap loss. Some studies suggest a perioperative pause of tamoxifen which is oncologically safe.

8.2.2 Intraoperative Management

Unfortunately there is little evidence-based data on intraoperative management in free flap surgery. Generally it is recommended to elaborate standard operative procedures (SOP) with the anaesthesiologists to maintain the standards with changing personnel. Besides basic points such as sufficient intraoperative warming, Foley catheter and two peripheral venous catheters (ideally foot/ankle), the fluid management (crystalloids) should not exceed 3.5–6 ml/h/kg BW. Higher administration can lead to increased free flap complications. Colloid fluid substitution was not examined regarding free flap surgery. Haemoglobin level should not fall under 10 g/dl and HCT (haematocrit) under 30%. However, a transfusion should only be considered with clinical problems or a haemoglobin below <7 g/dl if no other morbidity requires an earlier intervention.

A further parameter is duration of surgery. Recent studies show that short operation times lead to fewer intra- and postoperative microsurgical complications. This might be connected to body temperature, blood flow and relaxation in the operation.

8.2.3 Flap

The flap should be cut from its nourishing vessels at the donor site if the recipient vessels are ready for anastomosis. This keeps ischemia time as short as possible. Although most perforator flaps are tolerant to ischemia as they mostly consist of skin, subcutaneous tissue local flap problems like fat necrosis or a now-reflow phenomenon are more likely with longer ischemia time.

After harvest the flap should be stored cool. It is weighted to correlate flap weight with the mastectomy weight. Then the flap vessels are dissected under the microscope. Normally it is sufficient to separate the artery from the vein for a short distance. Then the artery and vein are dilated with a dilator or the blunt branches of a microneedle holder. Visible clots can be rinsed away with a heparin solution (5000–10.000 IE heparin per 100 ml isotone saline). We flush the flap gently through the artery with 10 ml heparin solution until clear solution comes out of the vein. For flushing we use a syringe armed with a lacrimal cannula. Then the vein is anastomosed first followed by the artery.

8.2.4 Blood Flow and Blood Pressure

After the connection to the recipient vessels is established, the flap needs a substantial blood flow. As blood flow cannot be well monitored, and the blood pressure (BP) is used as parameter. We aim a mean arterial pressure of >70mmHG or a systolic pressure of ≥120mmHG. The flaps need a good flow and a good flow, is considered to open the so-called choke vessels in the flap which is supposed to enlarge the flap volume.

There is no uniform procedure to manage BP during the operation. In our hands noradrenaline proved of value. Of all catecholamines it seems to have the least effect on the flap capillary bed, thus it is considered to have only a minor risk of spasms within the flap. We start noradrenaline using a perfusor after the flap was harvested. Dosing depends on the BP.

To avoid local spasms of the flap vessels and recipient vessels, we use papaverine, which is a cAMP-phosphodiesterase-inhibitor and relaxes the smooth muscles within the vessel wall. Dilation and higher perfusion is usually seen after 5 min. It is sparingly drizzled over the vessels. If applied with heparin solution, it precipitates without causing problems. Always store papaverine on the operating table in a syringe that cannot be used for vessel injections to avoid a mix-up.

> **Tip**
>
> After anastomoses the mean arterial BP should be around >70mmHG. Noradrenaline can be used to manage BP. Spasms are avoided by papaverine. Store papaverine in a syringe that cannot be used for vessel injections to avoid a mix-up.

8.3 Anastomoses

Harvesting and shaping of the flap are the key steps in breast reconstruction. The microsurgical focus however are the anastomoses and the vessel dissection. Both require microsurgical expertise. You will need a microscope, quiescence and training. Microsurgery appears to be easy especially for vascular or heart surgeons but requires special techniques and extensive training; it is a complete transplantation of a "de novo made"organ and not only a re-vascularisation; veins are also sutured, usually not performed in other specialties, and complication management is also different with regard to thrombosis or no-reflow phenomena.

We will describe the usual techniques, special problems such as end-to-side anastomoses or anastomoses with intima lesions or intima calcifications are subject to microsurgical teaching.

8.3.1 Flap Pedicle

The flap pedicle should be properly dissected. The main steps should be performed when the pedicle is still in place. Veins and artery are to be separated at the later anastomosis site. It is easily done if only one artery and one vein are present. At the anastomosis site no branches should be seen. If two veins are present, one is usually the leading: it is larger and transports more than the other. In almost all flap pedicles, both veins are connected. Thus the leading vein is usually sufficient, and only one venous anastomosis is needed. The second can be clipped out gently. However, if a venous congestion occurs, the clip can be removed, and the vein can be used for a second anastomosis.

If the separation is not possible in situ, or requires special instruments/techniques, it can be done after the flap was harvested under the microscope. At the anastomosis site the vessels should be dissected over a short distance under the microscope. Assistance can be of help. The adventitia around the artery should be cut to avoid an interposition and obstruction of blood flow.

The vessels should be gently rinsed with heparin solution to remove clots. The vessels should be dilated with a dilator or the blunt branches of a microneedle holder. We flush the arterial leg with 10 ml heparin solution until the solution comes clear out of the vein.

8.3.2 Venous Anastomoses

The vein should be anastomosed in a zone without valves as they promote thrombosis. The recipient vein is clamped with a bulldog, and the distal end is clipped. The vein is rinsed and clots are removed. Before anastomosis the branches and all the connections to the accompanying vein (rami communicantes) in that zone are clipped. Otherwise the branches can cause a kinking if the pedicle is moved resulting a venous congestion.

If the vein is manually sutured, the technique is the same like in an arterial anastomosis. However, the sutures do not have to be set as close because the intraluminal pressure is lower. A 8–0 to 10–0 nylon suture with a small needle is preferred. When finished the clamp is removed, and venous flow is possible.

We use a mechanical coupler device consisting of a reusable device that holds a single use ring with six pins. The flap vein and the recipient vein lumen are put over the pins. The device then presses the rings together. The closed coupler remains in the patient. The lumen should be large enough for this technique. A small diameter lumen below 1.5 mm is difficult to handle. Additionally the device needs some space for proper handling. A narrow approach to the anastomosis site makes it difficult to perform. A vessel-measuring gauge allows to measure the vessel and to use the right coupler size. If the vessels are not scarred, they always can be dilated. The IMV and their perforator veins usually require a 2–3 mm coupler. Before coupling place the ends of the veins without twisting. Then ends should lie like the pedicle is planned.

Start to put the more flexible flap vein on the coupler ring and then continue with the recipient vein. The flap vein is pulled with a micro forceps through the ring and then put on the best available pin. With the coupler forceps the vein is squeezed on the ring. The intima is now everted. The next pin is the 120° pin from the first one and so on. If required the vessels are rinsed with heparin. Then the recipient vein is put into the device in the same manner. The device has to be held close to the recipient vein as it is usually shorter than the flap vein. Care should be taken that no tension is applied with the device to avoid a tearing of the veins. After final rinsing the device is closed and additionally pressed together with a curved haemostat. Then the ring is ejected from the device and again gently pressed together with the haemostat. Then the bulldog clamp is removed and the arterial anastomosis is started.

If a coupling is not possible or not successful, simply convert to a handsewn anastomosis to avoid long ischemia times.

Tip

Avoid venous valves at the anastomosis site; avoid twisting of the veins which will cause thrombosis. When ejecting take care that the artery is not trapped in the device.

8.3.3 Arterial Anastomosis

The arteries are still hand sewn. We use nylon from 8–0 to 10–0 with a small needle (e.g. Ethilon 9–0 BV-4 needle) using an interrupted suture technique. Only in large matching vessels a running suture is recommended for each frontal and back side of the vessel. We do not need approximators; we found them not useful. In the following we describe two classic anastomosis techniques. After the bulldog clamp is set on the artery, the distal part is clipped, and the artery is cut. The adventitia is removed from the artery to avoid obstruction from adventitia interposition.

Using the *flip-over technique*, the flap is placed this way that it can be turned/flipped with its pedicle about 180° (horizontal/upside down). This manoeuvre allows to suture the respective frontal side of the vessel under view. The flap lies caudal of the recipient vessels. The arteries are placed in front of each other. The surgeon starts the anastomosis at the point which is most distant. The following sutures are placed towards the surgeon. As the back side is open, the risk to grab the back wall is low. After this side is finished, the flap is flipped over 180° cranially. The back side is now visible and can be sutured using the same technique. The last two sutures are tied later to see the inside of the lumen.

Then the bulldog clamp is removed and the flow is released. Within 30 s the flap should be perfused, and a flow through the vein should be visible. A milking test on the vein can be used to control the flow from the flap. The vein distal to the anastomosis is gently held with two micro forceps. The surgeon occludes the vein with the first forceps distal to the anastomosis. The blood is then transported distally with the second forceps. The vein between the two forceps is now freed of blood. Now the second forceps occludes the vein, and the first one is opened. If positive the vein is filled with blood from the flap. This test shows good inflow and outflow, thus a vital flap. With good perfusion the flap can be inset and shaped. Take care that the pedicle is not twisted or kinked.

In the *backhand technique*, the flap is fixed, e.g. caudally from the breast, and the pedicle is placed in front of the recipient vessels without any tension. The surgeon starts to sew the back side of the vessel at the most distant position and puts the next suture towards the surgeon (◘ Fig. 8.1a and b). If the back side is finished, the surgeon starts again at the most distant position and places the next suture towards

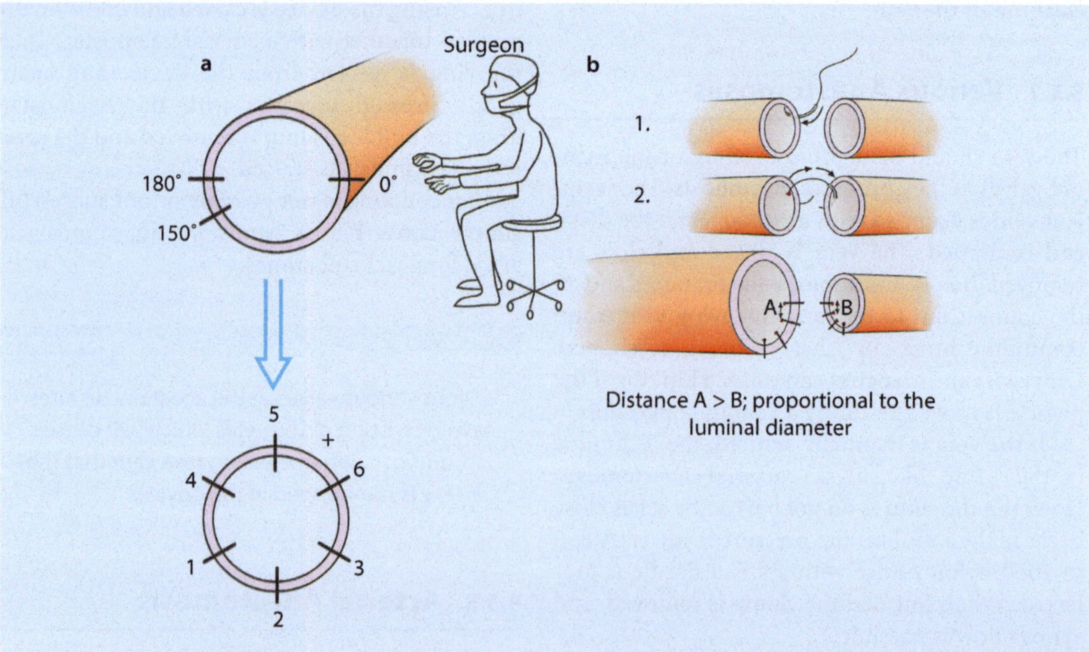

◘ **Fig. 8.1** **a** Shows the backhand microsurgical technique of vessel anastomosis. The surgeon is relaxed, and the vessel lies horizontally in front of him. Anastomosis is started with suture 1, approx. at 150° of the vessel. This is the most distant and less visible part of the anastomosis. Then the back wall is completed (2 and 3). The suture is then continued from the distant part of the front wall (4) to the surgeon (5 and 6). The last two stiches are tied after the both are placed to see the lumen. If necessary the number of stiches can be increased, depending on the luminal diameter. The anastomosis should be leak-proof in the first place. **b** 1 and 2. Backhand suture for a right-handed surgeon. The needle passes at the 150° point of the vessel on the left side from external to the inner lumen and then on the right side from the inner lumen to the outer part. The knot is then made externally. The back wall is continued using this technique. The front side is closed with regular sutures from external right to inner right and then from inner left to outer left. Lower vessel: If the vessels show a mismatch (e.g. IMAP to long pedicled deep inferior epigastric artery lumen), we found it possible in most cases to use and distribute the suture placement proportional to the luminal diameter on the respective side. In these cases an additional stich may become necessary after the clamps are released and the flow shows a leakage. It is strongly recommended to use a suture with a small needle him. The last two stiches are tied later to look into the lumen and avoid obstruction. It is more difficult to place the first stiches using this technique, but if the pedicles (flap and recipient) are short and not flexible (e.g. TMG-flap or in a rib-sparing approach), this technique is very easy and reliable.

8.4 Postoperative Management

As soon as the patients are stable, they can get up and are mobilized. This is usually at the day of operation or the first postoperative day. A special anticoagulation is not necessary besides the regularly used low molecular heparin (LMH) therapy for prophylaxis if the patients have no history or evidence of coagulopathy. We use a single prophylactic dose in the evening (e.g. enoxaparin, Clexane 40). Additionally we start a 100 mg Aspirin dose from the first postoperative day at noon. Patients with coagulopathy should be treated with a therapeutic dosage of LMH, and a specialist on coagulopathies should be consulted. The anticoagulants are used to prevent flap loss and other possible lethal embolisms. On the other hand anticoagulation therapy should have the operation and postoperative bleeding in mind. In Germany an anticoagulation therapy is recommended after discharge until the patient is fully mobilized.

To monitor flap perfusion, an intensified control is recommended in the first 24 h. We prefer visible skin monitors. If flap skin is not regularly used for reconstructive purposes, we use the inset of a temporary skin island which can be removed after 48 h.

Others use implantable probes, monitor with a handheld Doppler or do not monitor at all.

Postoperative hypotension (mostly by drugs) should be avoided. If patients have a hypertension medication, a pause can be considered according to BP monitoring. Local warming in the first hours (e.g. a Bair Hugger) might improve flap perfusion.

8.5 Vascular Complications and Management

The detailed microvascular complication management should be learned from microsurgical teaching books. Here we list possible solutions for situations special to breast reconstructions.

With proper dissection most vascular problems are seen if the patients have (1) a coagulopathy (see history), (2) the flap is not well perfused (white flap) or congested (purple) at the donor site, (3) the recipient vessels show a reduced inflow or outflow or (4) intraoperative management of blood flow and BP is inadequate.

Pedicle exposition can cause vessel spasms, which can be well treated with papaverine. Careful drizzling over the vessels can resolve the spasm. We have not seen any rebound phenomenon from this medication. Increasing BP can also be of help in flap perfusion.

▪▪ Decreased perfusion

In most cases decreased perfusion is a result of a thrombosis at the anastomotic site. If verified, redo the anastomosis. The clamps are set and the former anastomotic area is resected. The ends are inspected and completely cleared from clots using a forceps or dilator. The flap should be flushed. If this is easily possible, there might be no clot inside the flap. The anastomosis can be redone.

If the flow from the recipient is doubted, open the bulldog clamp and assess the flow. If the flow is reduced, another artery should be tried. First one should check the distal clipped artery. In some cases there is a sufficient flow from the distal end. If not, one can change from the IMA to the subscapular vessels or vice versa. In some cases one can switch from the IMA to a cranial IMA-perforator. If the pedicle is long enough, this will work well. The use of thrombectomy catheters (e.g. balloon catheter according to Fogarty) makes only sense on the flap or the subscapular artery. We do not use the catheter on the IMA because a rupture of the artery underneath the ribs is dangerous. A possible bleeding cannot be controlled properly.

If a thrombosis is evident within the flap, an isolated administration of drugs that resolve the thrombosis (e.g. tPA, tissue plasminogen activator) is recommended. To avoid a systemic action, one should open the vein to avoid a lytic activity within the rest of the body. Alternatively or additionally an intraoperative application of i.v. aspirin can be considered.

If the flap was badly perfused at the donor site, a complex manipulation at the recipient site would not bring the flap back. In fact an increased perfusion from the recipient vessel can improve blood flow; however, if the perforators within the flap are too weak or too little, the flap will not survive in the long run.

Congestion

If the flap was not congested at the donor site but is after anastomosis, the reason is the venous anastomosis or an obstruction from the recipient vein outflow. In some case a valve can induce a thrombosis. Then a redo will eliminate the problem. Only rarely a reduced influx is the reason for a reduced outflow. However, this possibility should be excluded.

If the pedicle has two veins, and one cannot be used anymore, the other should be tried.

Some patients show a venous obstruction in the recipient vein due to tumours or prior surgery. In these cases the vein should be explored more cranially, or the distal vein can be examined, or the second accompanying vein can be used, or the flap is hooked to a different arterial/venous system, such as a cranial perforator or subscapular vessels. Although the coupling devices have proven to be safe, a handsewn anastomosis can be tried after recurrent thrombosis.

If the flap is completely dissected and only bound through the pedicle in the donor site and then congested, one should consider if the flap is too big and a congestion is due to venous pooling within the flap. If so, reduce the size and see if the flap recovers. If not, a second vein within the flap (in most cases a superficial one) should be carefully dissected and planned for additional anastomosis. If this is done, one should draw a flap template and mark the new vein. Use the gauge to identify the area around the recipient site to look for a second vein. Often a IMV-perforator can be found and used. The transposition of the cephalic vein was also described as alternative.

Early haematoma around the flap

An early haematoma can result from the mastectomy cavity, but it can also be an early symptom of venous occlusion. In a venous congestion due to a kinking or thrombosis, the flap can "open" other veins if the arterial inflow is still intact. The resulting haematoma is of dark purple colour. This haematoma is often earlier than a change of the monitor skin island. An early revision is recommended.

Interposition grafts

Vein grafts can be used for bridging arteries or veins. These grafts should match the vessel calibre. For arterial use the vein grafts are used against their natural flow, and for venous use they are used with their natural flow direction. Venous vein interposition grafts can be coupled. Veins can be harvested from the lower arm and the thigh (saphenous vein when using a TMG-flap). In rare cases the veins can be used from the caudal abdominal incision, from the superficial epigastric vessels (SIEA) or from the contralateral deep epigastric vessels (artery! and vein).

Every revision shortens the pedicle length. This can change flap position and the aesthetic result. This can also influence beforehand fitted skin islands. In these cases the flap should be inset according to vascular purposes. If the flap is vital after some days, a skin graft can be considered.

In revisional surgery the surgeon should not only see the flap but the entire patient, duration of surgery and the number of revisions. It is always worthwhile to fight for the flap, but in some cases it might be better for the patient to resect a poor or not functioning flap in better time.

8.6 Aesthetic Considerations, Complications and Radiation Therapy

Breast reconstruction aims an aesthetic and symmetric outcome. Inset and shaping of the flap have to meet these criteria. If it is previously clear that symmetry is only possible if the contralateral breast is included into the planning, this should be discussed with the patients.

Shaping has also to take in consideration that the perfusion stays safe. A necessary shaping that influences flap vascularity should be postponed. Inset does not only comply with the aesthetics (placement and shape of volume) but also with pedicle length, recipient vessels and vascular situations.

When the flap is insetted, the IMF should be symmetrical. If possible the upper medial volume (décolleté) should be reconstructed symmetrically as later corrections in that area are difficult. It is helpful to bring the patient in a sitting position intraoperatively. Surplus skin should also be shaped within this operation if possible. In secondary or delayed reconstructions or conversions from implant to autologous tissue scars, NAC malpositions and other situation can implicate further surgery to improve the aesthetic outcome.

Parts of the flap that are poorly perfused or congested should be removed even if the desired volume or shape cannot be achieved. Problems from vascular origins are difficult to manage. If a radiation therapy is necessary after reconstruction, the entire flap can be included into the radiation field (◘ Figs. 8.2, 8.3, and 8.4). We have not seen any long-term complications and significant aesthetic problems when flap perfusion is stable. Recent studies underline this concept.

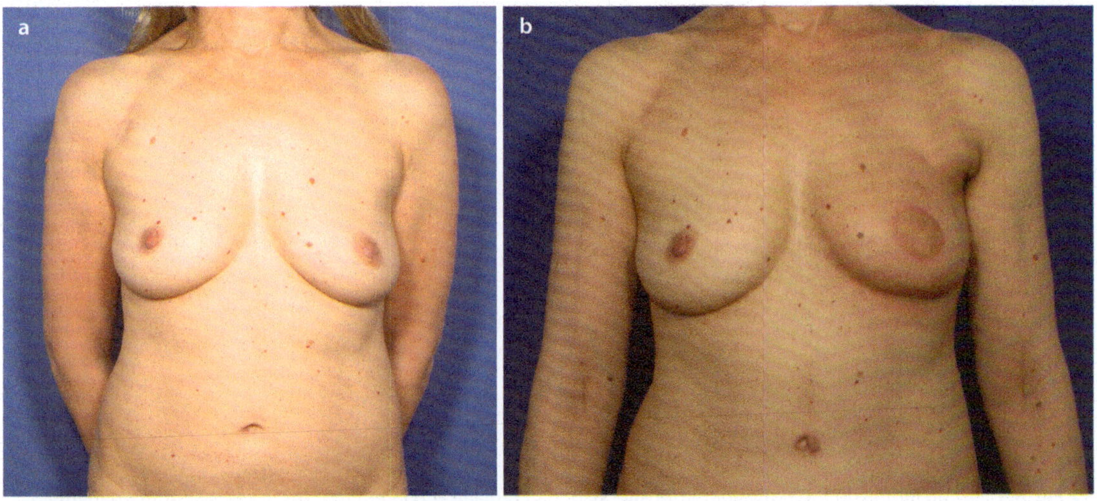

◘ **Fig. 8.2** **a** Carcinoma on left side. SSM and DIEP-flap. **b** Outcome after directly after radiation therapy. Oedema and redness of the skin are visible. This reaction is more extensive with the mastectomy skin than the flap because it is less perfused compared to the flap

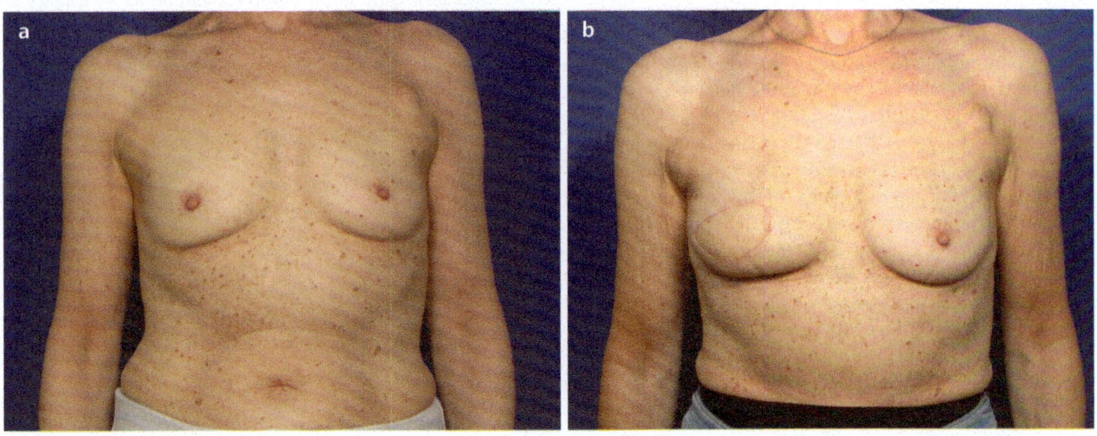

◘ **Fig. 8.3** **a** Carcinoma on the right side. Periareolar SSM and DIEP-flap. **b** One year after radiation therapy without any visible radiation sequelae

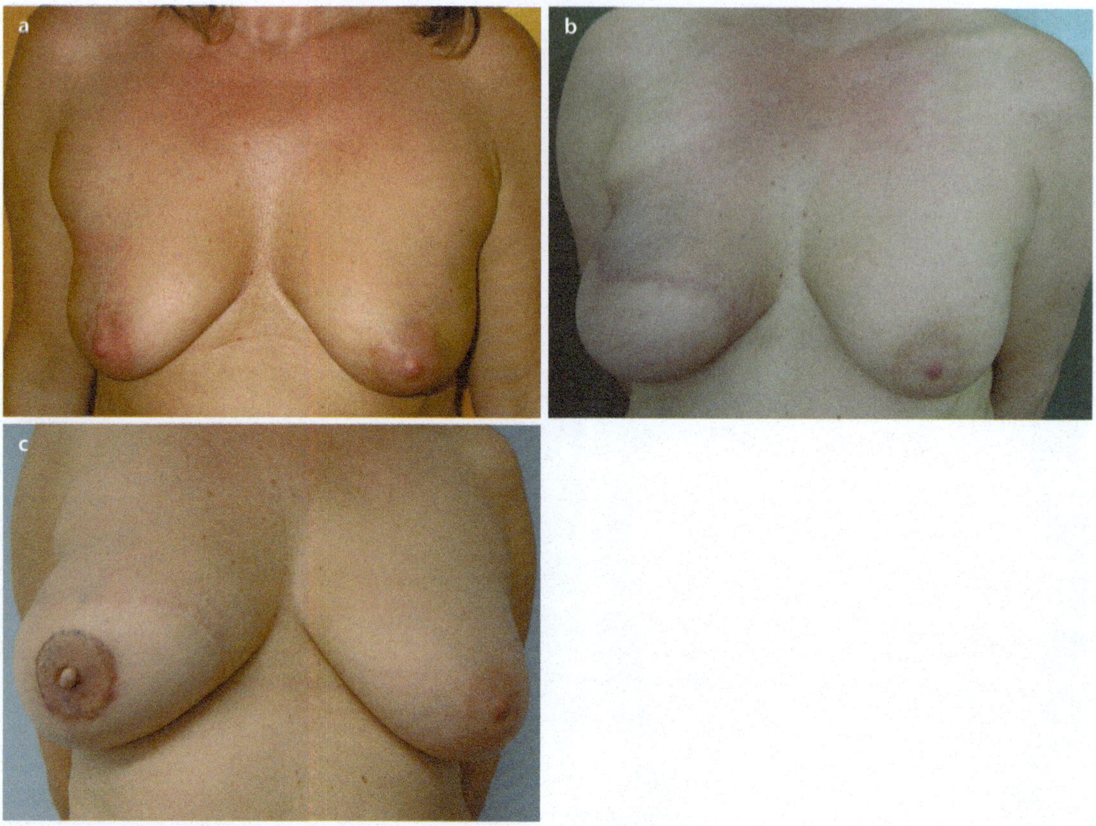

■ **Fig. 8.4** **a** Carcinoma on the right side. Extensive skin resection and DIEP-flap. **b** Directly after radiation therapy. The borders of the radiation fields are clearly visible cranially and laterally. **c** Three years later the patient demanded a nipple reconstruction. No volume change or flap shrinkage is visible

Literature

1. Billig J, Jagsi R, Qi J, Hamill JB, Kim HM, Pusic AL, Buchel E, Wilkins EG, Momoh AO. Should immediate autologous breast reconstruction be considered in women who require postmastectomy radiation therapy? a prospective analysis of outcomes. Plast Reconstr Surg. 2017;139:1279–88.
2. Chen C, Nguyen MD, Bar-Meir E, Hess PA, Lin S, Tobias AM, Upton J 3rd, Lee BT. Effects of vasopressor administration on the outcomes of microsurgical Breast reconstruction. Ann Plast Surg. 2010;65:28–31.
3. Hyza P, Streit L, Schwarz D, Kubek T, Vesely J. Vasospasm of the flap pedicle: the effect of 11 of the most often used vasodilating drugs. Comparative study in a rat model. Plast Reconstr Surg. 2014;134:574e–84e.
4. Kneser U, Horch RE, Lehnhardt M. (Hrsg.) Grundkurs Mikrochirurgie. Hrsg. Springer Verlag Heidelberg 2015.
5. Pont LP, Marcelli S, Robustillo M, Song D, Grandes D, Martin M, Iglesias I, Aso J, Laloumet I, Díaz AJ. Immediate breast reconstruction with abdominal free flap and adjuvant radiotherapy: evaluation of quality of life and outcomes. Plast Reconstr Surg. 2017;140: 681–90.
6. Vyas K, Wong L. Intraoperative management of free flaps: current practice. Ann Plast Surg. 2014;72: S220–3.
7. Warnecke IC, Kretschmer F, Brüner S, Frerichs O, Fansa H. Hereditäre Thrombophilie bei mikrochirurgischen Lappenplastiken. Handchir Mikrochir Plast Chir. 2007;39:220–4.
8. Zhong T, Neinstein R, Massey C, McCluskey SA, Lipa J, Neligan P, Hofer SO. Intravenous fluid infusion rate in microsurgical Breast reconstruction: important lessons learned from 354 free flaps. Plast Reconstr Surg. 2011;128:1153–60.

Recipient Vessels

H. Fansa, C. Heitmann, *Breast Reconstruction with Autologous Tissue*,
https://doi.org/10.1007/978-3-319-95468-4_9

Proper recipient vessels are one prerequisite for free flaps. Standard recipient vessels are nowadays the internal mammary artery (IMA) and internal mammary vein (IMV). In the following we will use IMA even if we mean both artery and vein. The perforators from the IMA (IMAP) are also artery and vein, sometimes also a nerve.

If possible we nowadays prefer the anastomosis to the perforators, which pass through the intercostal muscles and the pectoral muscle and then enter the breast. In some patients the IMA or IMAP are not suitable due to scarring from radiation or capsular fibrosis. Alternatively the thoracoacromial artery, the lateral thoracic artery or the subscapular vessels with their branches to latissimus dorsi muscle (thoracodorsal artery) or serratus anterior muscle are used. Normally a microsurgically experienced surgeon can use any vessel with a good flow. However, the aesthetic needs have to be considered too, such as positioning and volume.

Vessel dissection requires fine instruments and loupe magnification or a microscope.

> The recipient vessel selection is essential for a vital flap. All vessels have advantages and disadvantages. From our point of view, the following vessels are best (in order):
>
> 1. IMA perforators (IMAP). They are superficial, have a good flow and are dissected fast. The vein can be couplered. The arterial anastomosis needs more concentration.
> 2. IMA. It is a constant, reliable vessel. It lies deeper in the thorax than the IMAP: dissection can cause more trouble.
> 3. Subscapular vessels. They are the thoracodorsal artery and the branch to the serratus anterior muscle. In a mastectomy with axillary dissection, they are visible. The flow is lower compared to the IMA; medial positioning of the flap always requires long pedicles. Venous coupler ring is more difficult due to the narrow approach. Using the thoracodorsal vessels loses the latissimus dorsi muscle as backup.
> 4. Thoracoacromial artery, thoracic lateral artery or perforators from the Würinger septum are more a kind of backup vessels if others are not suitable.
> 5. Contralateral IMA and interposition graft.

9.1 Internal Mammary Artery, IMA

IMA arises from the subclavian artery and runs on the pleura within the thorax from cranial to caudal. At the level of the caudal sternum, the IMA branches into a vessel for the diaphragm and the superior epigastric artery (nourishing the pedicled TRAM flap and anastomoses to the deep inferior epigastric artery). The IMA can be dissected on both sides of the sternum. The left one is frequently used in bypass surgery (◘ Fig. 9.1).

IMA dissection is obvious as (1) it has a good flow, (2) it has a constant anatomy and (3) it is located within the wound after a mastectomy. No additional incisions are necessary. The more cranially the IMA is dissected, the larger are the vessels. Ideally the IMA is dissected between the second and fourth intercostal space (ICS).

The pectoralis major muscle is dived parallel to its fibres above the desired ICS close to the sternum. A wound retractor is used. In a sufficiently large ICS, a *rib-sparing approach* can be chosen (◘ Fig. 9.2). A length of 1–1.5 cm for artery and vein is sufficient for anastomosis. If the ribs have a narrow distance, cartilage removal is recommended (◘ Fig. 9.3).

Dissection in the ICS is best done with a fine bipolar forceps. The external and then internal muscle is removed. In some cases third muscle is encountered dorsally, transverse thoracic muscle, which also has to be removed. The muscles should be removed completely to allow a convenient anastomosis. The intercostal nerve that runs parallel to the rib can be

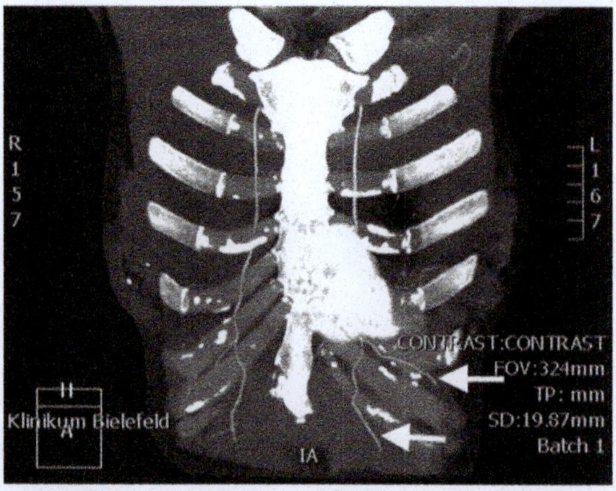

◘ **Fig. 9.1** Coronal CTA. The bilateral course of the IMA is clearly seen. Caudally it divides into two branches. One is the epigastrica superior artery that nourishes the cranial rectus abdominis muscle and is the pedicle for the cranially pedicled TRAM flap. The right arrow shows the branch to the diaphragm

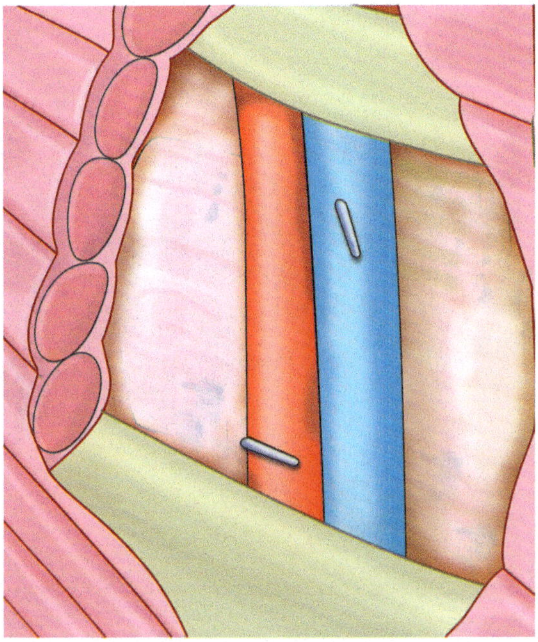

■ **Fig. 9.2** Rib-sparing approach to the IMA. The sternum on the right side. In the ICS the intercostal muscles are resected. The muscles should be removed completely to have enough space for the anastomosis. Pleura is dorsal

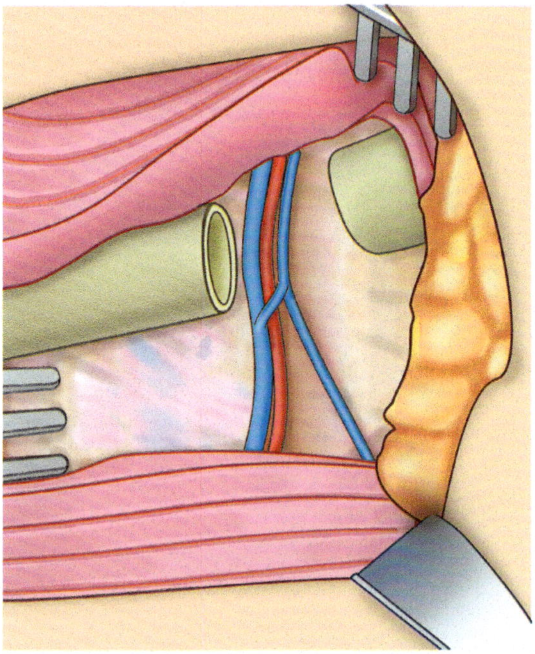

■ **Fig. 9.3** IMA dissection with cartilage resection. IMA lies in between two IMVs. In a narrow ICS, the rib cartilage can be removed above the vessels. First the ventral periosteum is cut along the rib. The cranial periosteum is folded cranially while the caudal caudally using a raspatory. The cartilage is the removed with a Luer bone rongeur. The dorsal periosteum should be kept intact. If the cartilage is removed over a distance of 1–2 cm, the dorsal periosteum can be removed carefully. This is done safer if the vessels are dissected in the ICS beforehand. The vein often is stuck to the periosteum, and rough handling can lead to bleeding

saved. Dorsal to the muscles, there is a thin membrane. Dorsal to this membrane, the vessels and the lymphatic structure are located. The membrane has to be incised carefully. The vessels can be now dissected. The artery is located between the veins. In the cranial ICS, the veins run parallel; in the more caudal ICS, the veins have multiple connecting branches, which are often seen on top of the artery. In some cases only one vein is evident (■ Fig. 9.4).

Tip

Vessel dissection is best performed with a fine dissecting forceps (e.g. a fine Overholt forceps) and a fine bipolar forceps. Microclips can clip even little branches fast and reliably. Proactive haemostasis is mandatory as bleeding should be avoided in any case due to the high blood flow. Uncontrolled bleeding can lead to reactions that can impair the vessel suitability. In an uncontrolled bleeding, the vessels should be temporarily clamped with a bulldog clamp. Then the source of bleeding is located and haemostasis is performed. If this is not possible, the vessel is clipped or ligated. The IMA is then dissected in a more cranial ICS.

If the ICS is too small or longer recipient vessels are needed, rib cartilage is removed above the IMA. We prefer to dissect the IMA first in the ICS and then to remove the cartilage under sight. However, the opposite approach is also possible.

First the ventral periosteum is cut along the rib. The cranial periosteum is folded cranially while the caudal caudally using a raspatory. The cartilage is the removed with a Luer bone rongeur. The dorsal periosteum should be kept intact. If the cartilage is removed over a distance of 1–2 cm, the dorsal periosteum can be removed carefully. This is done safer if the vessels are dissected in the ICS beforehand. The vein often is stuck to the periosteum and rough handling can lead to bleeding.

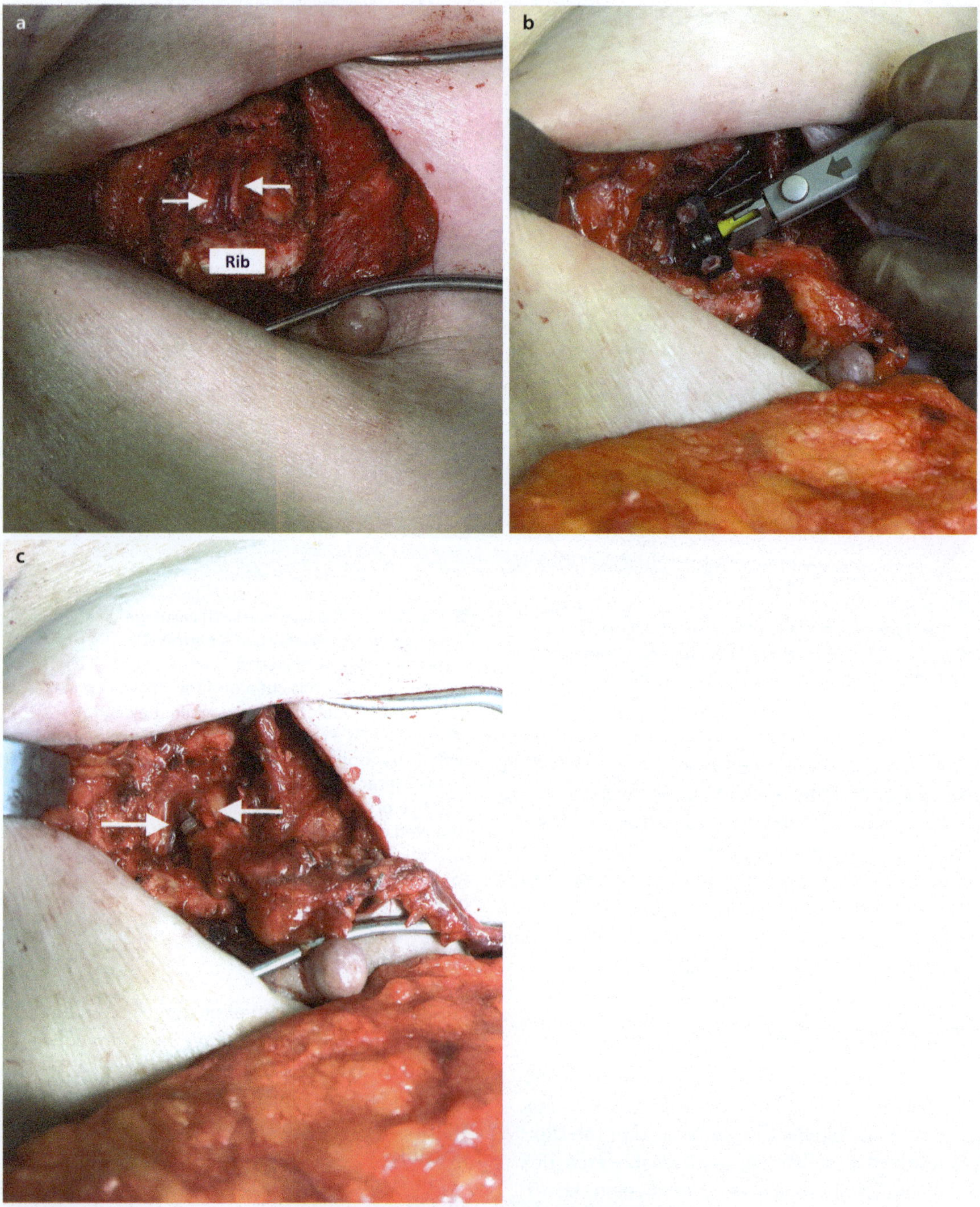

Fig. 9.4 **a** Anastomosis of a flap vessel to the left IMA and IMV in a rib-sparing approach. The ICS muscles are removed. IMA (right arrow) is accompanied from a branching vein (left arrow). The pleura lies dorsally. The vessels have to be dissected meticulously and all the branches have to clipped off. **b** First the flap vein (below) and then the recipient vein (top) are put over the respective ring. The black bulldog clamp is on the cranial recipient vein. The caudal part is clipped. **c** Left arrow indicates the venous anastomosis; the right arrow indicates the arterial anastomosis (9-0 sutures)

! The pleura is located dorsal to vessels. It should be left intact. An injury to the pleura can be sutured if possible or closed with a fascia or muscle strip and fibrin glue. The anaesthesiologist should be informed immediately. In severe cases a thoracic surgeon should be consulted. In most cases a chest tube is not needed.

9.2 Internal Mammary Artery Perforators, IMAP

Until recently the IMAP were rarely used. Meanwhile the strong cranially located IMAP are used for IMAP-flaps and have proven as excellent recipient vessels. We used them not only for breast reconstruction but also as recipient vessels for head and neck cases. They are located medially within the mastectomy wound. Injuries to deeper structures (bleedings from the IMA or injuries to the pleura) are avoided. The IMA is kept for later bypass surgery. Anastomosis is more delicate, but the IMAP are matching the flap vessels of shorter pedicle flaps (TMG-flaps or short pedicle DIEP-flaps).

Meanwhile we use the IMAP in more than 45% of all our breast reconstructions as recipient vessels, not only in primary reconstructions but also in delayed cases. Their use does not reduce the breast skin perfusion (▫ Fig. 9.5).

IMAP have a strong blood flow and nourish the sternum and the breast. They arise from the IMA and perforate the intercostal muscles and then the pectoralis major muscle (▫ Fig. 9.6). The largest are in the first to third ICS. They can be used for anastomosis if the lumen measures from 0.7 to 1 mm. The veins are more fragile than the IMV and have more valves. However, their calibre is sufficient for venous anastomosis (▫ Figs. 9.7, 9.8, and 9.9).

In thin or light-skinned patients, the venous course is seen in the cranial ICS beforehand and can be marked. During mastectomy the IMAP are seen medially and can be saved or if "caught" clipped and dissected later on. Like all perforators they tend to react with a vasospasm. In our experience we rely on the "first sight". If the IMAP appears good (pulsating artery and filled vein) when first encountered, they can be used (▫ Figs. 9.10, 9.11, 9.12, 9.13, and 9.14). A thin vein at the first encounter usually stays thin. Such IMAP should not be used. If a large IMAP becomes spastic, papaverine can reliably resolve the spasm.

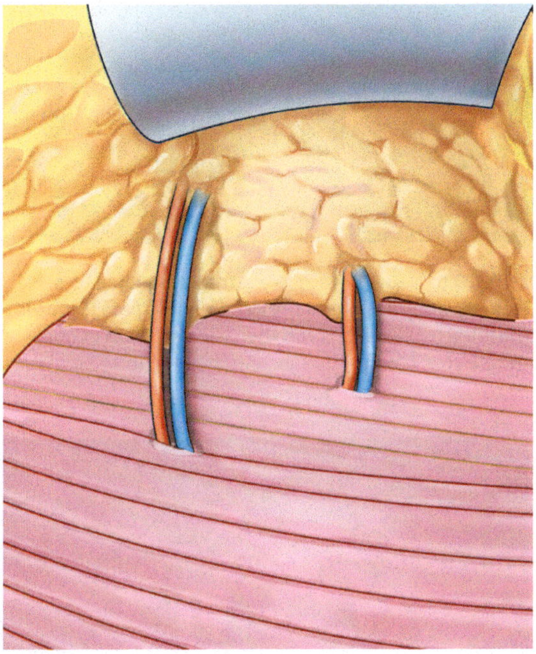

▫ **Fig. 9.5** Example for IMAP at the medial dissection border of a mastectomy. The cranial IMAP are stronger than the caudal ones

If IMAP dissection is undertaken in a delayed reconstruction, the IMAP should be dissected at the ICS. In most cases, a length of 1.5–2 cm is enough. IMAP are very variable; mostly a sensitive nerve runs together with the vessels. Sometimes only one vein and artery exist, and in other cases strong IMAP are encountered when dissecting the way to the IMA (▫ Figs. 9.11, 9.12, 9.13, and 9.14).

Tip

Starting with the mastectomy medially allows to dissect and then save the IMAP. If injured they can be clipped and used later. If one doubts the IMAP quality as recipient vessel or an IMAP is not found at first go, use the IMA. Additionally the position of the IMAP in relation to flap position and flap pedicle has to be considered. A very cranially located IMAP and a flap with a short pedicle will possibly result in a too cranially positioned breast. In these cases a more caudal IMA anastomosis is preferred.

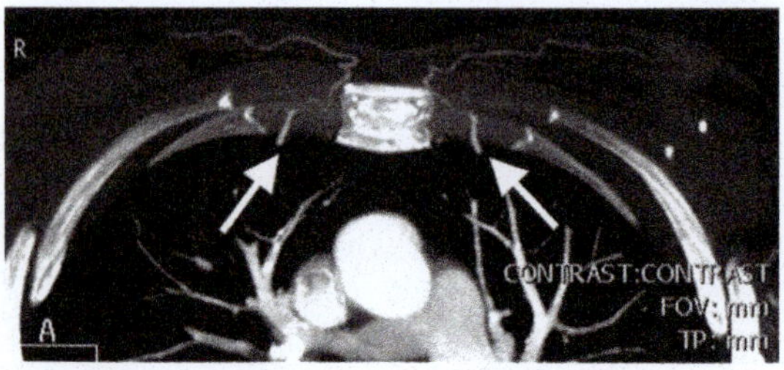

■ **Fig. 9.6** Axial CTA. Showing the IMAP, gland and sternum. They arise from the IMA (arrows), pass through the intercostal muscles and then the pectoralis major muscle towards the sternum and then run into the gland

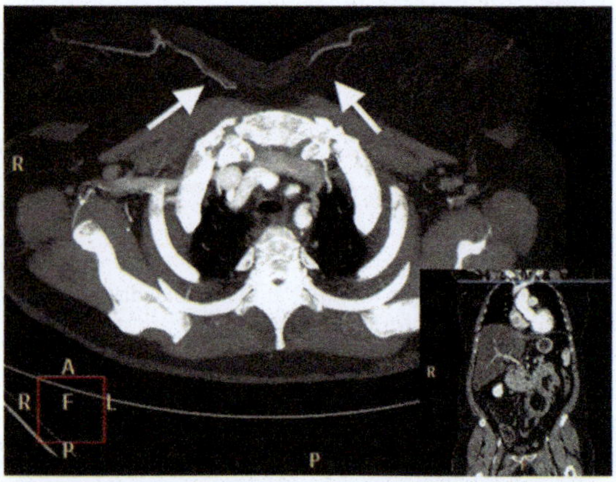

■ **Fig. 9.7** Axial CTA. The strongest IMAP are located in the first to third ICS (here first). The large arteries are accompanied by large veins in this patient

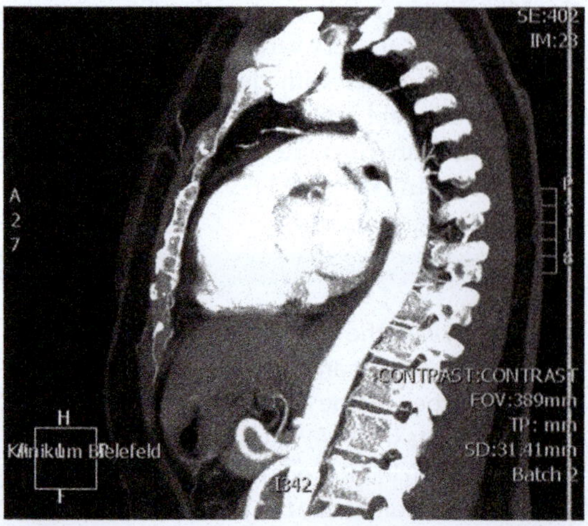

■ **Fig. 9.8** Sagittal CTA. Strong arterial and venous IMAP for a secondary reconstruction

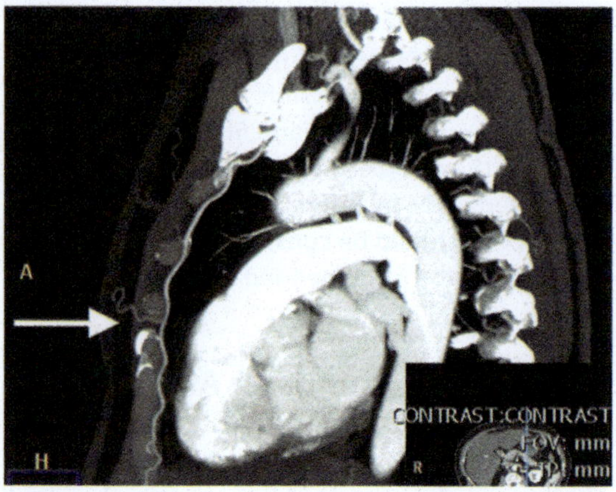

■ **Fig. 9.9** Sagittal CTA. Here a strong IMAP is existent in the fourth ICS. CTA shows no vein. Intraoperative evaluation has to determine if a vein is present. See the wide ICS. If the IMA is used, a rib-sparing approach is justified

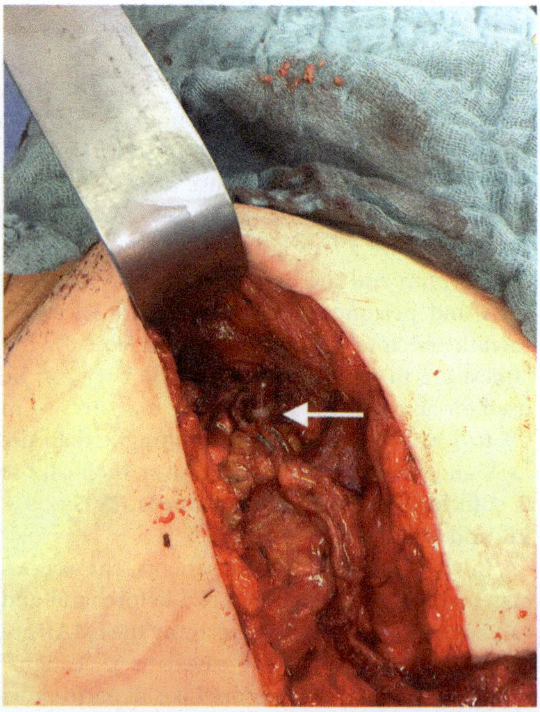

■ **Fig. 9.10** DIEP-flap is hooked to a IMAP (arrow). IMAP are on the top; the flap vessel runs down

9.3 The Subscapular Vessels

If the IMA or IMAP cannot be used, anastomosis is performed in the axilla. This was the standard procedure over years. Meanwhile the axillary

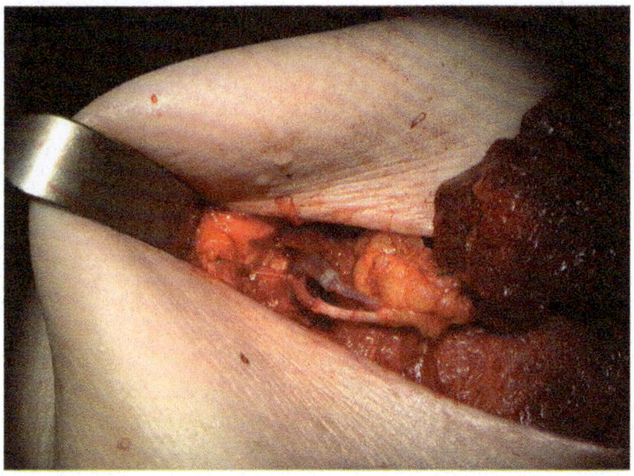

Fig. 9.11 Ms-TRAM flap to IMAP (left, flap vessels run to the right). Artery lumen is between 0.5 and 1 mm. The IMAP artery has to be dilated. The epigastric artery should not be dilated

anastomosis is an exception. However, it is used as backup technique. Points against an axillary anastomosis are:

1. Long pedicles are needed to place the breast in adequate medial position. This increases morbidity in DIEP-flaps.
   Short pedicled flaps may need interposition grafts.
2. Blood flow is initially lower in the subscapular vessels.
3. In secondary cases, the incision has to be lateral or a second incision at the axilla is needed.
4. After an axillary dissection or radiation, the dissection is very tedious and complex; in some cases an arm lymph oedema can occur.
5. Dissection and handling under the microscope are more difficult in the axilla.
6. Using the thoracodorsal vessels excludes the use of the latissimus dorsi muscle as a backup procedure.

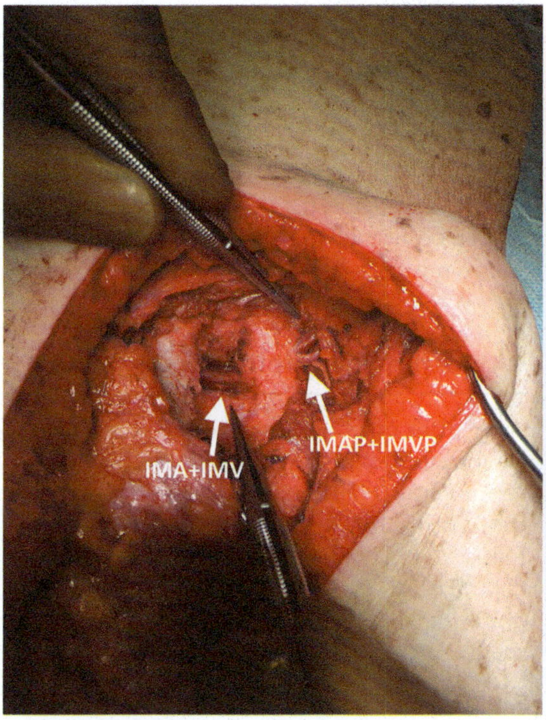

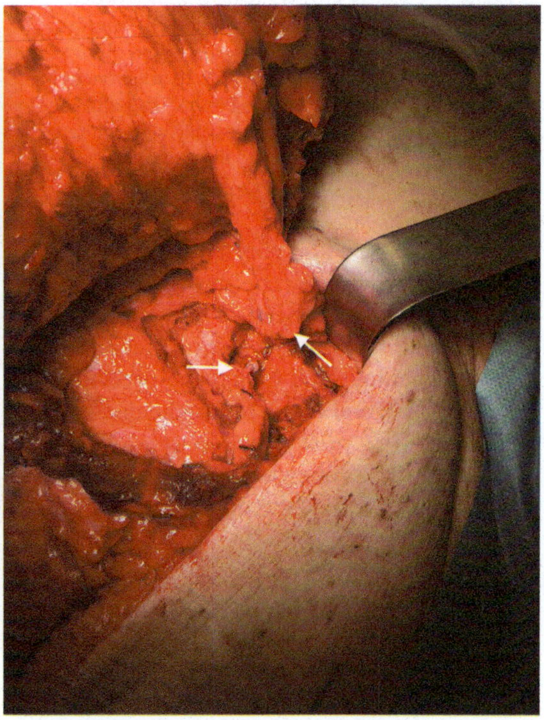

Figs. 9.12 and 9.13 Special situs. IMA (rib-sparing approach) and IMAP are dissected. In this case the DIEP-flap needed an additional venous outflow. Fig. 9.13. The pedicle is connected to the IMA and IMV (left arrow); a superficial flap vein (SIEV) is hooked to the perforator vein (right vein). A vein dissection out of the mastectomy site is avoided

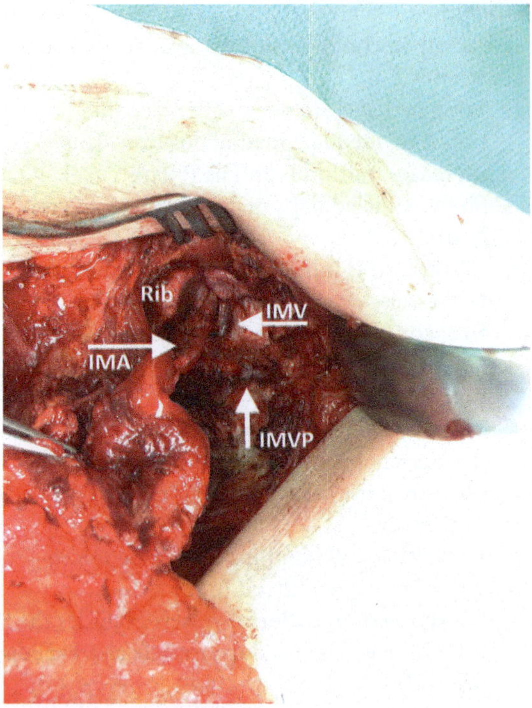

Fig. 9.14 Special situs in a patient with severe capsular contracture after radiation therapy. IMA was approached by removing rib cartilage (the sternum to the right). The IMA was dissected, but due to adherences the vein was not removable from the pleura. Thus, the venous anastomosis to the IMV was not possible without harm. Therefore, the flap was hooked to the IMA and perforator vein

However, there are also reasons for axillary anastomosis. For example, the vessels are exposed during an axillary dissection and can be used, which requires a primary reconstruction. Using the SLN technique will reduce the need for axillary dissection, and in the future the dissection is reduced anyway.

The terminal branches of the subscapular artery are suitable: thoracodorsal branches and branches to the serratus anterior muscle. Dissection is best started at the frontal muscle border. Here the scarring is less pronounced if the axilla was dissected beforehand. The thoracodorsal vessels enter the muscle together with the nerve from underneath cranially. The vessels can then be dissected from caudal to central. A vessel loop can facilitate the handling. The peripheral branches are ligated or clipped. Approximately at the level where the thoracodorsal vessels enter the latissimus muscle, the *branch to the serratus anterior* muscle is found. If this branch is used, it can

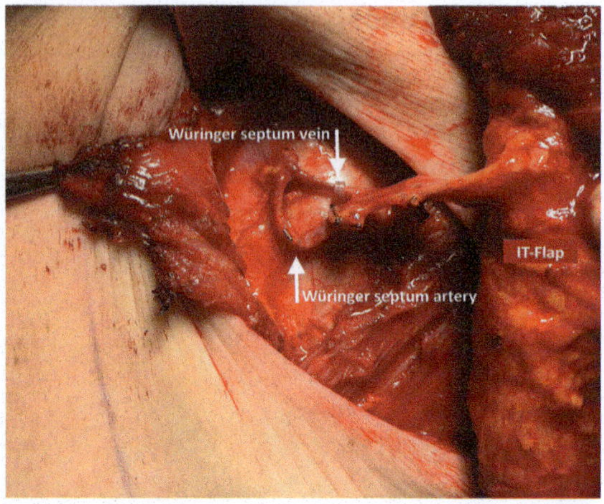

Fig. 9.15 Inner thigh flap anastomosed to a perforator from the Würinger septum left side. The vessels arise from the upper rib. These perforators are not always suitable. But the lumen size matches the TMG vessels

be dissected from here. The long thoracic nerve must be kept intact. The branches are usually very tiny and may not be used in any case. However, like in IMAP dissection, papaverine can be used to dissolve vasospasms.

Tip

If the approach to the axilla is difficult under the microscope, the entire operation table can be inclined to the opposite side to allow a more relaxed handling.

9.4 Other Recipient Vessels

After prior operations, in second flaps and aplasia, or after excessive resections, alternative vessels might become necessary. The perforators of the Würinger septum (Fig. 9.15) can be used but also the thoracoacromial vessels. Also the contralateral IMA can be used. Interposition grafts can be also planned primarily. However, these approaches are reserved to nonroutine cases.

Literature

Fansa H. Supermikrochirurgie. In: Kneser U, Horch RE, Lehnhardt M, editors. Grundkurs Mikrochirurgie. Heidelberg: Springer Verlag; 2015.

Fansa H, Schirmer S, Cervelli A, Gehl HB. Computed tomographic angiography imaging and clinical implications of internal mammary artery perforator vessels as recipient vessels in autologous Breast reconstruction. Ann Plast Surg 2013;71:533–7.

Haddock NT, Teotia SS. Five steps to internal mammary vessel preparation in less than 15 minutes. Plast Reconstr Surg. 2017;140:884–6.

Sacks JM, Chang DW. Rib-sparing internal mammary vessel harvest for microvascular Breast reconstruction in 100 consecutive cases. Plast Reconstr Surg. 2009;123:1403–7.

Vollbach FH, Heitmann CD, Fansa H. An appraisal of internal mammary artery perforators as recipient vessels in microvascular breast reconstruction-an analysis of 515 consecutive cases. Plast Reconstr Surg Glob Open. 2016;4:e1144. https://doi.org/10.1097/GOX.0000000000001144.

Autologous Reconstruction: Free Flaps

H. Fansa, C. Heitmann, *Breast Reconstruction with Autologous Tissue*,
https://doi.org/10.1007/978-3-319-95468-4_10

10.1 DIEP-Flaps, ms-TRAM Flaps and SIEA-Flaps

DIEP- and ms-TRAM flaps are the workhorse free flaps in autologous breast reconstruction. The first TRAM flaps, transverse rectus abdominis muscle flaps, were cranially based on the rectus abdominis muscle and transposed to reconstruct the breast. Perfusion arises from the superior epigastric artery. The main disadvantage is that the lower abdomen is mainly perfused from the deep inferior epigastric artery and not the superior. The network between both of the arteries lies within the muscle and is very variable. It is not always sufficient to nourish the desired amount of tissue. Harvesting the muscle can result in weakness of herniation of the abdominal wall leading to pain or additional mesh stabilization surgery.

Improvement in microsurgical techniques and better understanding of anatomy then resulted in the first free TRAM flap that was microsurgically transplanted to the breast. Firstly the TRAM included the entire lower rectus abdominis muscle with the deep inferior epigastric vessels. After understanding the concept of perforator vessels, the muscle and fascia parts included were reduced to the necessary vessels. The classic TRAM became a muscle- and fascia-sparing (ms) flap.

The perforator concept then allowed to harvest the lower abdomen purely based on the perforator vessels without a significant amount of muscle or fascia. The DIEP-flap, deep inferior epigastric artery perforator flap, is the standard flap nowadays. The perforator consists of one artery and one or two accompanying veins, sometimes a nerve. The diameters can vary. An artery without a vein or a vein without an artery is very rare but will most likely result from prior operations.

One good perforator is usually enough to perfuse a flap. In all other cases, additional separated perforators or a small part of the muscle that includes some perforators is used. The goal is to have both a safe well-perfused flap and minimal donor site morbidity. DIEP- and ms-TRAM flaps usually do not harm the muscle significantly and allow a primary closure of the fascia in almost all cases. This is of importance especially below the arcuate line. The DIEP-flap is favoured over the pedicled TRAM flap as (1) the perfusion is better and (2) donor site complications are lower.

In the following we will mention only the DIEP-flap for simplicity. We will also only mention the perforator, although it consists of artery and vein.

The SIEA-flap is nourished from the superficial inferior epigastric artery. The harvested tissue is the same like in DIEP-/TRAM flaps, but the vessels are different.

10.1.1 Indications

Breast

Autologous tissue from the lower abdomen can often be used. The volume is enough to reconstruct one breast that matches the contralateral side. In bilateral reconstructions this technique does not have to respect the existing size as it creates two new symmetric breasts. If necessary a mastopexy technique has to be added to reduce the skin envelope. The new size has to be communicated with the patients prior to surgery.

Immediate reconstructions in SSM or NSM are best because they leave the breast skin intact. Secondary reconstructions require a visible skin inset from the flap. If a different skin type is not desired, an expander can be placed prior to autologous reconstructive surgery. In these cases the expander is placed epipectoral. The DIEP-flap can also be used with defects after BCT to replace volume. In these cases the DIEP can be used with only one perfusion zone.

Donor site

Mostly the patients have enough tissue at their lower abdomen. Only slender patients with a tight abdomen are not suitable. The tissue that can be harvested can be assessed with a pinch test and roughly compared to the breast volume. In many cases patients with less abdominal tissue have small breasts and thus being suited for this technique. If the lower abdomen and thigh are possible as donor sites, the site should be chosen according to the patient's desire and the surgeon's expertise. Scars from a caesarean section, appendectomies, rectus muscle diastasis, or an umbilical hernia do not exclude a DIEP-flap.

In the beginning of DIEP-flap surgery, it was not common to include patients with a BMI larger than 30. Nowadays we now that these patients benefit from this technique over an implant reconstruction. And, if the abdomen is handled gently, the complication rate is acceptable.

10.1.2 Contraindication

Patients after a liposuction in the donor site should be carefully examined if prior surgery (scars, dents, loss of tissue) is a contraindication. In our patients a DIEP was possible in many of those cases. A prior abdominoplasty is a contraindication. Median laparotomies can be a contraindication if the tissue from one side is not enough. However a reduction of the contralateral breast or the transplantation of both flaps on separate pedicles can be considered. Present hernias or repaired hernias are a contraindication. CT scan or MRI angiography (CTA or MRA) may allow a prior assessment of the abdomen.

Overview DIEP-flap
Indication: all breast shapes

Skin island:
- Transverse, rarely vertical (then VRAM)
- Size 30–40 cm width and 10–20 cm height, depending on the abdomen

Pedicle:
- Deep inferior epigastric artery and veins and their perforators
- Source: external iliac artery or femoral artery and vein
- Pedicle length, depending on the entering of the perforator into the flap up to 20 cm

Overview SIEA-flap
Indication: all breast shapes

Skin island lower abdomen:
- Size: 20–25 cm width and 10–20 cm height, depending on the abdomen. In most cases the ipsilateral SIEA does not perfuse beyond the midline. This has to be considered for planning. SIEA-flaps are therefore more suitable for smaller breasts or bilateral cases.

Pedicle:
- Inferior superficial epigastric artery and veins.
- Source: femoral artery; length max. 5–7 cm; the artery shows a small diameter. Note for inset that the pedicle enters from lateral into the flap (axial flap), while in a DIEP-flap (island flap), the pedicle enters from below.

Specials:
- Approximately 15% of all patients have a SIEA that can be used as pedicle for a flap and that perfuses a hemi-abdomen.
- The SIEA-flap does not require a perforator from the rectus muscle. The rectus sheath stays intact and is not injured. Donor site morbidity is decreased significantly.
- The pedicle enters from caudal into the flap. Therefore its placement is best to an IMAP which runs on the pectoral muscle.
- Flap shape and pedicle suggest the following: the pedicle in a right SIEA-flap enters caudally right. If turned 90° clockwise, the flap is best used in the left breast and anastomosed to an IMAP. Thus there is no vessel mismatch and the pedicle fits in length.

10.1.3 Characteristics

10.1.3.1 Perfusion

The DIEP-flap has characteristic arterial and venous properties. Perforator vessels perforate the rectus sheath, enter the fat below Scarpa's fascia and then the fascia itself to the subcutaneous tissue and then form a vascular plexus underneath the dermis. Therefore the fat underneath Scarpa's fascia can be resected in the flap periphery if needed without harming the perfusion.

This vascular plexus perfuses over the midline. If, for example, the perforator is located on the left side, the right side is perfused via this plexus. However there is a perfusion gradient. The best perfused zone is around the entrance of the perforator; the less perfused zone is the most distant on the contralateral side laterally. The classification into four zones, initially published by Hartrampf, was modified by Holm: zone 1 is located around the perforator, zone 2 lies on the same side like the perforator, zone 3 is located on the contralateral side next to the midline and borders to zone 1, and zone 4 is contralateral lateral. Mostly the perfusion beyond the midline is stable, so that zone 1–3 can be used safely. Zone 4 can be removed to avoid complications from decreased perfusion areas.

The flap should always be well perfused. Areas that are not well perfused should be removed. It is better to transplant a smaller flap that is well perfused. This technique avoids fat necrosis, revision surgery and bad outcomes after radiation therapy. If more volume is desired, a later lipofilling or implant should be considered.

Normally the superficial venous system of the flap corresponds with the deep system. The superficial veins drain into the deep system and then into the deep epigastric vein. In rare cases this network is not sufficient. The flaps show a venous congestion at the donor site and turn purple after dissection. It is difficult to find out beforehand which patients have insufficient connections between both systems. A well-executed CTA can add some evidence but also the fact that with the caudal incision large superficial veins or a significant superficial inferior epigastric system is encountered. In these cases it may be better not to use one single perforator but to include more large perforators or to harvest a ms-TRAM flap. One should also consider to dissect the superficial veins and to integrate them into the flap for backup. In some cases the superficial veins can be anastomosed additionally. Alternatively the volume reduction to only zone 1 and 2 can be another option.

In the *SIEA-flap*, the superficial inferior epigastric artery arises from the femoral artery, through the saphenous opening, and runs cranially. The pedicle enters from the caudal into the lower abdomen. It can run below or above Scarpa's fascia (▫ Fig. 10.22). The pedicle usually halves the inguinal ligament and is accompanied by some lymph nodes.

10.1.3.2 Tissue Characteristics

Tissue from the lower abdomen is soft and pliable and can be shaped well. The feel is like the involuted breast and lies like breast tissue within the skin envelope. Caudally the lower abdomen is thinner than periumbilical. This detail should be considered when the flap is inset.

The colour of the abdomen is lighter than the colour of the breast skin. In some patients the region can carry hair. As most of the flap is usually de-epithelialized, it is not relevant. However if hair remains at the breast, they can be later removed by laser or other permanent techniques.

The flap stays volume stable. Shrinkage was not seen in our patients when the body weight remains stable. If a radiation therapy becomes necessary, the entire flap can be included into the radiation field if flap vasculature is stable. In our patients we saw no significant shrinkage, aesthetic impairment or any flap loss. Recent studies confirm this result.

10.1.4 Informed Consent

The disclosure of general and special risks should be documented with standardized and evaluated forms. Infection, haematoma and wound-healing complications can occur. The risk of complete and partial flap loss should be mentioned, as well as wound-healing complications at the donor site like abdominal wall weakness and hernia. In rare cases a partial or complete necrosis of the umbilicus can occur. Seroma formation and visible scars can result. In mastectomy cases loss of sensitivity to the breast skin and the NAC is often. Loss of sensitivity can also occur at the donor site. A skin necrosis and NAC necrosis can occur and may require a reoperation. Smaller wound-healing problems can remain conservatively treated.

A lymph oedema of the breast and thoracic wall is possible in rare cases. The patient should be aware that breast shape, colour and symmetry are altered. Aesthetic change can result in psychological problems which may require psycho-oncologic consultation.

The incisions should be visualized in a drawing. The indication for a SSM or NSM should be discussed carefully. Scarring can distort the NAC in an NSM. Fat necrosis can occur. In most cases it shows no symptoms but can be detected by ultrasound. Second operations should be mentioned if histopathology is unclear or wound-healing problems occur or a contralateral mastopexy/reduction is required. A significant change after radiation is not likely to occur if the flap is well perfused; however it should be mentioned. If the patient does refuse recommended surgery or parts, this should also be documented.

If a bra and compression garments are recommended, the patients should be informed prior to surgery. Also the after treatment should be explained.

10.1.5 Planning and Preoperative Markings

10.1.5.1 CT Angiography (CTA) and Other Preoperative Imaging Techniques

The course of the epigastric vessels and the position of the ideal perforator are anatomically variable. Security can be increased if anatomy can be visualized beforehand. We found that the CTA is currently the best method to visualize the vessels. Duplex sonography and handheld Doppler can also show the vessel course, but they are highly dependent on the examiner, and they do not always give a sufficient overview. MR angiography also a proper technique; however duration of examination, costs and direct perforator imaging are not always sufficient and have limited use.

Once established CTA is a valuable planning tool. The image can be done in all planes, sagittal, axial and coronal, and of course as 3D image. The CTA scan shows also umbilical hernias and rectus diastases. The position of the umbilicus allows a good orientation. It is worthwhile to introduce the CTA with an interested radiologist and to focus on this cooperation. This ensures the necessary scan quality.

The use of contrast agents and the needed radiation dose are unfavourable. However when thoroughly planned, the CTA can be also used for staging purposes. CTA eases the search for the ideal perforator and can reduce harvest time. Especially in teaching situations, the CTA can facilitate learning to harvest the flap. The teacher, the fellow and the patients have a more relaxed situation. While experienced surgeons do not necessarily need a CTA in a single DIEP, in a bilateral DIEP, the CTA supports even the experienced surgeon.

CTA shows how the deep inferior epigastric artery enters from caudal/lateral into the rectus muscle. The coronal plane demonstrates a branching of the artery within the muscle (◘ Fig. 10.1). Ideally, but unfortunately rarely, the perforator arises with a short course within the muscle from the epigastric artery and perforates the rectus sheath. Mostly however the epigastric artery branches into 2–3 branches within the muscle. Moon and Taylor described these branches in 1988. The perforators then arise from these branches (◘ Fig. 10.2). Thus, if equivalent perforators are evident, the one with the least dissection effort can be chosen.

Sagittally the course of the epigastric artery is seen with regard to the muscle. It is evident whether the vessels run below or within the muscle. But also the superficial veins and the SIEA are demonstrated (◘ Figs. 10.3, 10.4, and 10.5). A high-quality CTA shows the detailed course of the SIEA within the flap and thus allows assessing if it runs more medially or laterally in the hemi-

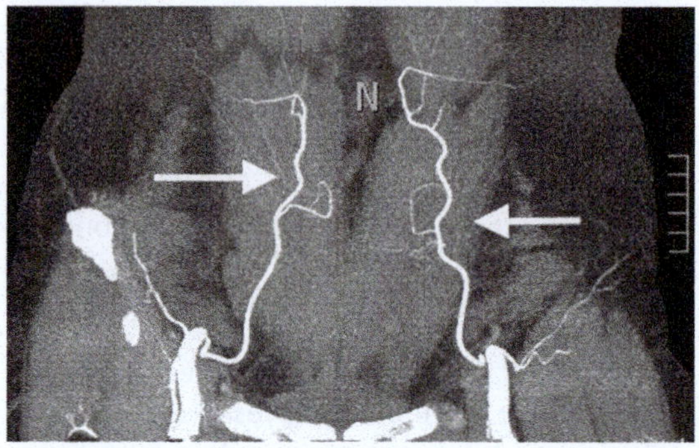

◘ **Fig. 10.1** Coronal CTA. Deep inferior epigastric artery enters from lateral into the rectus muscle. Here the artery does not branch. The perforator around the umbilicus (N) is the terminal branches of the artery

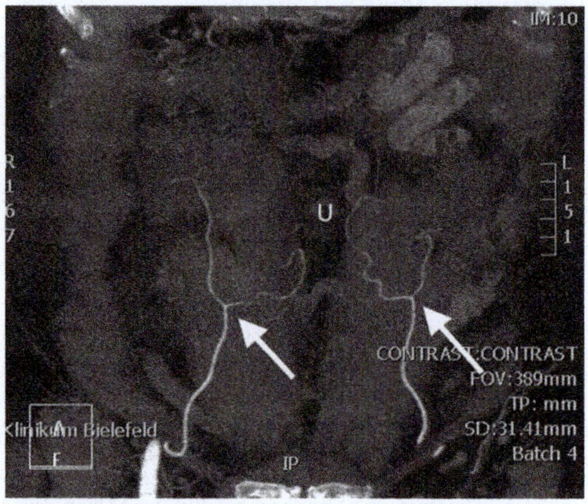

◘ **Fig. 10.2** Coronal CTA. The artery is not so strong compared to ◘ Fig. 10.1. The artery has two branches running medially and laterally

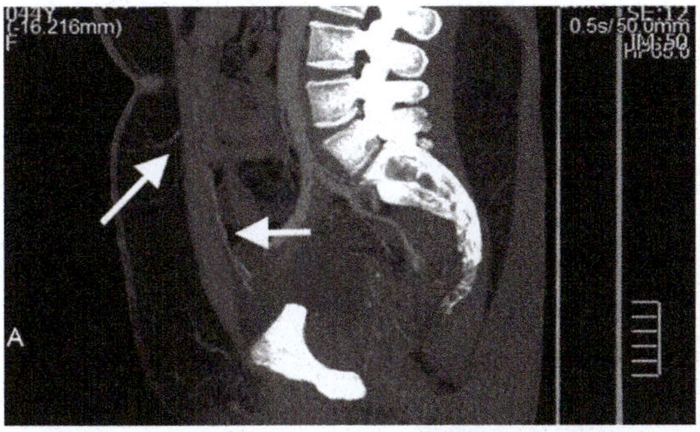

Fig. 10.3 Sagittal CTA. The deep inferior epigastric artery runs underneath the muscle (right arrow) and gives off a perforator (left arrow) after a short intramuscular course. The umbilicus is 2 cm higher

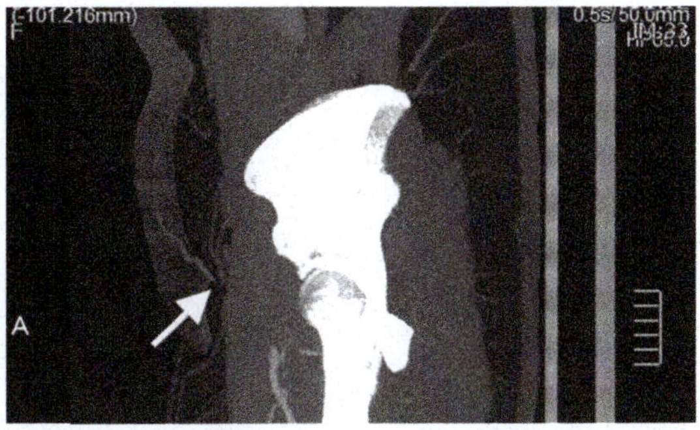

Fig. 10.6 Sagittal CTA. The SIEV (arrow) is present. Dorsal small branches of the SIEA are seen and some lymph nodes

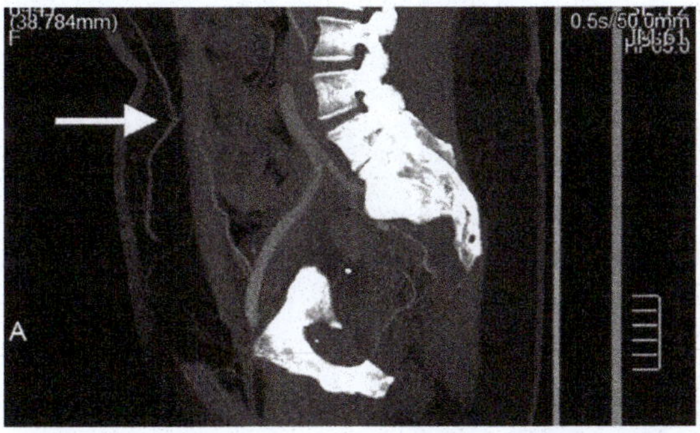

Fig. 10.4 Sagittal CTA. The venous perforator shows a connection with the superficial veins of the subcutaneous tissue. Thus the superficial is connected to the deep venous system

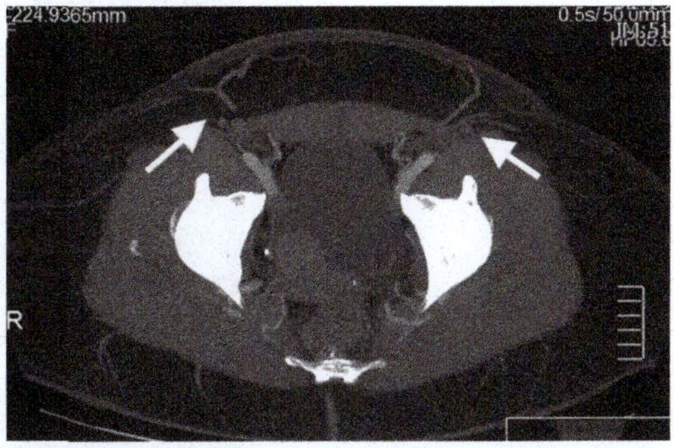

Fig. 10.7 Axial CTA, same patient like Fig. 10.6. SIEV is seen on both sides. Left, the SIEA branches are seen. They run more laterally, away from the flap volume. Thus a SIEA-flap is not suitable in this case

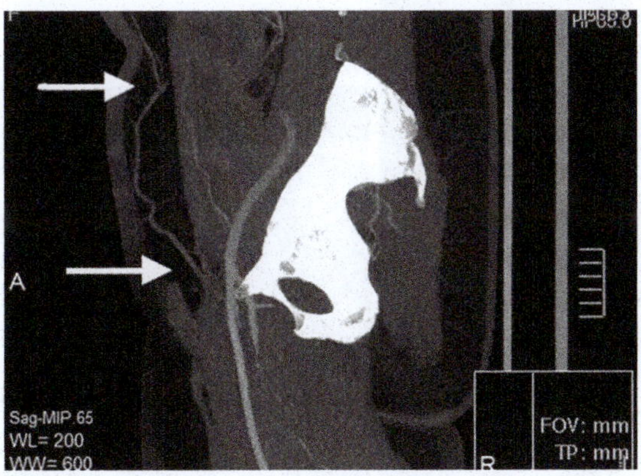

Fig. 10.5 Sagittal CTA, same patient like in Fig. 10.4. Communication between the two venous systems is present

abdomen (Figs. 10.6, 10.7 and 10.8). A SIEA that is visible in a CTA can mostly be used regarding its calibre.

Axially the perforators are seen best. The arterial phase allows assessing the arterial calibre, but also the venous drainage is seen (Fig. 10.9). The perforators exit the muscle and the rectus sheath. In many cases they exit at the tendinous intersections. If the course within the muscle is unclear, other CTA planes can help to assess it. A very pronounced superficial venous system can indicate an unincisive connection between the superficial and the deep venous system. Mostly the venous phase of the CTA can offer some evidence about the venous drainage.

Duplex sonography, handheld Doppler and recent thermal detections (e.g. thermography, Flir

Fig. 10.8 Sagittal thoracic and abdominal CTA. This figure shows that the ventral torso is basically perfused by a connected vascular system. The upper arrow shows a right IMA perforator in its arterial and venous phase; it can be used as recipient vessel. The middle arrow shows the IMA course dorsal caudal. The lower arrow shows a deep inferior epigastric artery perforator

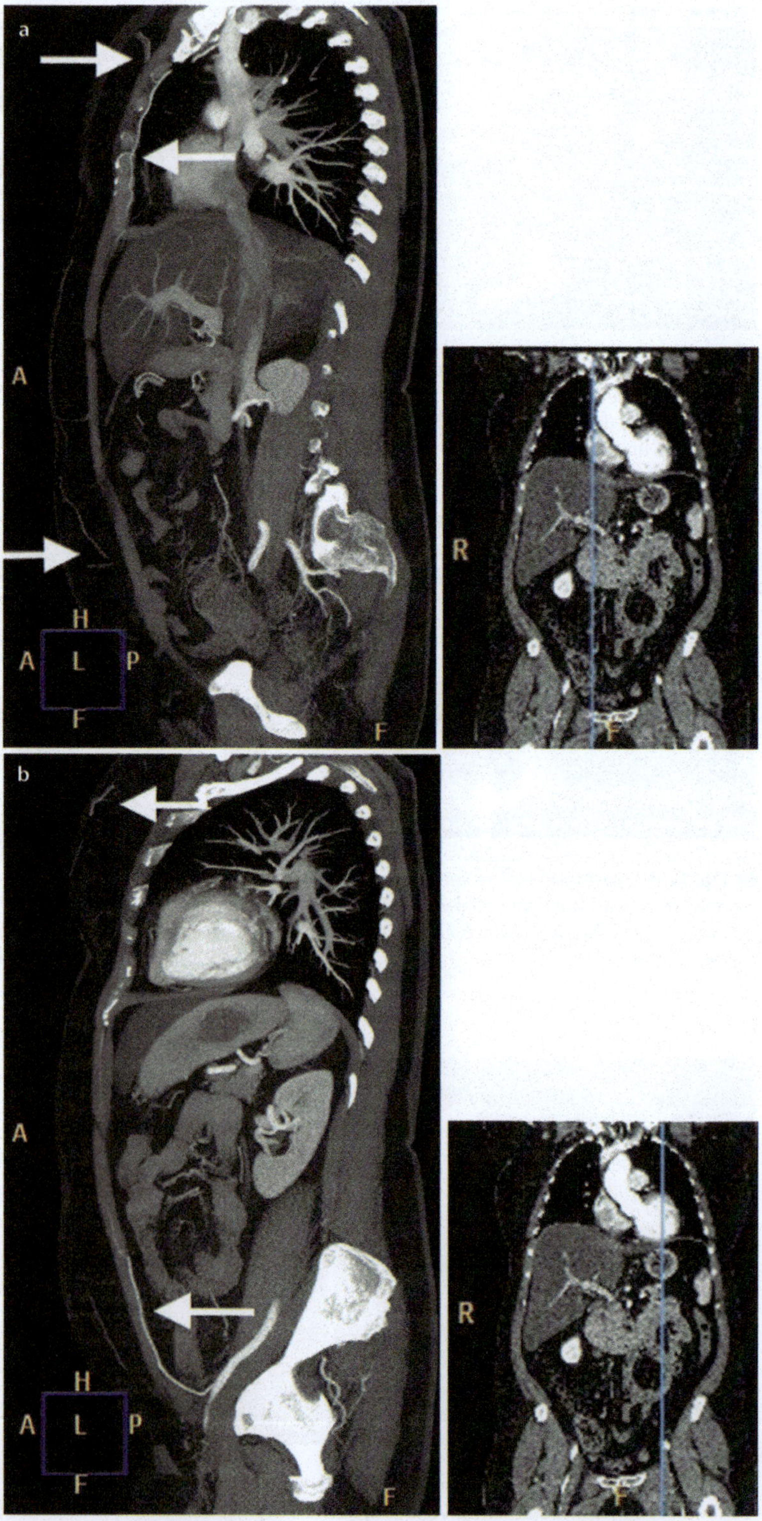

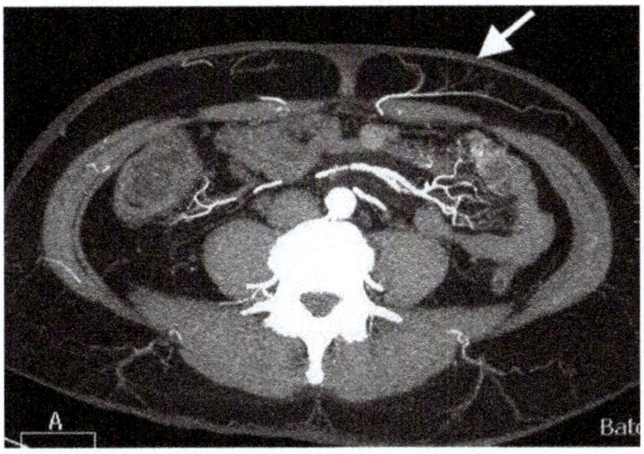

Fig. 10.9 Axial CTA. Significant periumbilical perforator with branches into the adipose tissue (arrow) in its venous and arterial phase. The perforator branches directly from the medial deep inferior epigastric artery. Harvesting does not cause a significant harm to the muscle. Note the strong lumbar perforators

Systems, USA) can also show the distribution and quality of the perforators. In opposite to a CTA, they do not have a radiation dose. However their sensitivity depends on the examiner. Some information like the course of the vessels within the muscle and the branching are better seen in the CTA.

Conclusion

CTA shows the course of the deep inferior epigastric artery and their perforators in all planes. This can reduce duration of the harvesting.

- CTA shows the course of the deep inferior epigastric artery and veins. In the sagittal plane, the superficial veins and the SIEA are seen.
- Coronal planes show the branching of the epigastric vessels within the muscle.
- Axial planes demonstrate the perforators clearly. The arterial phase shows the calibre, but also the venous drainage is usually visible.

10.1.5.2 Preoperative Markings and Measures

Tip

A scar from a prior caesarean section is not a contraindication for a DIEP-flap. It can be included as caudal DIEP incision, or if it is located too caudally, the DIEP incision can be placed cranially. This double incision does usually not cause any wound-healing problems but facilitates abdominal closure.

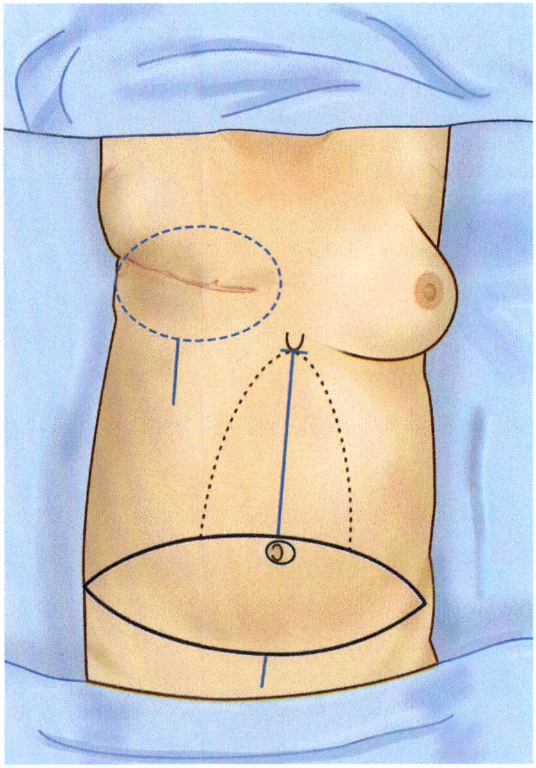

Fig. 10.10 Marking in a delayed reconstruction. The breast borders and the midline are marked. The mastectomy scar is used. At the abdomen the midline is marked as well as the incision, in this case ellipsoid-shaped

Markings are done with patient in upright position. The breast is marked. In secondary reconstructions the breast borders are marked with regard to the contralateral breast. The upper border and the IMF are landmarks. For centring the volume, the midline should be marked too (Fig. 10.10). If a mastopexy or reduction is planned with the contralateral breast, it should be also marked.

The main volume from a DIEP-flap is located periumbilically. The tissue around the umbilicus should therefore be included into the flap. This places the scar higher than in an aesthetic abdominoplasty. If enough volume is located below the umbilicus and a suitable perforator is present below the umbilicus, the upper incision can be placed more caudally, allowing a lower scar. This is a so-called low DIEP-flap.

The abdomen is marked like an abdominoplasty. If the skin is elastic and a surplus of tissue is evident, the lower incision can be placed at the border between the pubic eminence and the lower

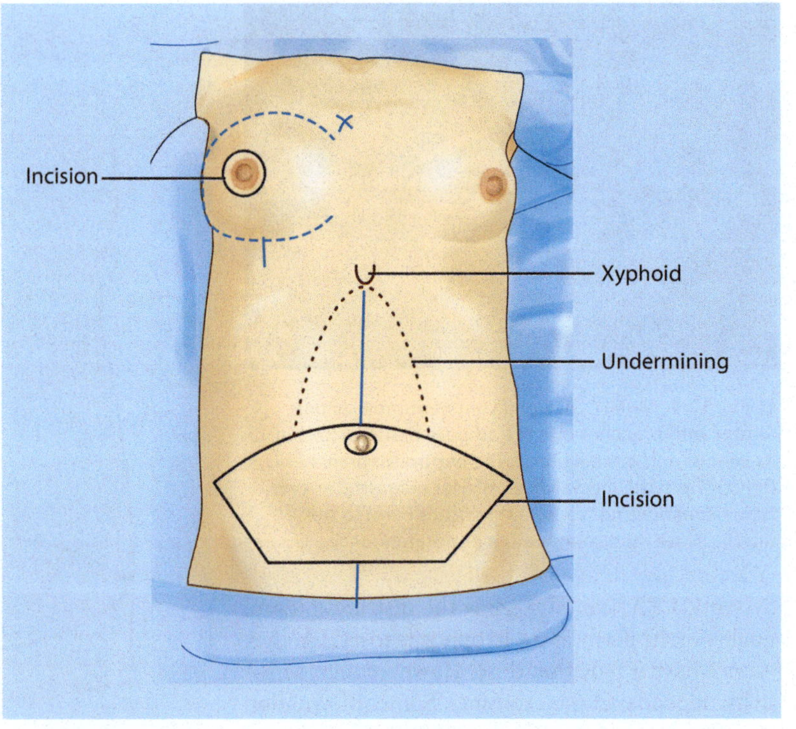

Fig. 10.11 Marking in a primary reconstruction. A periareolar mastectomy is planned. The breast borders and the midline are marked. The cross indicates an IMAP as a recipient vessel. At the abdomen the midline is marked as well as the limited Lockwood undermining. The flap is harvested with a trapezoid incision

abdomen. In a very tight abdomen, the scar should be placed higher to allow a tension-free closure. To place the lower scar in the relaxed tension lines, one can let the patient sit after marking to assess the marking. The cranial incision follows the existing volume and the needed volume. In most cases it is located periumbilically and will form an ellipse or a trapezoid running to the lateral ends of the incision (Figs. 10.10 and 10.11).

If a CTA was done beforehand, the main perforator can be marked, and the incision can be planned according to this perforator.

In bilateral DIEP-flaps, the midline is marked. To increase the flap volume, the lateral flap borders can be shifted laterally.

Preoperatively the patients should have a light diet, and a laxative can be considered to relieve the lower abdomen postoperatively.

Anatomic borders of SIEA- and DIEP-flaps

- Cranial: transverse incision above, at or below the umbilicus.
- Lateral: area around the anterior superior iliac spine (ASIS) on both sides.
- Caudal: transverse incision in transition to pubic eminence, approx. 6–8 cm lateral to the midline on both sides, and then forming an ellipse laterally cranially. The lower incision can be placed higher if the abdomen cannot be closed tension-free.

10.1.6 Technique

10.1.6.1 Positioning on the Operation Table, IV Lines

Patient is placed supine (Fig. 10.12). The table must be inflective at the hip and knee region. Arms are adducted by 45–30° in the shoulder. The elbows are placed on little arm pads, and the hands are placed under the lumbar region. In a two-team approach, simultaneously two electrosurgery devices with two electrodes are required. A Foley catheter is recommended. The patient's body temperature can be managed with a convective warming device (e.g. Bair Hugger). Two peripheral lines are sufficient, preferred at the ankle/feet. The anaesthesiologist is located at the foot. Breast and abdomen are prepared.

10.1.6.2 Operation

Flap harvesting is best performed under loupe magnification with a headlight. A microscope is necessary for anastomosis. Harvesting is per-

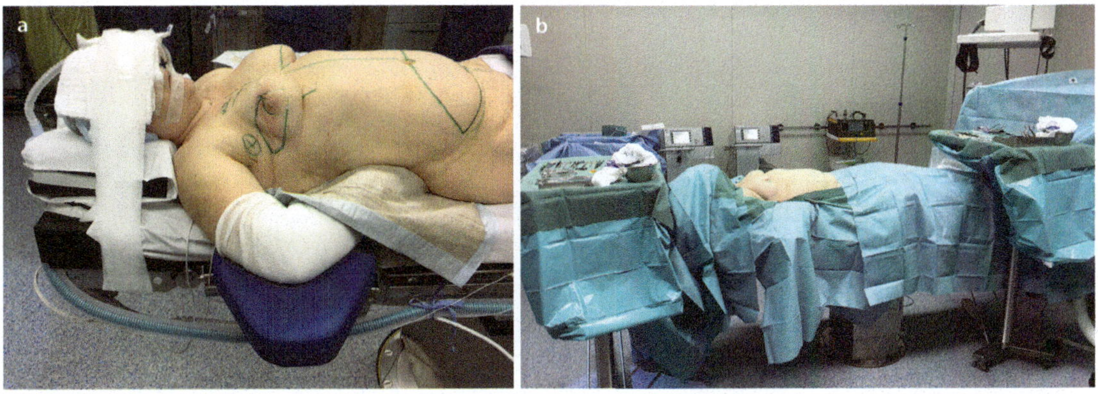

Fig. 10.12 **a** Positioning on the operating table for a DIEP-flap. The patient receive two peripheral IV lines at the foot/ankle. A central line or an arterial monitoring is not necessary in otherwise healthy patients. Ventilation tubes are extended so that patient's head and torso are placed away from the anaesthesiologist. **b** Two operation tables are used. The anaesthesiologists can approach the patient from distal. If necessary they are allowed to control ventilation at any time. The same setting is used with the inner thigh flap

formed within 45–90 min if no complications occur. Dissection of the recipient site depends on type of reconstruction, immediate or delayed.

Dissection can be performed with scissors (Metzenbaum) or by electrosurgery. The latter however can lead to more seroma. Dissection of the pedicle should be done with bipolar forceps and fine scissors. A right-handed surgeon stands on the right side of the patient.

In the following we describe the most important techniques of harvesting. The perforator dissection however stays always the same.

Common and safe option

If there is no CTA, just incise caudally. This gives you the freedom to lower or higher the upper incision after the ideal perforator location has been selected.

After the dermis is cut, superficial veins, approx. 4–6 cm lateral of the midline, cross the incision perpendicularly. They can be dissected more caudally as a backup and clipped caudally. In our experience these veins are rarely needed, but they can offer an additional venous drainage if necessary.

More lateral, also perpendicular to the incision, the SIEA vessels are seen. Their course and calibre are very variable. They can be seen below or on Scarpa's fascia. The veins can run separated from the artery. In most cases the vessels are small and can be coagulated.

Once on the rectus sheath, the flap is elevated from caudal to cranial. The midline is the adherence zone at the linea alba. There are no significant perforators here. Smaller perforators can be coagulated and dissect further cranially. A strong caudal perforator should be kept. If they exist they usually have a favourable extra muscular run and perfuse the flap very well. In some cases the strong perforator is just "faked" by a strong sensitive nerve that travels with the vessels subcutaneously. Then the perforator should not be used.

Mostly there are two perforator rows, medial and lateral. Strong perforators are located mostly more cranially at the periumbilical level (Figs. 10.13 and 10.14). Most medially located perforators perfuse better across the midline than the lateral ones. However they can have a lower perfusion on zone 2. Lateral perforators leave the muscle less harmed when harvested (Fig. 10.14).

Patients after pregnancies can have a rectus muscle diastasis. The muscles are more apart than usual. This can make the lateral perforators appear too laterally. Accidentally these perforators can be coagulated or not included into the flap.

If the right perforator was not found by this approach, cut the umbilicus circularly. A stay suture is placed always in the same manner (we prefer a horizontal one) to avoid a twisting when the umbilicus is restored. The fascia around the umbilicus is cut, and the region around the umbilicus can be dissected very well by holding the stay suture and elevating the abdominal tissue with a little blunt hook (baby Langenbeck). If a goof perforator is located within the flap, the cranial incision can be made.

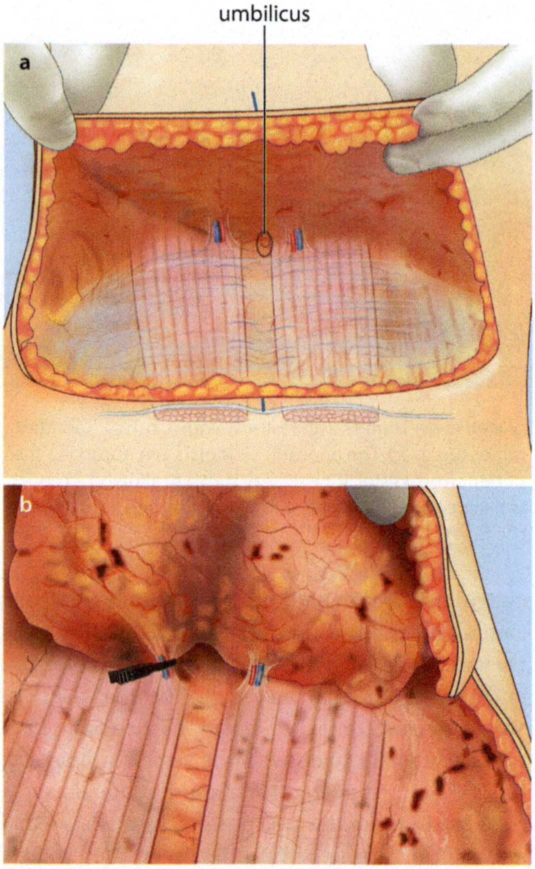

■ **Fig. 10.13** **a** After the caudal incision, the epifascial dissection leads to a sufficient perforator. The umbilicus is incised and freed and a stay suture is placed. It is held cranially. In this case two strong perforators are evident on each side (the rectus sheath is drawn transparently to show the muscle course). **b** One perforator is temporarily clamped with a bulldog. Thus the DIEP is only perfused from the selected one. It takes up to 5 min to finally assess the blood flow within the flap. If the perfusion from the selected perforator is not sufficient, remove the clamp from the first perforator and put it on the second. This technique allows a clinical assessment of flap perfusion (inflow, distribution within the flap, assessment of zones and outflow). The BP should be normal for this manoeuvre. An intraoperative Doppler signal does not indicate the perfusion within the flap. Pulsation can be palpated with fingers. If the perforators look the same, the one with the bigger vein and the less complicated intramuscular course (from CTA) should be used. In this case we use the left one

If several perforators are present, the ideal one or two can be selected by temporarily clamping the ones one do not intend to use. After approx. 5 min, the perfusion is based on the not clamped perforators, and one can assess the quality of the perfusion. If the flap bleeds light red from the

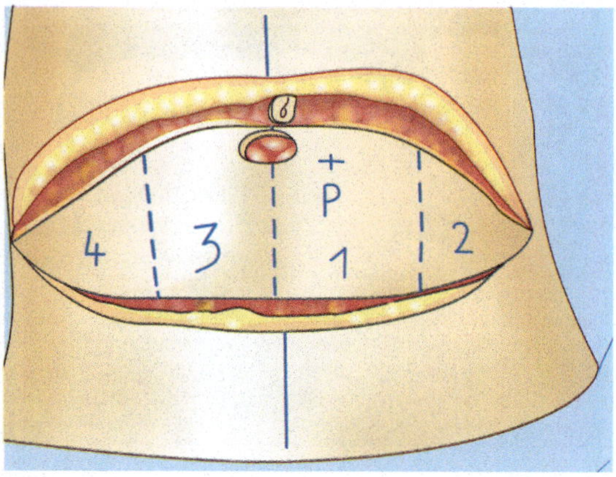

■ **Fig. 10.14** Zones of the DIEP-flap (according to Holm) in a left periumbilical perforator (P): around the perforator zone 1, same side adjacent 2, 3 adjacent across the midline and 4 is the most distant zone. Zone 4 can be resected in most cases. Only tissue that is well perfused should be transplanted, even if the flap becomes smaller than planned

edges, one can narrow down the perfusion to one perforator. If the flap is more whitish or purple, another perforator should be opened, or a complete different one should be selected.

10

Tip

Which perforator is the right one? If possible only one good perforator should be included. It facilitates dissection, preserves the muscle and allows a better inset into the recipient site. Selection should be decided clinically by means of flap perfusion. The good perforator has always a visible, well-filled vein. Its pulsation can be palpated if the BP is good. However the vein is the most important criterion. Almost always a well-filled vein is accompanied by a respective artery. In the opposite a good artery can have an insufficient vein in up to 35% of cases. Some perforators are "scared" by dissection and develop a spasm. Artery and vein appear thin. However the impression the surgeon has at "first sight" is mostly the right one. Leaving the perforator for a little period or applying papaverine allows reassessing the perforator. Another technique is to incise the rectus sheath and assess the perforator directly underneath the fascia. If the vein is well filled, the perforator is mostly suitable.

Perforator location. As stated there are two rows of perforators, medial and lateral. This refers to the rectus muscle. The most suitable perforators are around the umbilicus. But also caudal perforators can be suitable. Medial perforators are supposed to perfuse better across the midline than lateral ones. Theory is not always supported by clinical anatomy. The intraoperative clinical assessment should lead the decision for the right perforator, which is strong, has a well-filled vein and shows a good perfusion to the flap after temporarily clamping other perforators. If several good perforators exist, one should select the one that matches the breast shape best, prevents muscle injury and can be harvested faster. A CTA can be supportive.

If one perforator is not enough, two or three can be included into the flap. It is favourable over a ms-TRAM flap because only the fascia around the perforators is incised. Thus the rectus sheath is closed without tension. A ms-TRAM flap always includes more muscle and fascia without a well-defined perforator dissection.

While perforators are temporarily clamped, the upper abdominal dissection can take place. It is recommended to only release the adherence zones at the upper abdomen according to Lockwood: release medial over the midline up to the xiphoid and a little more laterally (◘ Fig. 10.15). This keeps enough lateral perforators intact to perfuse the abdominal wall. The wide dissection up to the costal arches is not needed in most cases.

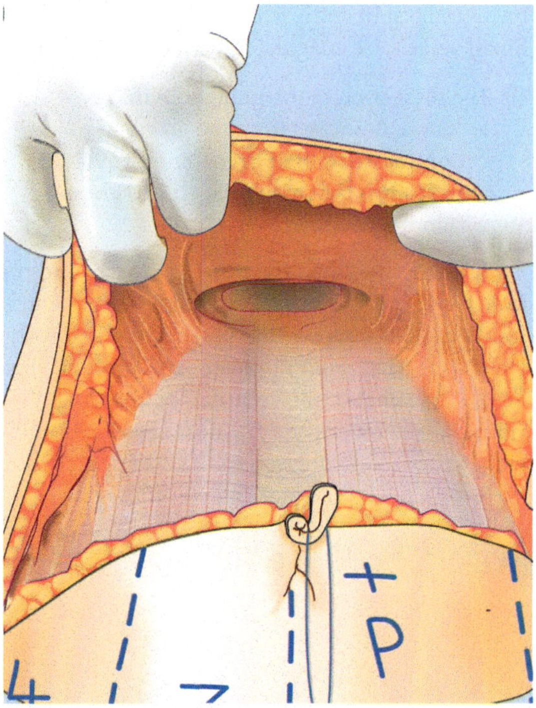

◘ **Fig. 10.15** After the perforator has been selected, the upper abdomen is dissected. A limited dissection is important to keep the perfusion of the abdominal wall intact and reduce wound-healing complications. The "high tension abdominoplasty" after Lockwood just releases the adherence zones at the midline and transversely central. Especially in patients with a high BMI or smokers, this can prevent complications. However a tension-free closure should be aimed after bringing the patient into the beach chair

▪▪ Incision of the rectus sheath

This manoeuvre is the same for all techniques. The incision is made with a knife. Initially the incision can be short, 5–6 cm. If needed the cut can be extended later on. A short incision is enough in most cases. A Roux or Langenbeck hook can help to follow the vessels. However this depends on the vessel course and anatomy. The shorter the incision the better the healing and stability of the rectus sheath, which is the important factor for preventing abdominal weakness. Especially below the arcuate line, the dorsal stabilization is missing. The risk for an abdominal weakness is low with DIEP-flaps or ms-TRAM flaps compared to pedicled TRAM flaps, but the longer the incision, the higher the risk for a weakness.

Almost always the perforator branches into several limbs before it enters the fat. They have to be coagulated or clipped carefully before they are divided. One now can follow the perforator into the muscle. We recommend fine DeBakey forceps and fine scissors (e.g. a Stevens Tenotomy). A blunt dissector, a fine Overholt forceps or a fine microdissector can support the dissection. Small and medium clips are useful for clipping the branches. Relaxation of the patient when dissecting the perforator can also be of help. A bipolar forceps is preferred for coagulation within the muscle (in lower effect and power if applicable).

If only one perforator is used, it can be followed from periphery to central. The muscle can be bluntly split with a dissector (◘ Fig. 10.16). Small vessels are coagulated with bipolar forceps.

The dissection of the pedicle should be accurate. Branches from the artery are clipped close to their branching to avoid long stumps that may cause turbulences within the vessels.

Pedicle length follows the need of the flap and the preference of the surgeon. The longer the pedicle is dissected, the bigger the vessels become. Mostly two veins that communicate are present. Just before they enter the femoral or external iliac vein, both veins merge. In most cases it is sufficient to use the stronger vein. If short pedicles are used, the vein that mainly drains the perforator should be used.

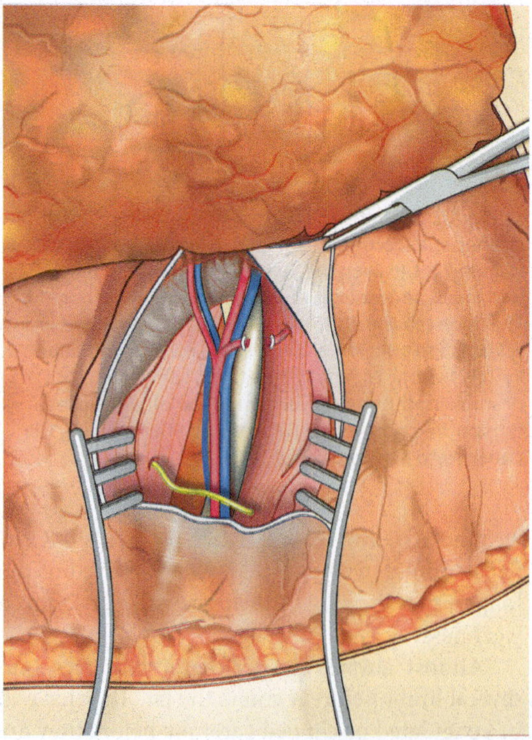

◘ **Fig. 10.16** After the rectus sheath is opened, the perforator is followed from periphery to central until the main vessel is seen. The muscle can be split bluntly with a fine blunt forceps (e.g. a Overholt forceps). Smaller vessels are coagulated with the bipolar forceps. The dissection has to be very accurate. Branches from the artery and vein should be clipped close to vessel to avoid turbulences within the vessels. The pedicle length follows the needs of flap inset. The longer the pedicle the stronger the vessels become. Usually two veins are present which communicate. Just before they enter the femoral or external iliac vein, both veins merge. In most cases it is sufficient to use the stronger vein. If short pedicles are used, the vein that mainly drains the perforator should be used

If several perforators are used, everyone has to follow to the main vessel. Using more than on perforator means that the segmental nerves that run from lateral to medial have to be divided and possibly re-coapted.

After dissection of the pedicle, the temporarily clamped perforators can be clipped. The flap now is based solely on this pedicle. Surplus tissue or not well-perfused parts can be resected. If flap position at the recipient site is determined, the parts that require de-epithelialization can be provided.

The final resection of the pedicle must be done accurately. A bleeding from the deep epigastric artery or vein is difficult to control. We use large Ligaclips. The flap is prepared for anastomosis now (◘ Fig. 10.17). The rectus sheath is primarily closed (◘ Figs. 10.18 and 10.19). If applicable the fascia can be closed caudally by doubling. We use a strong Vicryl suture with simple interrupted sutures to close the fascia roughly. The fascia is then closed with a barbed double-armed suture in a running technique (e.g. Quill size 2, polydioxanone). This usually leaves a strong hold of the fascia. If a ms-TRAM flap was harvested and the suture displaces the umbilicus to side of closure, the contralateral side can be gathered with the same suture to achieve a midline position of the umbilicus.

After the drains were placed, the abdominal closure can be done. The patient is placed in a "beach chair position". Below the umbilicus a 3-0 Vicryl is placed in the midline at the rectus sheath

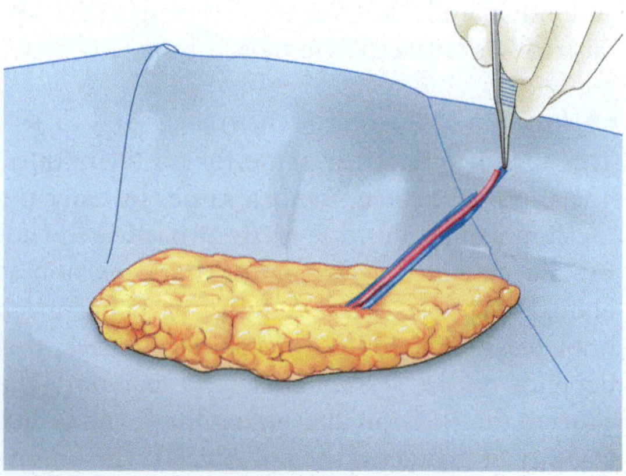

◘ **Fig. 10.17** Cut flap with pedicle. The pedicle is dissected under the microscope by separating the artery and vein and flushing the vessels with heparin solution

and then left together with the ends of the umbilicus stay suture. Suturing Scarpa's fascia with a strong resorbable interrupted suture closes the cranial and caudal abdominal wound. The subcorial suture is done with interrupted sutures (e.g. 3-0 Monocryl or Vicryl). The skin is closed with a running intracutaneous suture.

Before the abdomen is closed, the position of the umbilicus is determined. To allow a proper positioning, the skin should be closed centrally. Above the umbilicus a caudally pedicled U- or V-shaped flap is created. The umbilicus is taken out through the created hole with its stay suture. Some fat resection around the umbilicus and the flap can provide a better aesthetic result. The umbilicus is cranially fixed. Caudally a part is resected from the umbilicus that resembles the flap. The flap is then fixed to the abdominal wall using the provided Vicryl suture. This suture grasps the flap and the caudal part of the umbilicus. By this manoeuvre a more aesthetic result can be achieved. The circular suture around the umbilicus is done with a running intracutaneous suture.

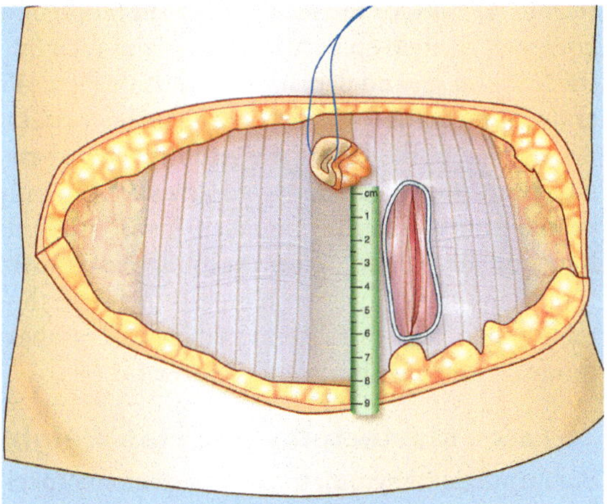

Fig. 10.18 The shorter the rectus sheath incision is made, the lower the risk of abdominal weakness or herniation. In a favourable vessel course and branching pattern, a 5–6 cm incision is usually sufficient. The caudal dissection is best made with a rectus sheath lifted upwards with a Roux or Langenbeck hook. A soft wad holds the dorsal sheath away from the dissection plane

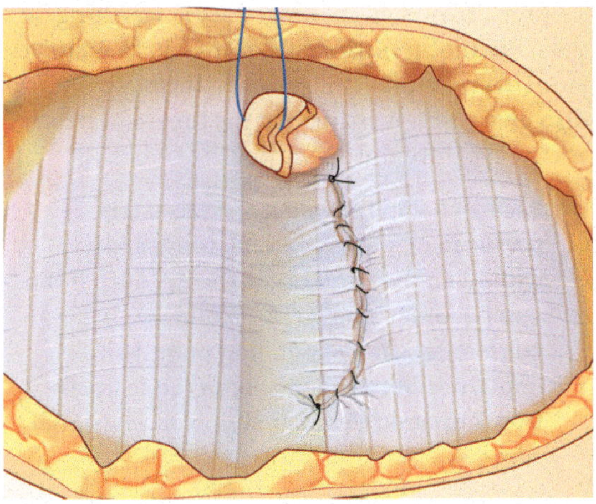

Fig. 10.19 The ventral rectus sheath is sutured with single interrupted strong Vicryl sutures; if applicable the fascia can be closed caudally by doubling. The fascia is then closed with a barbed double-armed suture in a running technique (e.g. Quill size 2, polydioxanone). This usually leaves a strong hold of the fascia

Harvesting with CTA

If a CTA was done beforehand, the selected perforators should be marked on the flap. If the CTA is reliable, the whole flap can be incised caudally and cranially. One can directly dissect the desired perforators. A contralateral backup should always be left and only resected after the dissection was successful. The pedicle dissection is done as mentioned above.

Bilateral DIEP-flap

A bilateral DIEP-flap is better performed with a prior CTA. Even experienced surgeons have a higher flap loss rate in bilateral flaps because both sides are not perfused identically well by the epigastric arteries. The CTA allows proper planning regarding the incisions and inclusion of perforators. The midline can be cut in the beginning allowing better access to the field. The perforators dissected from caudal and medial. The vessels are dissected as mentioned above. The rectus sheath should be closed as mentioned above. However if primary closure is not possible, a mesh can be used. It is recommended to use combined meshes from resorbable and non-resorbable material. The meshes should be placed and fixed on the muscle but underneath the rectus sheath. This reduces the palpation of sutures and scarring in thinner patients.

SIEA-flap

The SIEA halves the inguinal ligament. Variations are often present. The SIEA can run on or below Scarpa's fascia, depending on the incision. If a sufficient SIEA is seen at the caudal incision or in a prior CTA, it should be kept intact. After complete dissection the SIEA can be assessed by temporarily clamping the DIEP perforators. If the flap is then perfused at least to the midline and if no more volume than this is needed for the breast reconstruction, the SIEA can be considered. It is important to carefully assess the perfusion area, because in rare cases the SIEA can run towards the ASIS with almost no flow to the desired flap. In that case the flap is not perfused. Usually the pedicle can be dissected from the caudal wound. A little Langenbeck hook or Cottle hook can lift the skin up. Pedicle length can be 5–7 cm depending from the height of the caudal incision (◘ Figs. 10.22, 10.23, 10.24 and 10.25). At the femoral vessels, the vein plexus can become vulnerable and confusing. Consider to have a shorter pedicle than a messed up one.

▪ ▪ Special cases, venous

Some flaps require an additional venous drainage. This can be a result of a wrong perforator selection. Sometimes the superficial venous system does not communicate with the deep system at all. With proper planning these cases are rare. In many cases the resection of the venous congested flap parts can improve the situation. If this does not work and the flap is congested in the central parts, an additional venous anastomosis of a superficial vein is recommended. A congested flap fills the superficial veins automatically; thus it can be evaluated if they are suitable for an additional anastomosis. Additional recipient veins can be used at the subscapular vessels/axilla or caudal or cranial IMAP veins. The caudal IMV was also reported to be useful as additional vein although the direction is against the regular flow. The cranial/lateral cephalic vein was also described as recipient vein after it was harvested and transposed to the cranial border of the recipient site. This needs an additional incision. If venous interposition grafts are required, they can be harvested from the caudal abdominal wound. Longer grafts can be taken from arm, feet or lower leg. This leads to additional scars. The contralateral epigastric vessels were also described as grafts.

▪ ▪ Special cases, arterial

Mostly arterial perfusion is sufficient for zone 1–3. In cases where all zones are required (e.g. defect closure or if after median laparotomy both hemi-abdomens are needed), a second pedicle may secure perfusion. Usually the contralateral deep inferior epigastric artery and vein serve as second pedicle. However a sufficient SIEA can also provide a good pedicle. If the first pedicle is anastomosed to the IMA, the second can be anastomosed to the first pedicle, the subscapular vessels or a cranial IMAP. Anastomoses to the caudal IMA are also possible. The nicest way is to hook up the second flap to the first flap pedicle. In this case the cranial stump of the epigastric vessels of the first flap is harvested a little bit longer and temporarily clamped. This stump is then the recipient vessel for the second flap. The blood flow goes over the two epigastric arteries and then into the first and second flap. In our hands this is a safe and fast technique as a second recipient vessel is not needed at the breast site and the first epigastric artery has to be dissected anyway. The only prerequisite is that the cranial epigastric stump is long and large enough for a second anastomosis. If the flap should cover both breasts or a large thoracic wall defect, the second pedicle can be anastomosed to the contralateral IMA or IMAP.

10.1.6.3 Mastectomy and Flap Weight

For an adequate symmetry, the mastectomy specimen should be weighed. In a secondary reconstruction, the mastectomy specimen weight is usually documented in the histopathology report. After the flap is resected, it can also be weighed. Normally the gland and the DIEP-flap have a similar volumic density. Only if the gland is very dense and heavy, the weight is not a real indicator because the gland is then heavier despite a small volume. However in most cases, weighing is a valuable tool to estimate symmetry. In a conversion from implants/expander, their weight can also give a rough estimate if the breasts were symmetrical before the operation.

> **!** **Parts of a flap that are not adequately perfused or show a venous congestion should not be used but resected, even if the flap becomes smaller. A secondary augmentation by lipofilling or a small implant is better than a large fat necrosis from impaired vascular supply or revisional surgery.**

10.1.6.4 Shaping and Inset of the Flap, Buried Flap

Not required parts should be resected; not required skin should be de-epithelialized. Leaving the dermis keeps the subdermal vascular plexus intact, and perfusion is not harmed. Flap inset should follow the breast shape. The contralateral breast should be the breast that indicates the shape, or a contralateral mastopexy/reduction or even augmentation is planned. If the breasts have a ptosis or are large, this has to be integrated into the reconstructive algorithm. If unsafe parts of the flap are not removed, they should be placed lateral or caudal, where they can be better removed than in the décolleté of the breast.

The DIEP-flap is very versatile. It can be placed vertically or horizontally. The lower abdomen is thinner caudally. Therefore in a horizontal inset, the flap should be rotated by 180° (◘ Figs. 10.20 and 10.21). The flat part of the flap is located cranially and gives a natural result. In a vertical inset, the volume should follow the contralateral side. Shaping can also be done actively. Parts that are not needed can be removed; surplus fat underneath Scarpa's fascia can be removed with respect to the perforators, which allows better transition from thoracic tissue to the flap. Coning sutures can be applied to achieve projection. However the sutures should not impair perfusion and thus cause fat necrosis.

In secondary reconstructions with a transverse scar, the scar is excised, and the cranial part is elevated from the muscle. It can be done with the lower part too. The flap is then placed into this pocket. The skin island in this case is ellipsoid. If the skin is altered from radiation, the DIEP needs a long time to sag in its natural position. Especially in ptotic contralateral breasts, it is better to remove the caudal skin from the thoracic wall from the mastectomy scar to the IMF. The DIEP-flap is then de-epithelialized and cranially placed into the cranial pocket and is sutured with the abdominal skin left in place to the IMF. The décolleté has its original skin, and caudally the DIEP-flap is naturally shaped without any restrictions from scars or skin problems. This inset follows the aesthetic units of the breast. Unfavourable is the different colour of the abdominal skin compared to the original breast skin.

There are many concepts regarding the flap sutures. We think that the flap should at least be fixed medially and in the IMF to avoid dents and malposition and allow smooth transitions. Cranially and laterally sutures should be applied if the flap is better positioned and shaped. To avoid fat necrosis, the flap side should only be fixed at Scarpa's fascia or the dermis.

Bringing the patient into a sitting position intraoperatively can help to estimate the amount of needed skin, and its position on the flap in secondary reconstructions thus facilitates symmetry. If the mastectomy skin flap is not well perfused or cannot be assessed properly, the abdominal skin can be left on the flap. The mastectomy flap is placed over the flap. The flap is now buried. After some days viability of the mastectomy skin can be assessed. If the mastectomy skin has survived, the abdominal skin is removed in a short second operation; if not the mastectomy skin can be replaced by flap skin (◘ Figs. 10.42 and 10.43).

10.1.6.5 Anastomoses

The general technique has been described in ► Chap. 8. For a DIEP-flap, the anastomoses should be done at the IMA or IMAP vessels. IMA calibre resembles the epigastric vessels. Because long pedicles can be harvested for a DIEP-flap, the cranial IMAP can also be used as recipient vessels without hampering breast position or shape. The standard IMA approach is in the 3rd ICS. Perforator veins or the IMV can be coupled. The IMAP veins show more valves. At the anastomotic site, no valve should be present. IMAP veins are thinner than the IMV; thus gentle handling is required.

The arterial anastomosis to the IMA is usually easy. Anastomosis can be done in the preferred technique. In large vessels a running suture can be used for the back wall and the front wall of the vessel, respectively. Short pedicles can be best sutured with the backhand technique. Long pedicles can be done with a flip-over technique.

In a persistent calibre mismatch, the distance between the stiches on each side of the vessel should be proportional, thus wider at the larger side and narrower at the smaller sider. An 8-0 to 10-0 nylon should be adequate.

Generally the anastomosis can be done at the subscapular vessels, which requires a long pedicle. The recipient vessels are usually thinner. If the vessels are dissected due to an axillary lymphadenectomy, the anastomosis is feasible. However, due to the central position, the good blood flow, the possibility to use shorter pedicles and the fact that the anastomosis is more convenient at the IMA, we prefer the IMA system.

SIEA-flaps are best anastomosed to an IMAP. The calibre is matching and the positioning is easy. Due to the fact that the flap is "only" a hemi-abdomen, the subscapular vessels are not suitable for proper flap positioning.

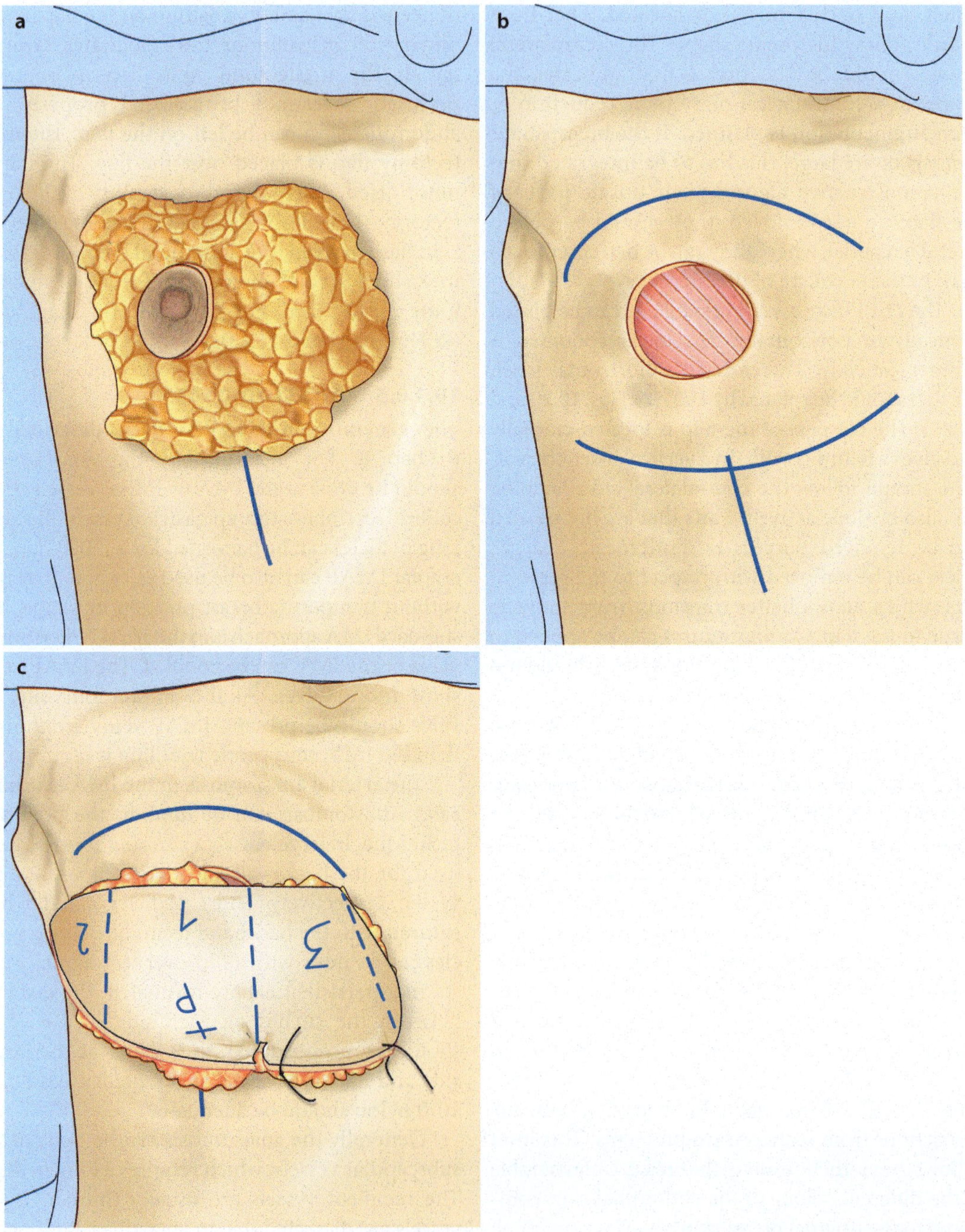

Fig. 10.20 **a** Mastectomy from a periareolar approach. **b** After mastectomy and dissection of the recipient vessels. **c** Temporary fixation of the flap for anastomosis. The mastectomy skin is lifted with a hook and the anastomosis is performed. The patient is placed in a beach chair position. The second team can close the abdomen. The flap is 180° rotated. The thinner part lays cranially and the thicker part caudally. By this manoeuvre the transition between the tissues is well hidden. In breasts which are wider than high, this technique gives good results. The marked midline can help to centre the volume. Refinements can be made by bringing the patient into a sitting position. The selected perforator was periumbilical left. Its entry into the flap now is caudal. Zone 4 is resected. A right-sided perforator would have shortened the pedicle. Alternatively the flap can be fit in vertically by 90°. The subcutaneous tissue should then be placed like in the contralateral side. Any flap positioning has to respect the pedicle length to the recipient vessels. No tension on the pedicle and anastomosis is allowed. A malposition of the flap due to a too short pedicle results in insufficient aesthetic results

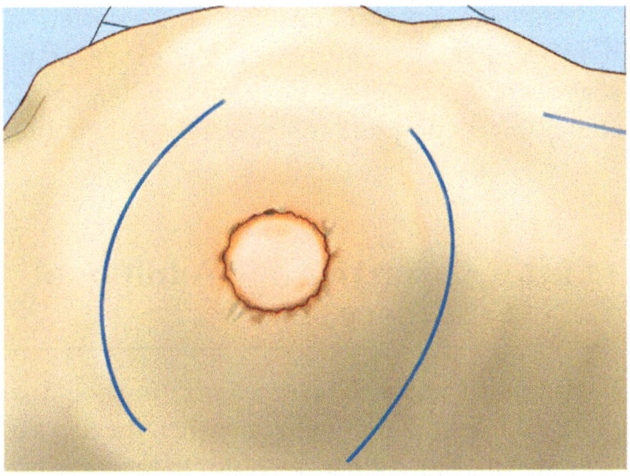

■ **Fig. 10.21** The flap is then de-epithelialized if the mastectomy skin is well perfused. The flap skin that replaces the NAC is left. We prefer to suture the flap medially and at the IMF (adherence zones of the breast). Cranially we put some stiches between the thoracic fascia and the flap (either Scarpa's fascia or the dermis). Lateral a suture between flap and thoracic wall can add some projection. All sutures should be buried and put with respect to the pedicle

10.1.7 Monitoring

After mastectomy and immediate reconstruction or secondary reconstruction, the decision has to be made if skin from the flap has to be used. If so the skin can be used to monitor flap viability. If no skin island is required, one should consider placing a temporary monitor island at the incision line to assess flap viability. A small, representative part is sufficient. If viability remains stable, the monitor can be resected after 2–5 days after flap transplantation. It can be done under local anaesthesia. The flap is de-epithelialized and buried under the mastectomy skin. A later resection is also possible but can impair the aesthetic outcome.

If the mastectomy skin cannot be assessed intraoperatively regarding its viability, the flap skin can be left temporarily underneath the mastectomy skin for some days. The flap is kept buried until the viability is clear. If mastectomy skin has to be resected, the resulting defects can be replaced by flap skin in a second operation short after (■ Figs. 10.42 and 10.43).

10.1.8 Aftercare

The patients are positioned in their bed in a beach chair position: upper part 15–45° up, legs bent in the hips and knees. If a direct transfer from the operating table into the bed is not possible, the legs should be elevated on a bolster until the patient is placed in her bed.

The patients are mobile as soon as they can get up. They should get up from the bed with relaxed abdominal muscles. They should be supported and instructed by PT or nurses when getting up the first times. The abdomen should be relaxed by bending the tummy when walking in the first days. The Foley catheter can be removed at the first postoperative day. A light diet is preferred the first 2 postoperative days. Bowel movement should be monitored. A bra that does not compress the pedicle can be used if necessary. A belt or corsage can stabilize the abdomen in the first postoperative days.

Thromboprophylaxis is recommended. Drains should be removed with regard to the fluid amount. Work and daily activities should be possible after 1 week and should not exceed the standard. Sporting, sauna and sun tanning should be avoided for at least 6 weeks.

A loss of sensitivity at the abdomen and the breast is usual. Seromas at the donor site can be punctured if necessary.

10.1.9 Complications

Complications are rare if surgery is properly performed. The vascular complications are similar for all free flaps (■ Fig. 10.44). Therefore these complications and their management are described in ► Sect. 8.5.

At the *donor site*, little haematomas can be tolerated; larger haematomas that cause pain, impair the aesthetic outcome or cause severe blood loss require revision. Necrosis of the umbilicus can occur, especially if an umbilical hernia is present. In most cases these wound-healing problems can be treated conservatively. A very rare complication is an abdominal compartment syndrome that was reported in some patients. In unrecognized abdominal injuries, an acute abdomen can occur. A visceral surgeon should be consulted immediately.

Seromas can be punctured and removed. Wound-healing problems can occur with smokers, patients with diabetes, and high BMI or immunosuppressed patients. These complications can be reduced with a limited abdominal undermining according to Lockwood. If conservative management is not sufficient, revisional surgery is necessary. If the wound cannot be closed primarily, a NPWT (e.g. VAC) can be applied for a few days, and then the wound is closed secondarily if it is clean. If a mesh was put in or the rectus sheath was closed under tension, a secondary abdominal weakness or hernia may occur. The later problem is not seen with SIEA-flaps. The rate of weakness complications is less for DIEP-flaps compared to pedicled TRAM flaps. If pain or discomfort is evident, a revision can become necessary.

Aesthetically the umbilicus can be distorted from the midline, or the abdominal scars can become asymmetric or bulging. In patients with a high BMI, adipose tissue can remain laterally, which can look noticeable.

Acute infections are evident after 2–3 days. The incision is red; the surgical site swells up. Lab work shows increased leucocytes and CRP. A wound swab and a surgical revision are necessary.

Chronic infection and seroma cause redness and delayed wound healing and lead to seroma or lymphatic discharge from the wound. In many cases local antiseptic treatment, wound punctures and systemic antibiotic treatment can support healing. Protein-rich diet and immobilization of the arm can help to reduce seroma production. If chemotherapy has started, the healing is very slowly. A surgical revision might become necessary.

Aesthetic complications include asymmetries, dents and skin irregularities. Shrinkage of the scar can distort the position of the NAC. Radiation therapy and their sequelae can amplify the symptoms.

10.1.10 Corrective and Additional Surgery

If additional surgery is necessary, it should be planned at least 3–6 months later then the flap surgery. If dents or irregularities occur in the transition zones between the flap and original tissue, they can be mildend by lipofilling; a secondary augmentation can also be done by lipofilling. A contralateral operation, if not done together with the reconstruction, can be planned at that time too. A secondary augmentation can also be done with an implant with respect to the flap pedicle because the flap does not achieve full vascular autonomy in most cases.

The reconstruction of the NAC is considered to be the last operation.

10.1.11 Pregnancy

Young patients who require a DIEP-flap frequently ask if they still can get pregnant after surgery. There is not much literature on this topic, but all show positive courses after DIEP- or pedicled TRAM flaps. Some of our patients became pregnant after a DIEP-flap. There was no situation to the abdominal wall in any case. Pregnancies are also possible after SIEA-flaps. In special cancer types, an oncological supervision might become necessary as well.

10.1.11.1 SIEA-Flap Intraoperative

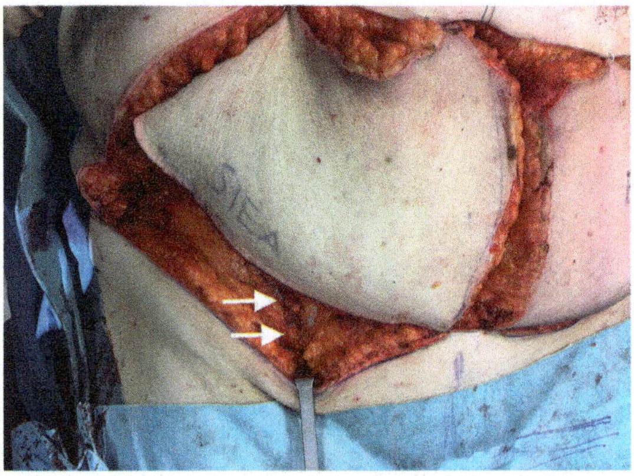

Fig. 10.22 The SIEA vessels are dissected from the caudal abdominal wound. The vessels run below, sometimes above Scarpa's fascia. They usually cut the inguinal ligament in half. If strong SIEA vessels are encountered, they should be kept intact. They can be used as flap pedicle or they can indicate that venous drainage is dominant from the superficial system. The SIEA only perfuses the ipsilateral hemi-abdomen. Thus the perfusion is not across the midline

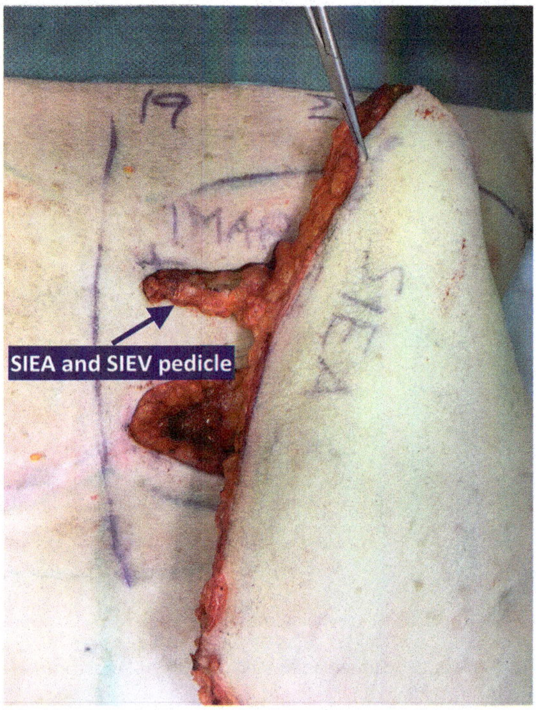

Fig. 10.24 Right SIEA-flap for delayed reconstruction left side. The flap is placed on the area where it is fit in later. It is turned 90 ° clockwise. The pedicle points to the sternum. In this case we planned the anastomosis to an IMAP (blue + on the skin). An IMAP is ideal for a SIEA-flap as it allows to place and form the flap easily

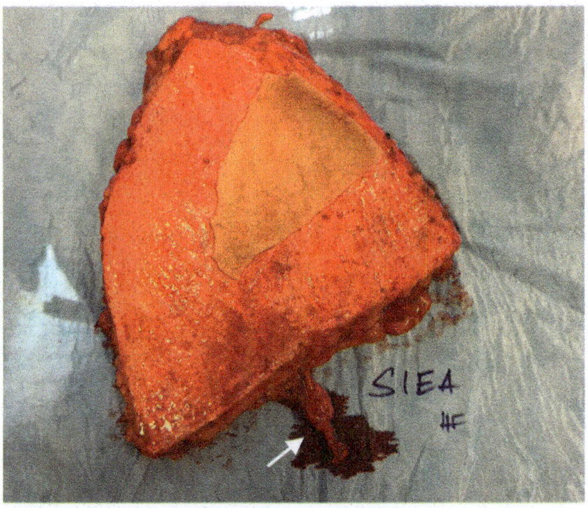

Fig. 10.23 Right SIEA-flap. The pedicle is not as long as a DIEP pedicle. Usually they measure about 5–7 cm depending on the position of the abdominal incision. This length is like with TMG pedicles. Different from a DIEP-flap, the vessels enter the SIEA-flap not from underneath but are excentric. Therefore the position of the flap with respect to recipient vessels and breast volume has to be planned meticulously

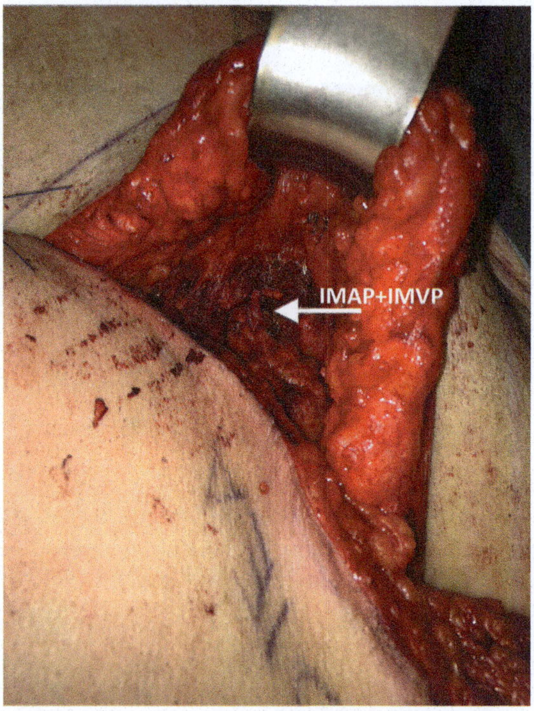

Fig. 10.25 Same flap as in Fig. 10.24. Anastomosis of the pedicle to an IMAP and its vein

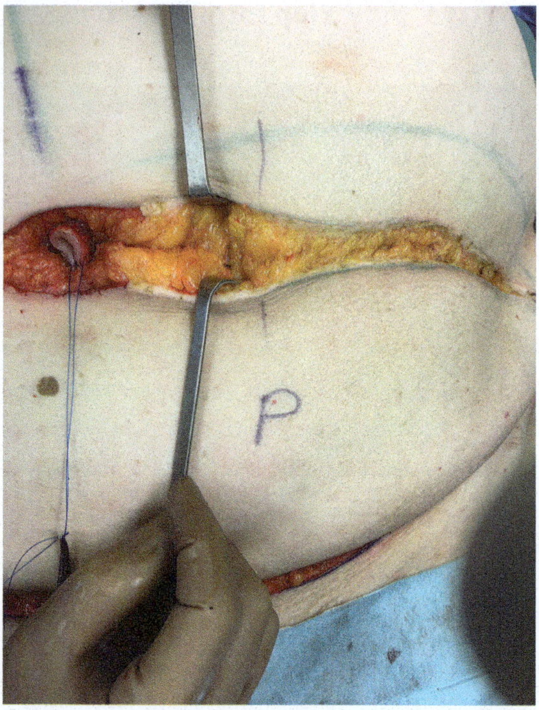

Fig. 10.27 Harvesting of a DIEP-flap. P is a perforator on the left side. Mostly you will find strong vessels at the cranial incision at the point where an imaginary line from the perforator to the cranial incision crosses the incision. If one encounters such vessels cutting the upper incision, the perforator is close

10.1.11.2 DIEP-Flap Intraoperative

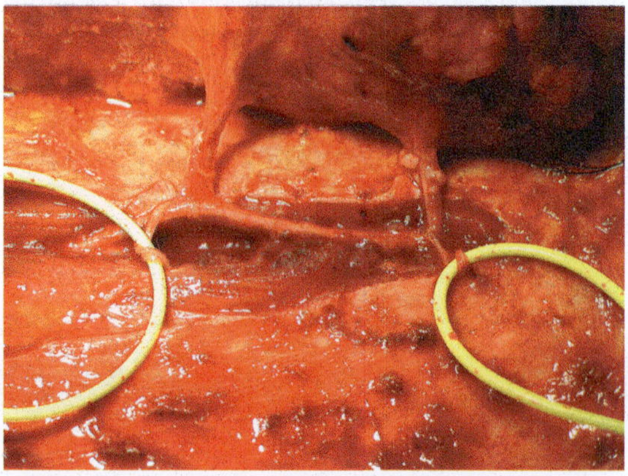

Fig. 10.26 DIEP-flap with two perforators. The segmental muscle nerves are looped (yellow). They run from lateral to medial. If two perforator flaps are harvested, at least one nerve has to be cut. The nerves can be sutured easily, but it remains unknown if these additional sutures improve recovery. The best is a strong single perforator

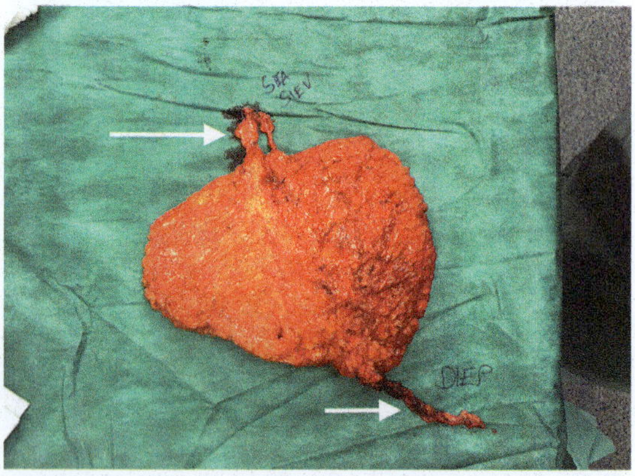

Fig. 10.28 In rare cases, if the flap has to be large or the superficial system does not communicate with the deep venous network, a superficial vein has to be added into the flap. In this case the SIEV was combined with a periumbilical DIEP perforator, because the flap showed venous congestion. Anastomosis see Figs. 9.12 and 9.13

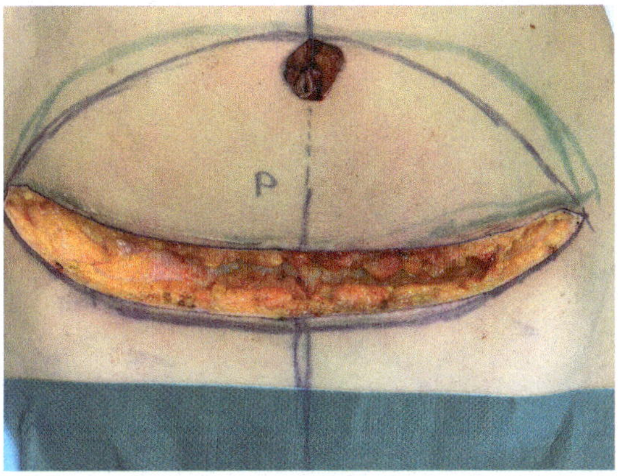

Fig. 10.29 Medial, caudal perforator (P) on the right side. These perforators are not always present, and sometimes they fake being strong by carrying a thick nerve. But if the vessels are good they can be used. They allow keeping the caudal incision low resulting in a better aesthetic result

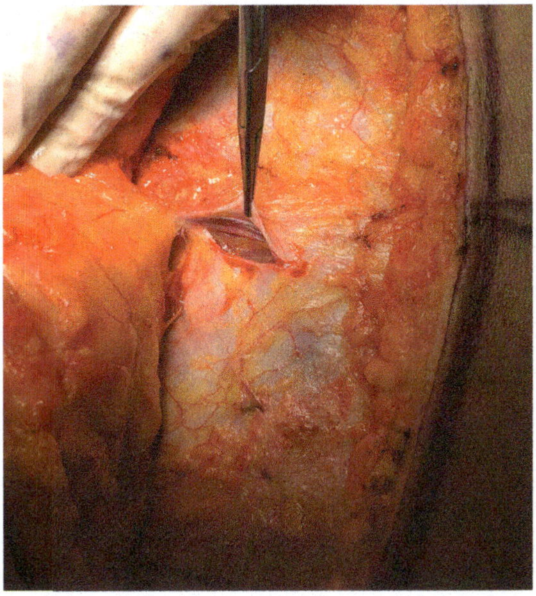

Fig. 10.31 The vessels often run on top of the muscle and their dissection causes less harm. If the rectus sheath is incised, the vessels can be injured if the cut is made too inattentive

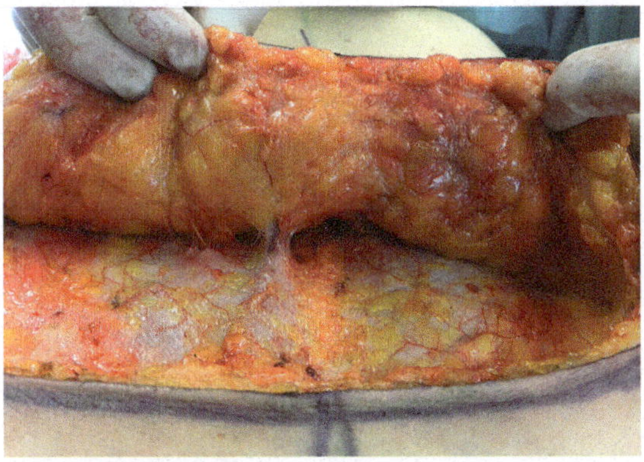

Fig. 10.30 In this case the vein is well filled; thus the perforator is a good choice

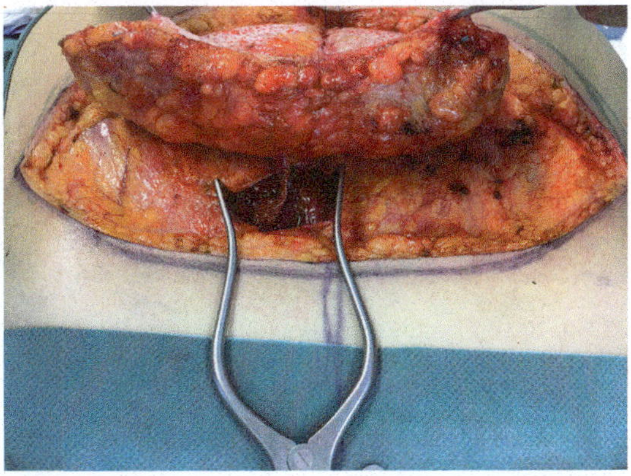

Fig. 10.32 Harvested flap with the caudal perforator

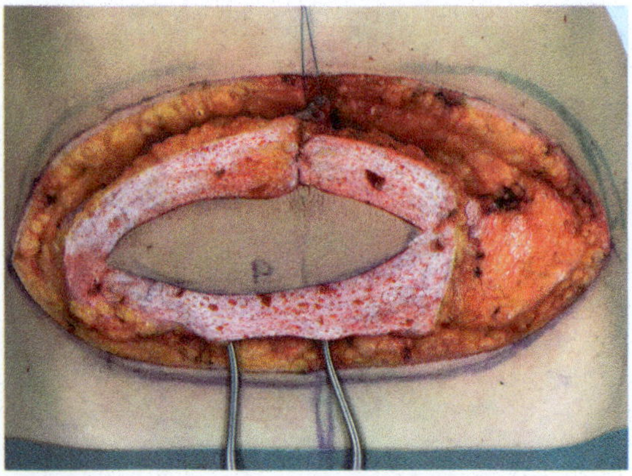

Fig. 10.33 The part where the umbilicus was is closed and zone 4 resected. The fat below Scarpa's fascia is resected medially and laterally. The flap will be turned by 180°. The parts that will be buried are de-epithelialized

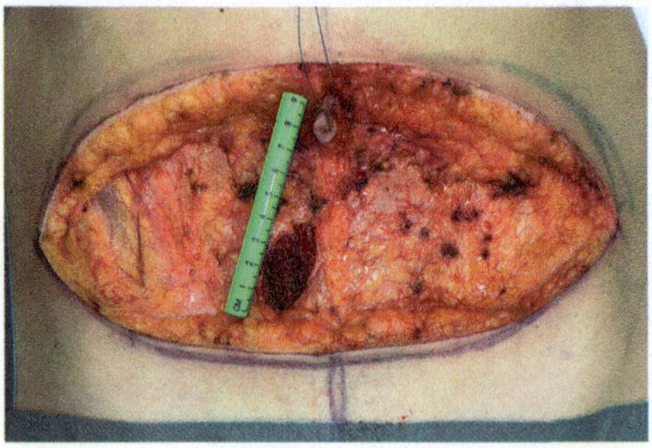

Fig. 10.34 Rectus sheath incision is 4 cm. This allows a safe harvest and a safe closure of the sheath, without any weakness

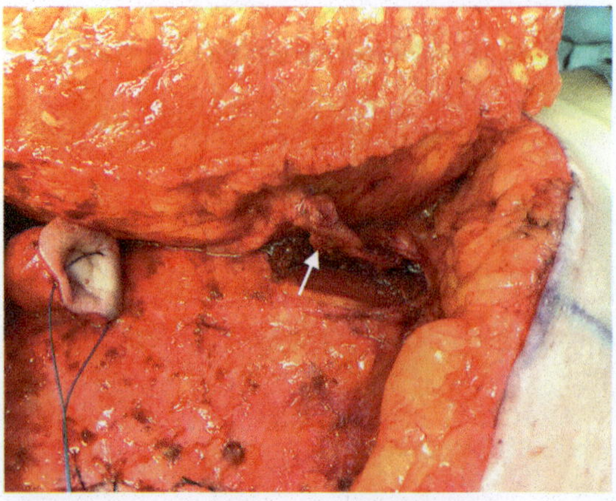

Fig. 10.35 Medial, caudal perforator on the left side. Again short incision of the rectus sheath

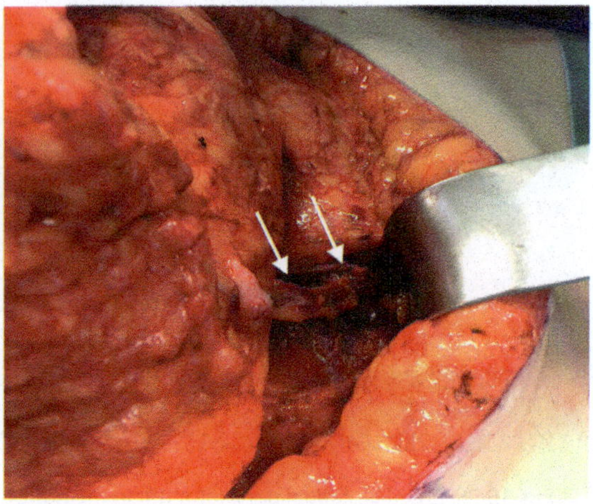

Fig. 10.36 A Roux hook allows to hold the muscle and fascia upwards after the first branches at the plane where the hook is placed are clipped. The epigastric vessels can be dissected by this manoeuvre from this hole. A headlight is helpful

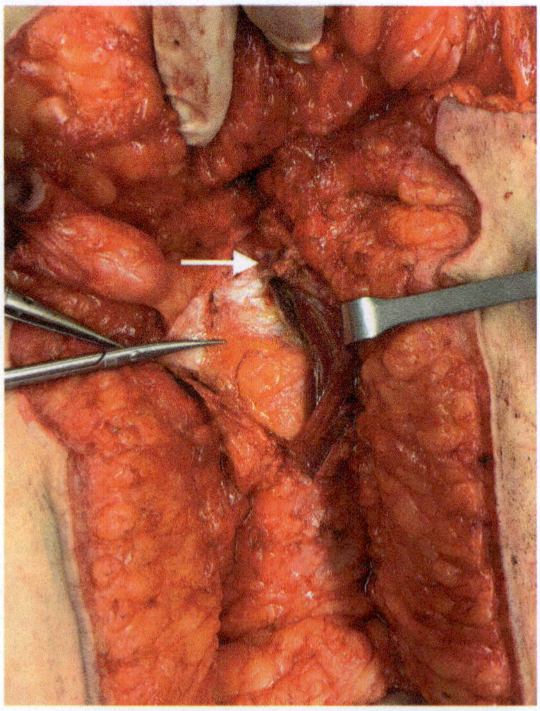

Fig. 10.37 Medial, periumbilical perforator left side (arrow) in a bilateral DIEP-flap. The umbilicus is freed and the dissection starts from medial. The scissors indicate the arcuate line. Caudally the dorsal part of the rectus sheath is missing. The very medial periumbilical perforators often run around the muscle medial to dorsal

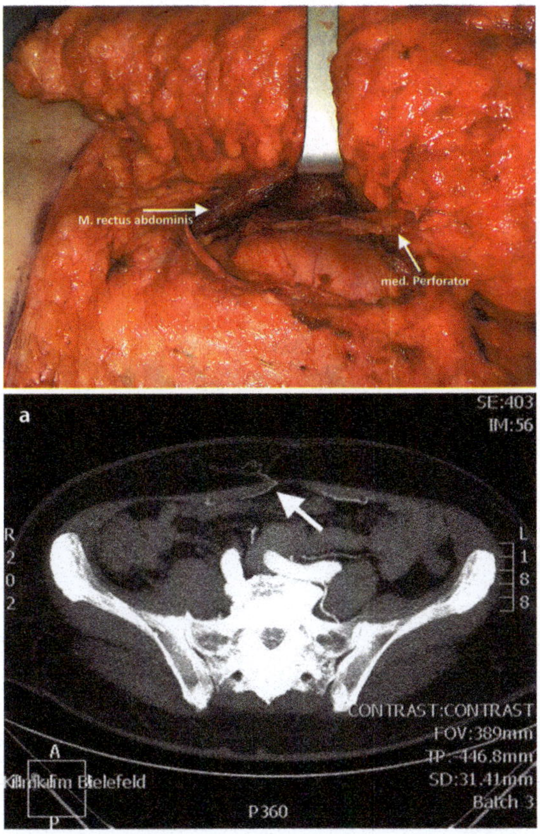

Fig. 10.38 Medial perforator right side. In this case caudal to the umbilicus, thus not directly periumbilical. Again the perforator runs from medial to dorsal around the muscle. Harvesting leaves the muscle intact. **a** CTA that matches such a course. The arrow indicates the typical medial course around the muscle

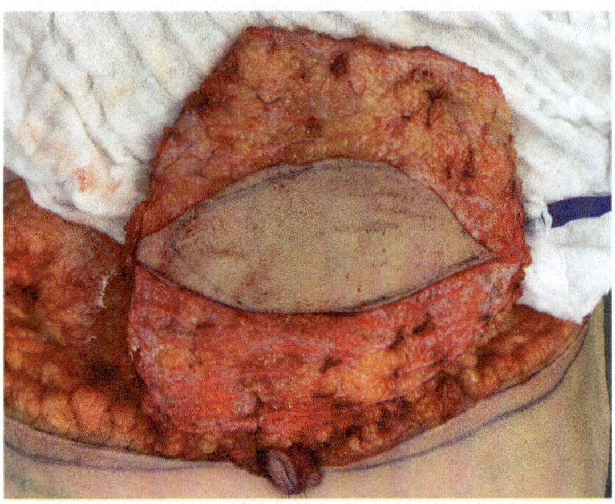

Fig. 10.39 Flap in situ. Zone 4 is resected and the skin that is not needed is de-epithelialized. The flap is fit by turning around 180°

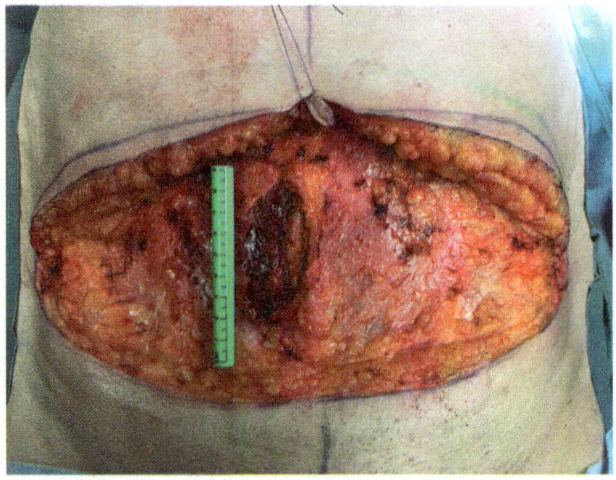

Fig. 10.40 Incision of the rectus sheath of about 6.5 cm

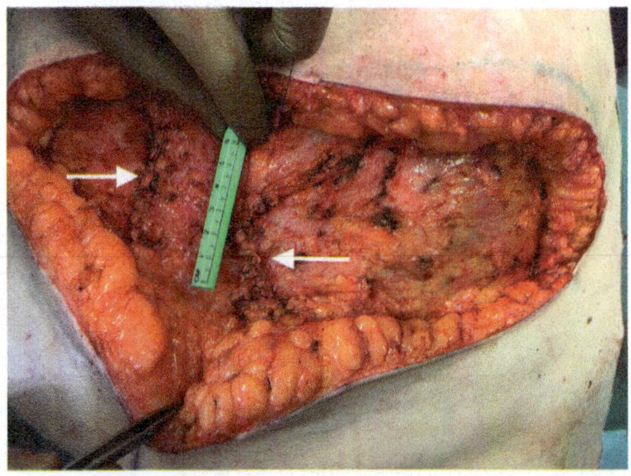

Fig. 10.41 Closure of rectus sheath in a bilateral DIEP-flap (arrows). The abdominal wall is closed tension-free without causing an umbilical malposition or the need for a mesh repair

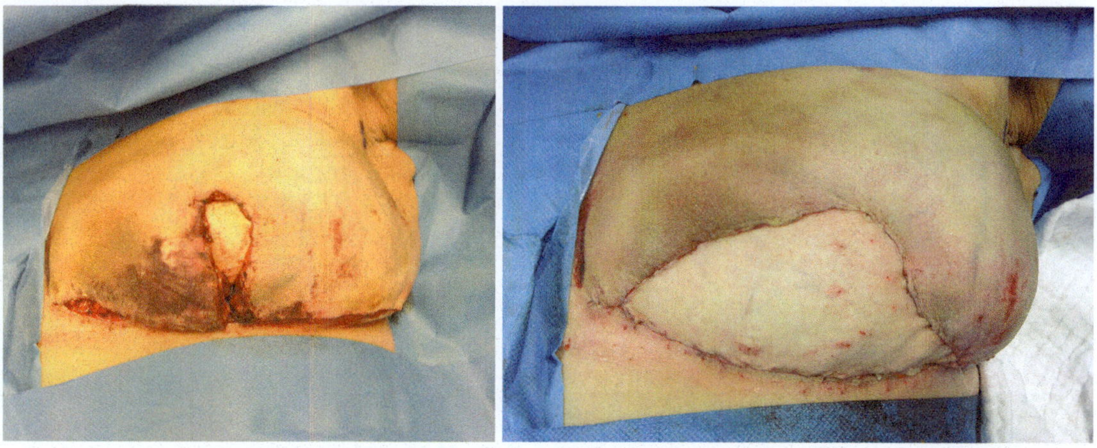

▫ **Fig. 10.42 and 10.43** Buried flap. Reconstruction of a left breast with a DIEP-flap after SSM and Wise-pattern incision. The DIEP-flap was not de-epithelialized in the parts where the mastectomy flap appeared to be impaired. After 4 days the medial skin is demarcated. The skin is removed and replaced by flap skin in a short operation

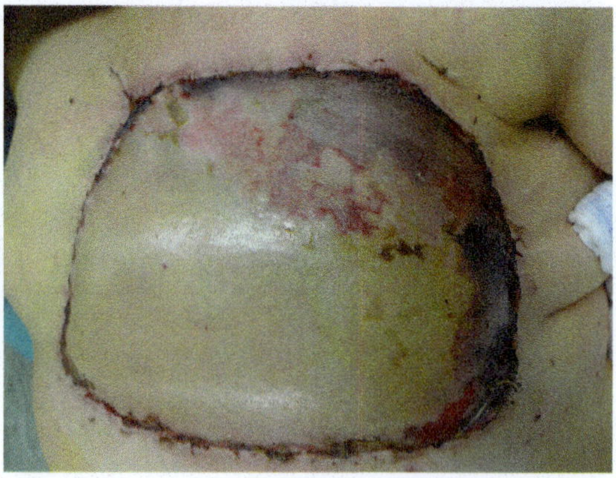

▫ **Fig. 10.44** Partial flap necrosis. The cranial and lateral aspects of flap rotated by 180° are not well perfused and partially necrotic. After demarcation the necrosis should be resected, and a new local or distant flap should be used to cover the defect. A conservative treatment takes very long, annoys patient and surgeon and usually results in a bad aesthetic outcome

10.1.11.3 Results After SIEA-Flap

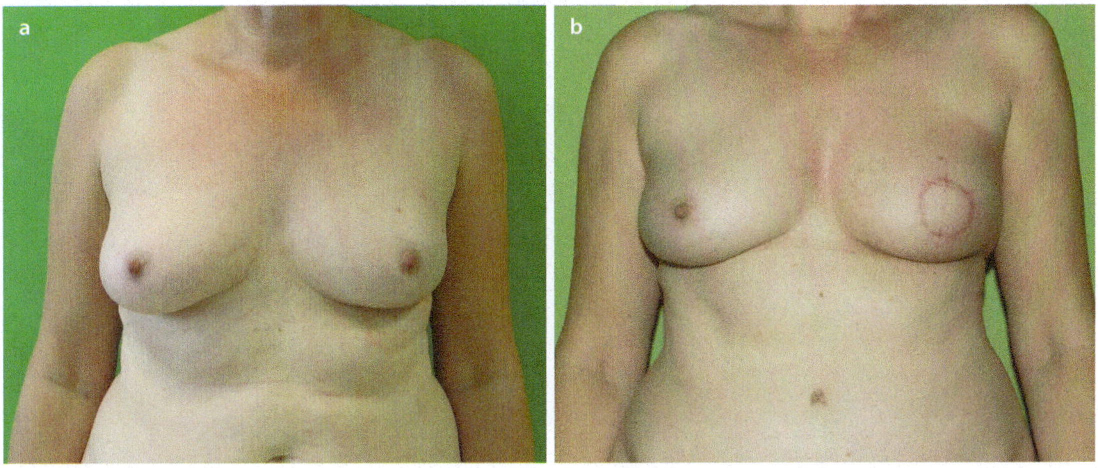

Fig. 10.45 **a, b** Invasive carcinoma left breast. Periareolar SSM and immediate reconstruction with a SIEA-flap. Immediately after radiation, 3 months postoperative

10.1.11.4 Results After DIEP-Flap

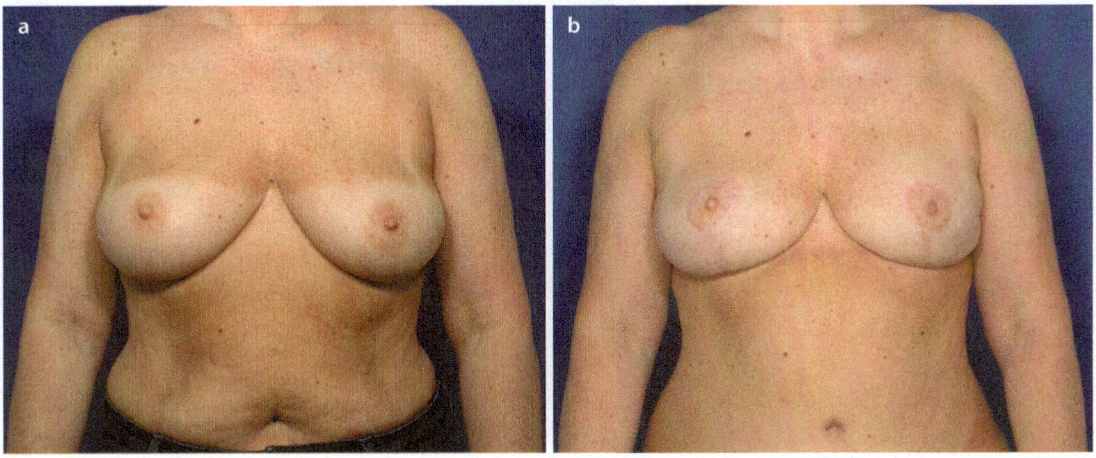

Fig. 10.46 **a** Immediate DIEP-flap left side (small invasive carcinoma and large 10 cm DCIS) with NSM and inverted T-incision, autoderm and reduction mammaplasty right. Initially little asymmetry and Nipple-Jugular notch distance of 24 and 23 cm. Nipple-IMF distance of 11 and 12 cm. Initial tightening of the skin usually leads to better results. **b** Result 3 months postoperative

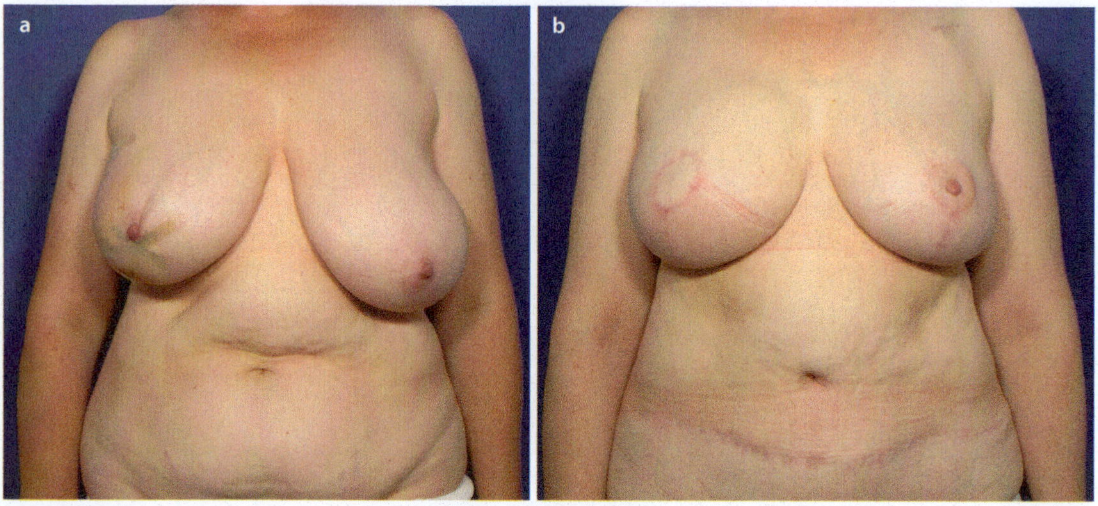

Fig. 10.47 **a** Immediate DIEP-flap right with inverted T-incision and SSM because of an invasive carcinoma. Reduction mammaplasty on the contralateral side. The DIEP-flap replaces the areola. **b** Result 7 months postoperative

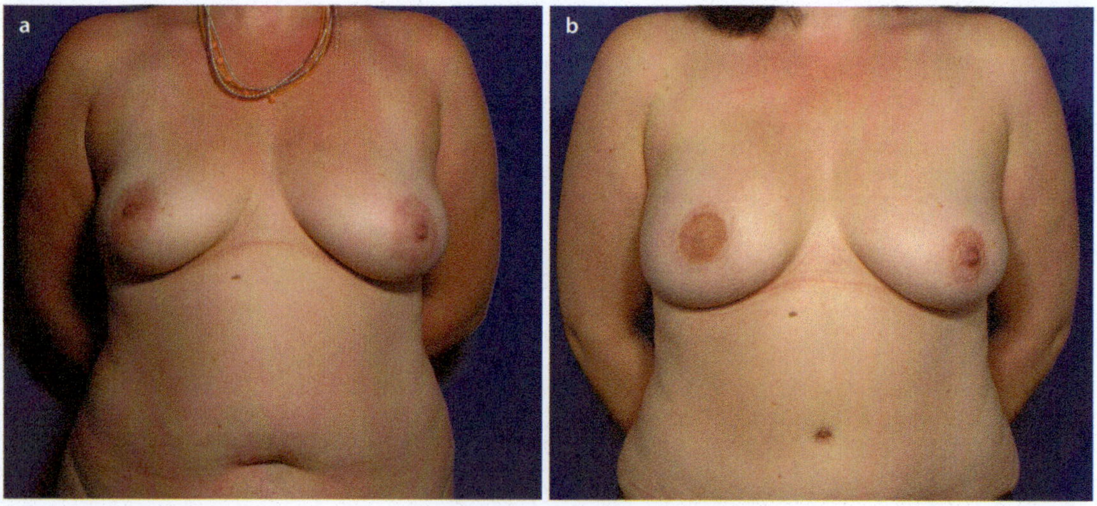

Fig. 10.48 **a** Immediate DIEP-flap right due to an invasive carcinoma. SSM with a periareolar incision. **b** Result after 12 months with nipple reconstruction with a C-V-flap and pigmentation of the areola

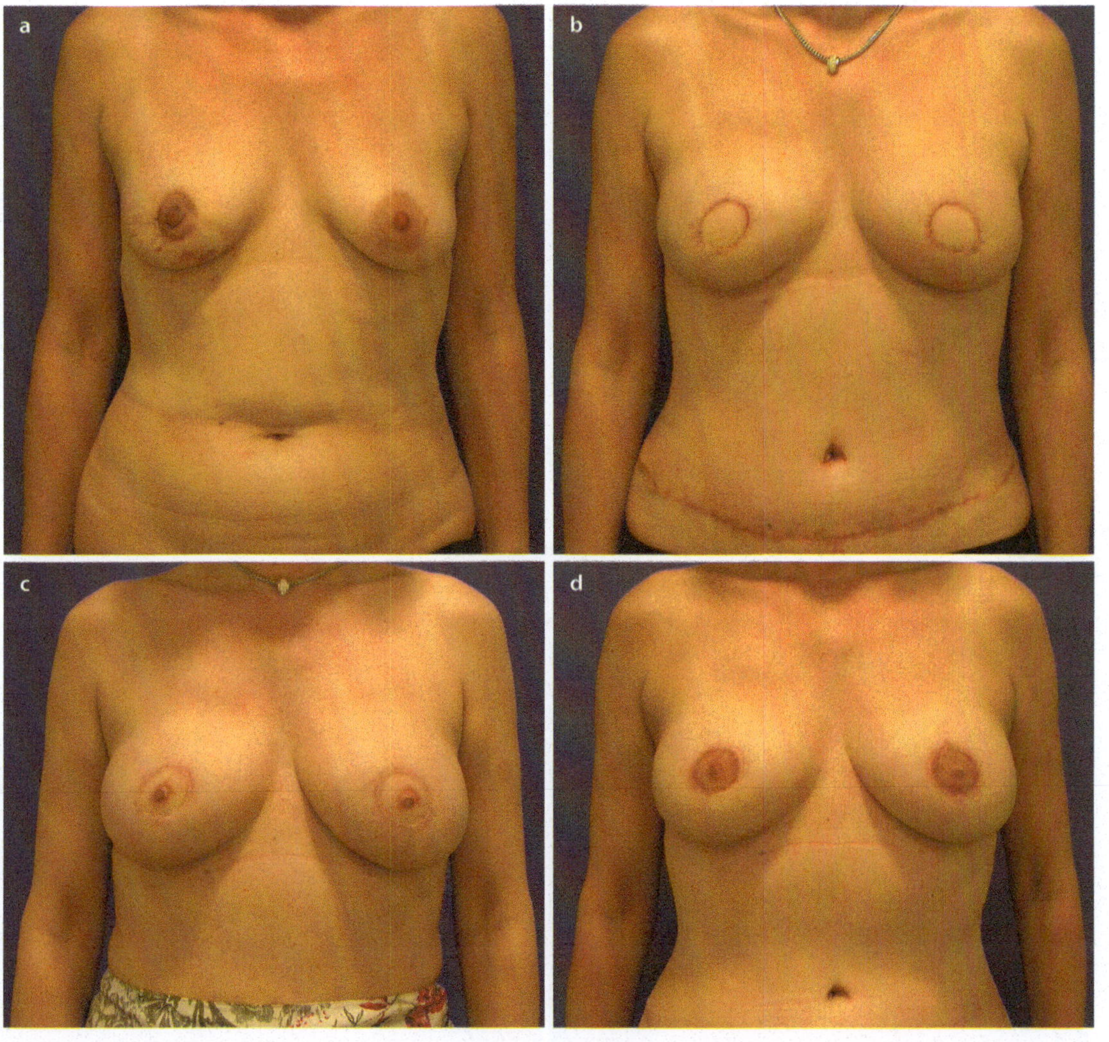

Fig. 10.49 **a** Bilateral SSM, invasive carcinoma right, preventive left. Immediate bilateral DIEP-flap. **b** Periareolar skin island bilaterally. **c** Nipple reconstruction with a C-V-flap. **d** Result after areola pigmentation after 15 months

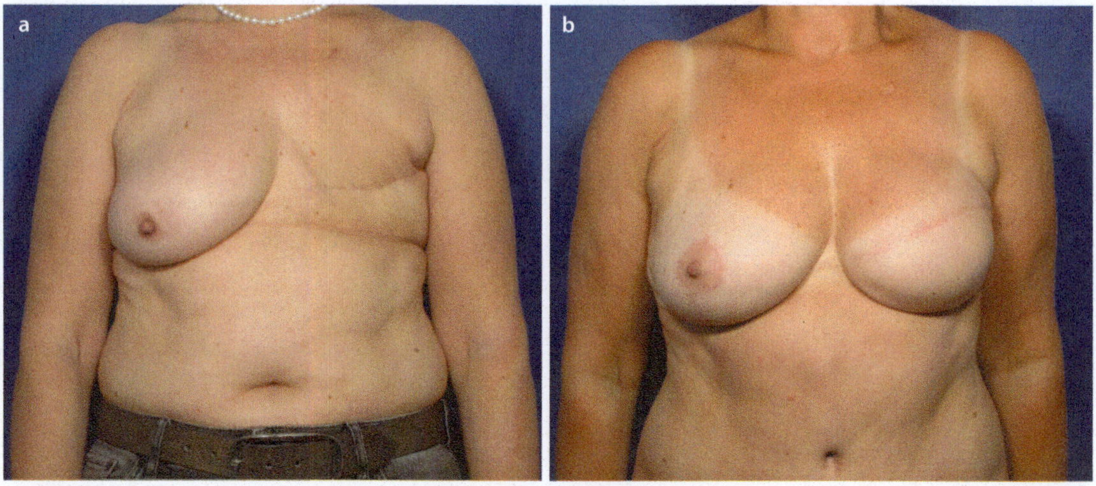

Fig. 10.50 **a, b** Secondary reconstruction after mastectomy and radiation left side with DIEP-flap. Ellipsoid skin island and reduction mammaplasty in the same operation. Result after 3 months

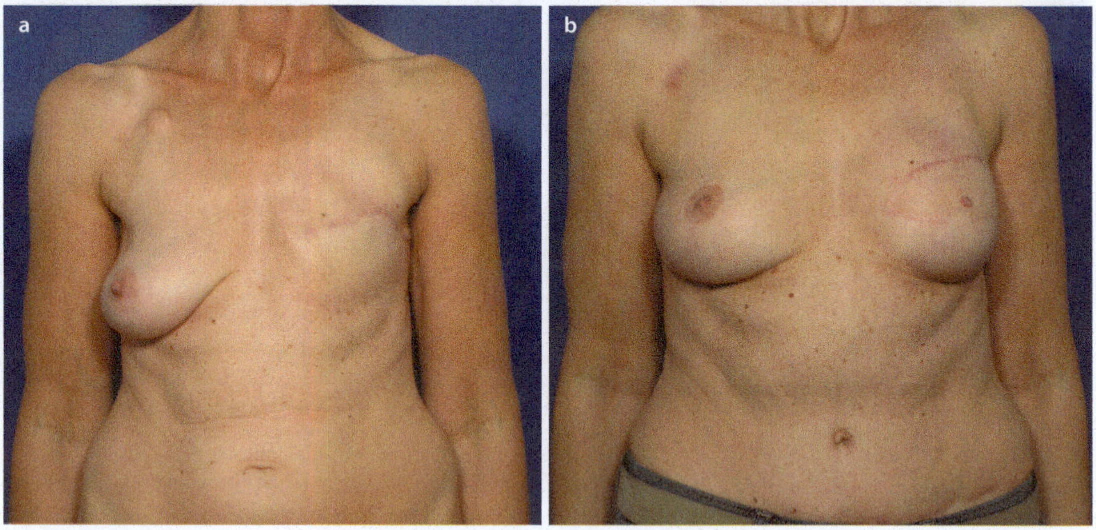

Fig. 10.51 **a** Secondary reconstruction after mastectomy and radiation with DIEP-flap. Ellipsoid skin island and reduction mammaplasty in the same operation. The very cranially located mastectomy scar is difficult. The flap is not very thick. Therefore is placed rotated by 90°, putting the volume centrally/medially with more projection to the breast. **b** Result after 6 months with nipple sharing from the contralateral side

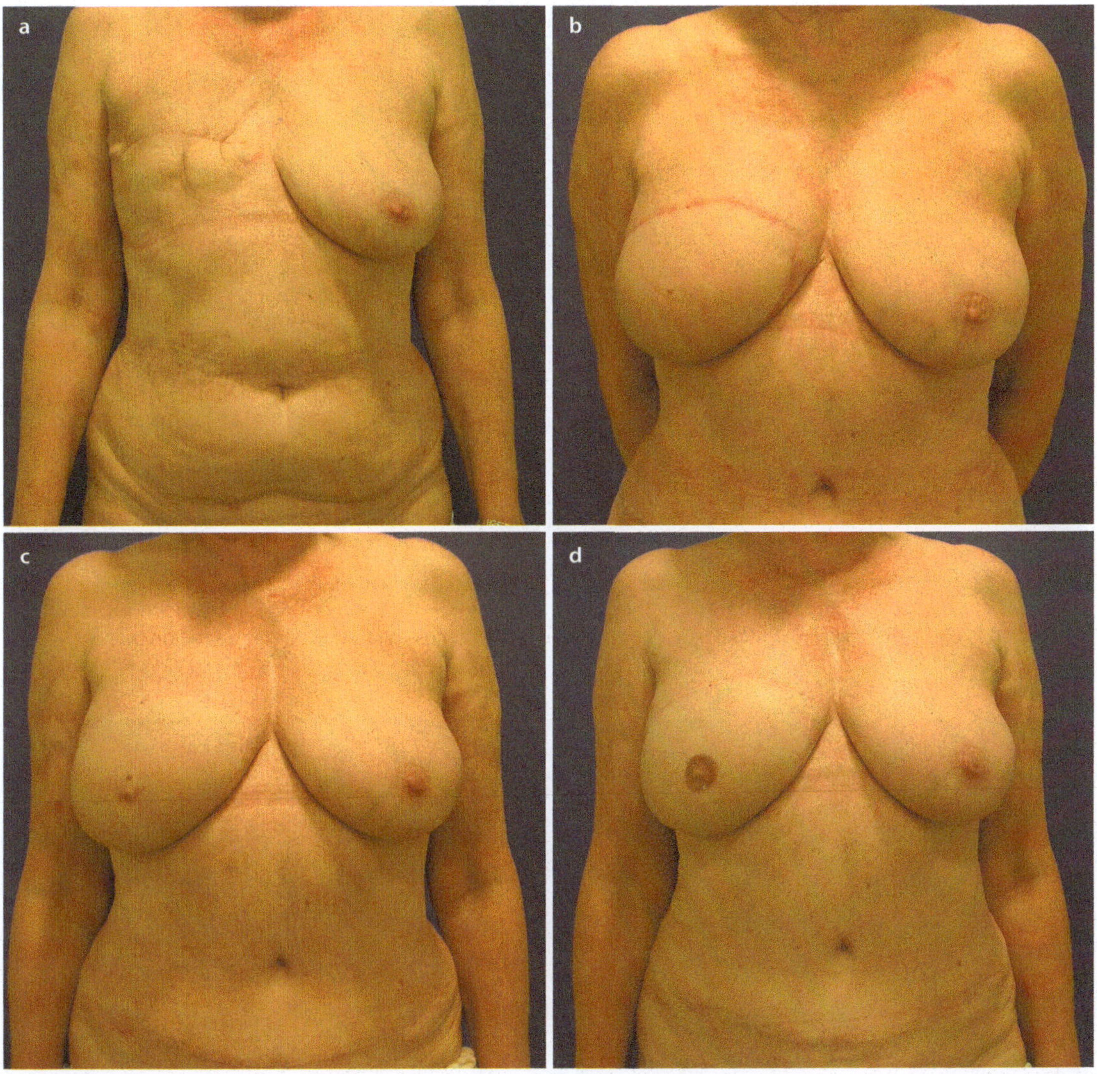

Fig. 10.52 **a** Secondary reconstruction after mastectomy and radiation right side with a DIEP-flap, inserted as aesthetic unit. The DIEP-flap is cranially placed underneath the mastectomy skin. The flap skin remains to the IMF. Thus the reconstructed breast falls more naturally. This technique requires much tissue from the abdomen. **b** Result after 3 months. **c** Nipple reconstruction by a local C-V-flap. **d** Final result after 18 months and pigmentation of the areola

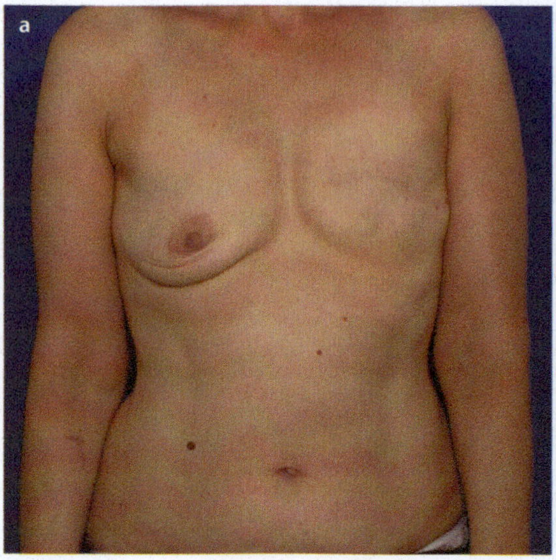

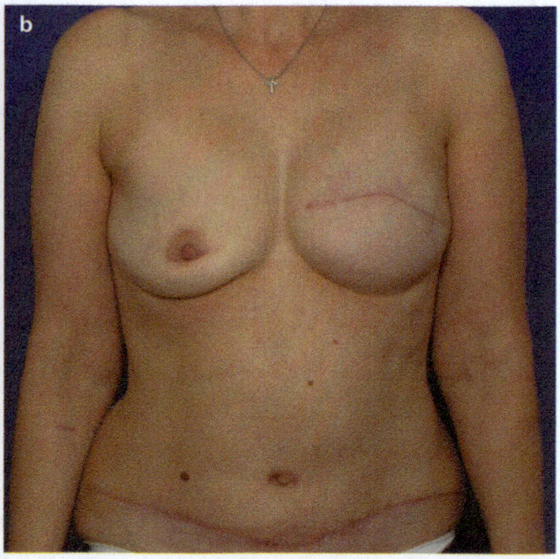

Fig. 10.53 **a, b** Secondary reconstruction after mastectomy and radiation left side with a DIEP-flap. The flap was buried because the skin was soft and elastic. A visible skin island is avoided. This can also be achieved with a prior expander implantation if the skin is not so elastic. Expander can also be used after radiation therapy

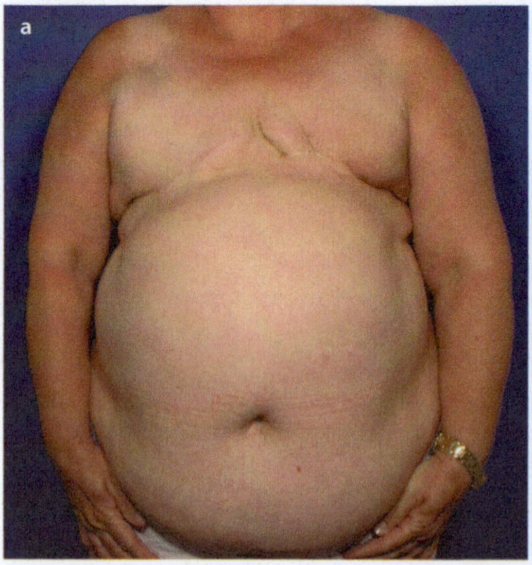

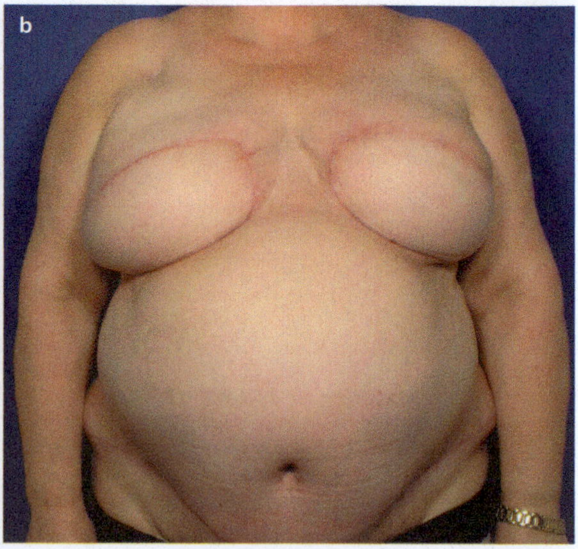

Fig. 10.54 **a, b** Secondary reconstruction after bilateral mastectomy with bilateral DIEP-flap (BMI > 40). Especially in these patients, an autologous breast reconstruction is the best solution; however the wound healing at the abdomen can be delayed and has to be monitored carefully. The "dog-ears" laterally can be corrected secondarily

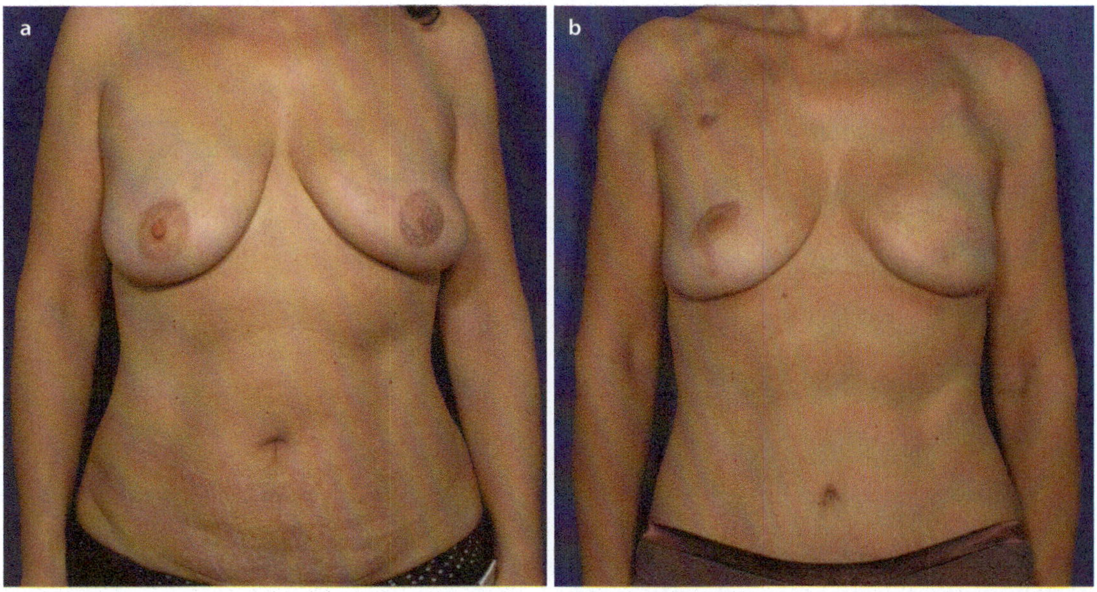

Fig. 10.55 **a, b** SSM left due to a local recurrence after BCT, radiation and nipple reconstruction (elsewhere). DIEP-flap reconstruction left and reduction mammaplasty right. The donor site is well hidden by the underwear. Result after 9 months

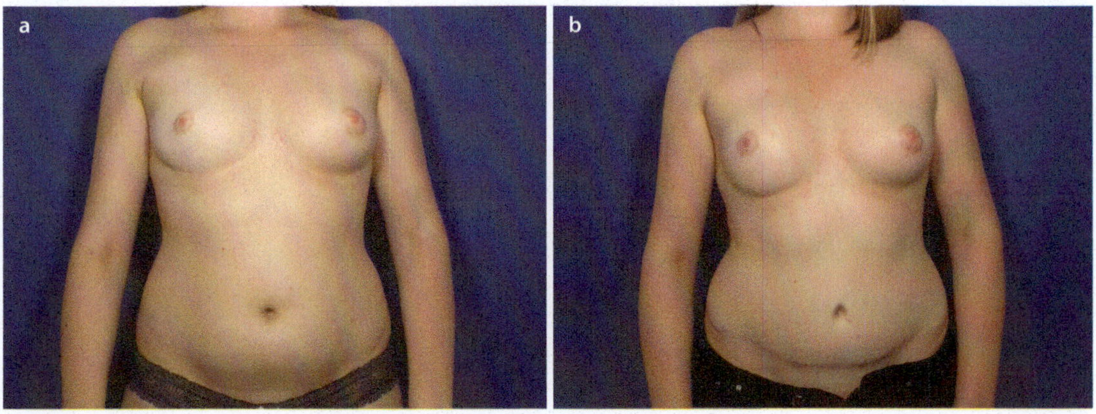

Fig. 10.56 **a** Capsular contracture right after implant after NSM. Resection of the capsule, removing of the implant and DIEP-flap reconstruction. **b** Result after 3 months

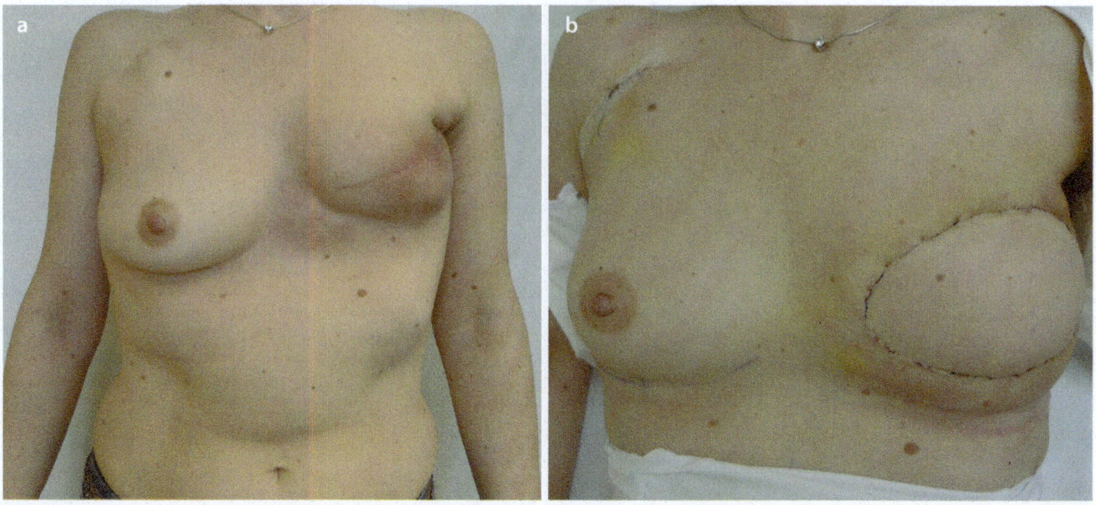

Fig. 10.57 **a** Infection after implant after mastectomy and radiation. Cranial displacement of the implant, loss of the IMF and thinning of the skin due the infection and mechanical situation. Single-stage implant and capsular resection and DIEP-flap. **b** Result at discharge

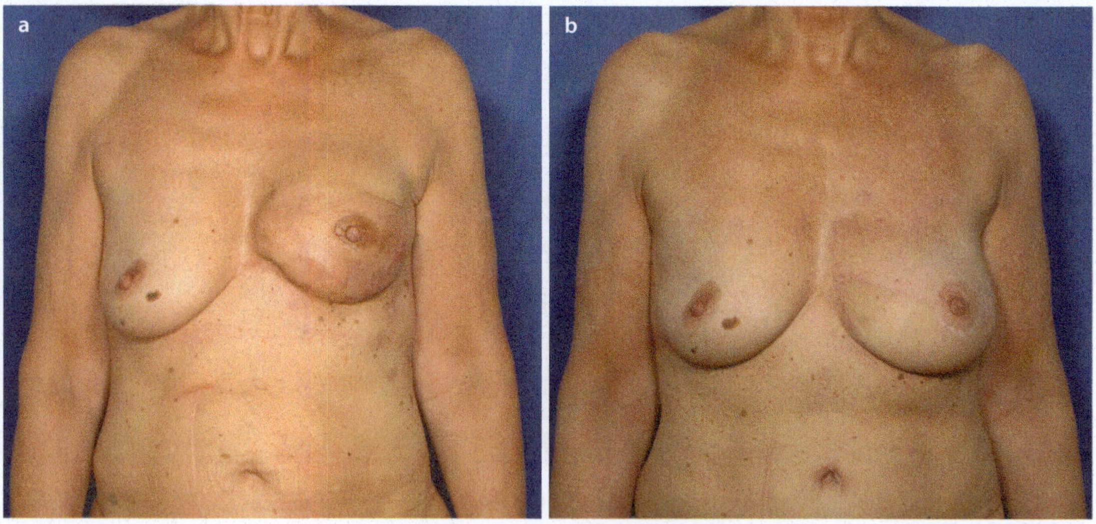

Fig. 10.58 **a** Capsular contracture left after NSM with implant and mesh placement and radiation therapy. Medial displacement. IMF is too cranial. Breast is rock hard. The skin caudal to the NAC shows an oedema and is very rigid. The implant and mesh are removed. The flap replaces the caudal skin. Here we were able to get the NAC more caudal. If the upper skin is also rigid, the NAC may not be moved. **b** Result after 6 months

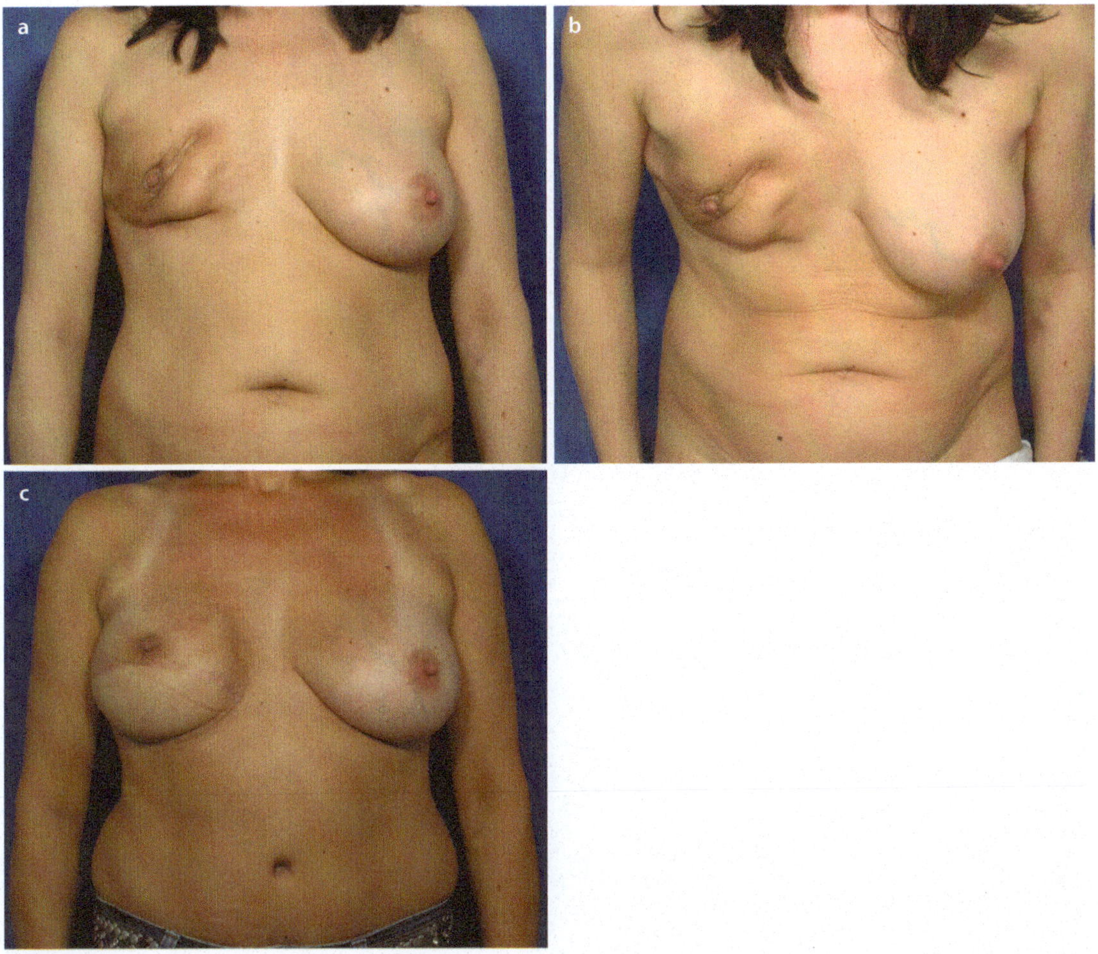

Fig. 10.59 **a–c** Patient with NSM after invasive carcinoma and radiation. Eight operations with implants did not work. A NPWT was applied and an infection was treated (elsewhere). The skin is stuck to the rest of the pectoralis major muscle, especially at the décolleté. DIEP-flap with skin replacement caudal to the NAC. Result after 4 months

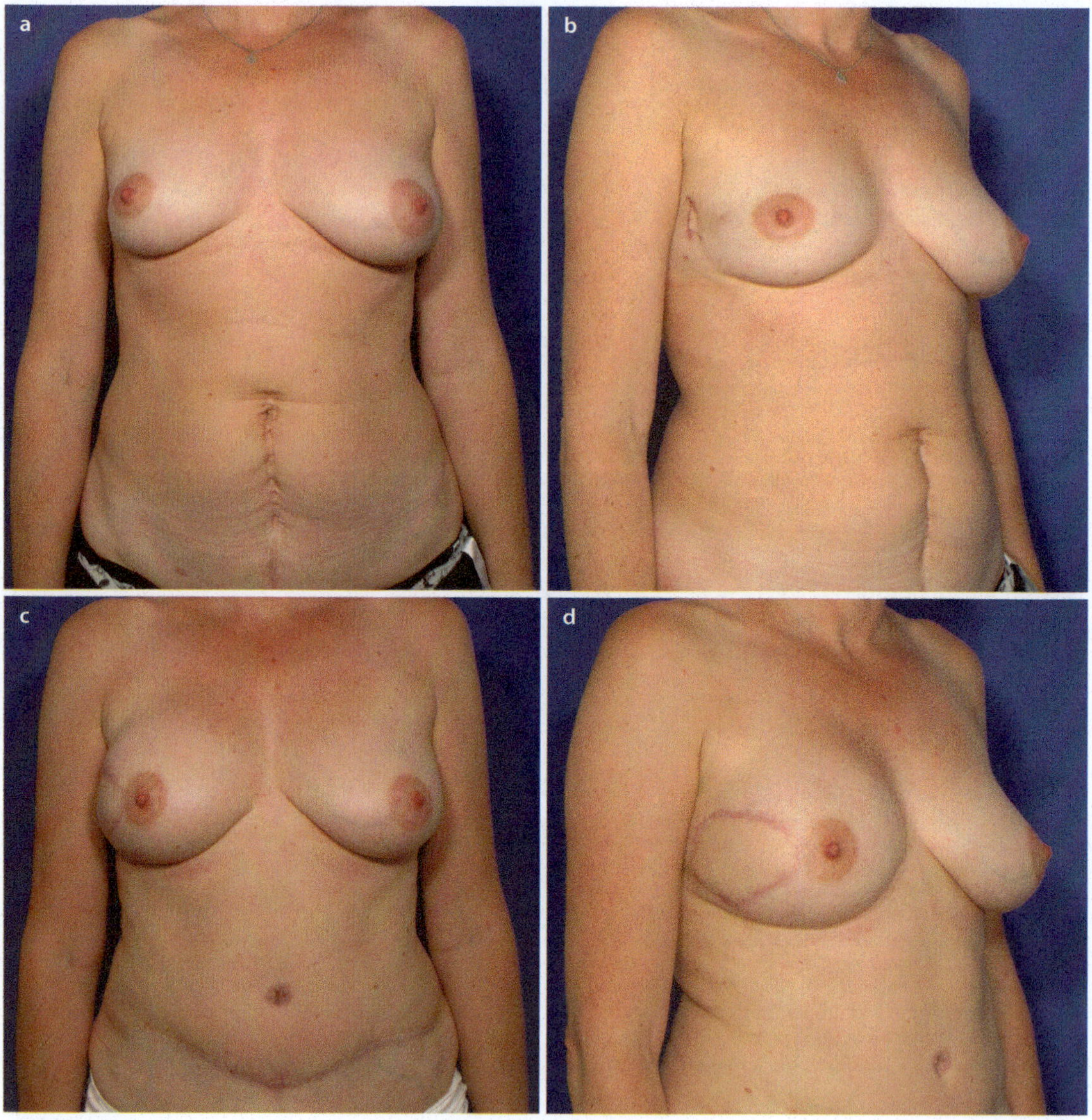

Fig. 10.60 **a–d** Patient after BCT right side, R1 resection (DCIS and invasive cancer). Displacement of the NAC laterally and asymmetry. Abdominal scar after median laparotomy due to Crohn's disease. NSM with immediate reconstruction from the hemi-abdomen. The flaps were positioned on top of each other (stacked flaps). The right flap was anastomosed to an IMAP; the left was hooked up to the cranial end of the right deep inferior epigastric artery. Result after 6 months without any adjusting surgery or refinements

Conclusion

The DIEP-flap is a routine procedure for autologous breast reconstruction. In specialized centres complication rate is low. The DIEP-flap is indicated in all patients with sufficient lower abdominal tissue without prior significant abdominal operations. The pedicle is very variable and can be hooked up to the IMA/IMAP or subscapular system. Anastomosis is usually not difficult. The patients have to know that they have a scar at their abdomen and some tension and loss of sensitivity are present in the first time at the abdomen. After 3–6 months, the final result can be expected.

10.2 Inner Thigh Flaps (IT-Flap)

The *inner thigh flap* (IT-flap) consists of skin and fat tissue from the inner thigh and lower medial gluteal fold. If the pedicle comes from the gracilis muscle and the skin island is oriented transversely, the flap is named *transverse upper gracilis (TUG)* or *transverse myocutaneous gracilis (TMG)* flap. The *vertical* shape is called "VUG". A combination of both designs that enlarges the flap volume is called fleur-de-lis shape. Some call a *bilaterally* harvested flap for one breast "BUG". As the gracilis muscle does not really contribute to the volume, we prefer the name *inner thigh flap*, which is the name we use in the chapter. Other pedicles are perforators from the profound femoral artery (*PAP-flap*), but the skin island is basically the same.

10.2.1 Indication

Breast

Autologous tissue from the inner thigh can often be used. The volume is enough to reconstruct a small- to medium-sized breast (A–C cup) with slender patients. In bilateral reconstructions this technique does not have to respect the existing size as it creates two new symmetric breasts. If necessary a mastopexy technique hast to be added to reduce the skin envelope. The new size has to be communicated with the patients prior to surgery.

Immediate reconstructions in SSM or NSM are best because they leave the breast skin intact. Secondary reconstructions require a visible skin inset from the flap. If a different skin type is not desired, an expander can be placed prior to autologous reconstructive surgery. In these cases the expander is placed epipectoral. The inner thigh flap can also be used with defects after BCT to replace volume. However it should be considered that the pedicle is not very long.

Donor site

Mostly the patients have enough tissue at their inner thigh. We think that the inner thigh flap is a full alternative to a DIEP-flap if anatomy allows selecting the donor site. Patients with contraindications for a DIEP-flap can be reconstructed with an IT-flap. The preferences of the surgeon and patients should be considered. The tissue that can be harvested can be assessed with a pinch test and roughly compared to the breast volume. In many cases patients with tissue on the inner thigh have small breasts and thus being suited for this technique.

10.2.2 Contraindications

Patients after a liposuction in the donor site should be carefully examined if prior surgery (scars, dents, loss of tissue) is a contraindication. In our patients an IT-flap was possible in many of those cases. A prior thigh lift is a contraindication. A prior saphenectomy can be a contraindication.

Overview DIEP-flap

Indication: small- to medium-shaped breasts

Skin island:

- Transverse, rarely vertical or fleur-de-lis
- Size 20–25 cm width and 7–11 cm height, depending on the thigh
- Bevelling allows taking tissue with the flap and leaving enough skin for thigh closure

Pedicle:

- Perforators from the gracilis muscle
- Source: lateral circumflex femoral artery or profunda femoris artery (deep femoral artery)
- Pedicle length: 5–7 cm
- Alternatively: perforators from the profunda femoris artery; pedicle length, 7–10 cm

10.2.3 Characteristics

Inner thigh tissue is pliable and can be shaped well. The feel is like the involuted breast and lies like breast tissue within the skin envelope. Ventrally the tissue is thinner than the dorsal/gluteal fold. This detail should be considered when the flap is inset.

The colour of the thigh is ventrally darker and lighter dorsally than the colour of the breast skin. In some patients the region can carry hair. As most of the flap is usually de-epithelialized, it is not relevant. However if hair remains at the breast, they can be later removed by laser or other permanent techniques.

The flap stays volume stable. Shrinkage was not seen in our patients when the body weight remains stable. If a radiation therapy becomes necessary, the entire flap can be included into the radiation field if flap vasculature is stable. In our patients we saw no significant shrinkage, aesthetic impairment or any flap loss. Recent studies confirm this result.

A single-sided reconstruction results in a thigh asymmetry. It is visible for the patients but well hidden if apparelled. If the patient desires a refinement, the contralateral thigh can be suctioned, and the aspirate can be used to undertake possible breast refinements. If the skin is not elastic, a thigh lift can be considered, if necessary after harvesting the fat for lipofilling.

10.2.4 Informed Consent

The disclosure of general and special risks should be documented with standardized and evaluated forms. Infection, haematoma and wound-healing complications can occur. The risk of complete and partial flap loss should be mentioned, as well as wound-healing complications at the donor site. Seroma formation and visible scars can result. In mastectomy cases loss of sensitivity to the breast skin and the NAC is often. Loss of sensitivity can also occur at the donor site. A skin necrosis and NAC necrosis can occur and may require a reoperation. Smaller wound-healing problems can remain conservatively treated.

A lymph oedema of the breast and thoracic wall is possible in rare cases. The patient should be aware that breast shape, colour and symmetry are altered. Aesthetic change can result in psychological problems which may require psychooncologic consultation.

The incisions should be visualized in a drawing. The indication for a SSM or NSM should be discussed carefully. Scarring can distort the NAC in an NSM. Fat necrosis can occur. In most cases it shows no symptoms but can be detected by ultrasound. Second operations should be mentioned if histopathology is unclear or wound-healing problems occur or a contralateral mastopexy/reduction is required. A significant change after radiation is not likely to occur if the flap is well perfused; however it should be mentioned. If the patient does refuse recommended surgery or parts, this should also be documented.

If a bra and compression garments are recommended, the patients should be informed prior to surgery. Also the after treatment should be explained.

10.2.5 Preoperative Markings and Measures

Tip

Use the ipsilateral thigh flap. The surgeon stands at the contralateral side and does not disturb the breast team. And the flap can be shaped to form an "anatomic implant" with optimal relation to the pedicle and recipient vessel.

Markings are done with patient in upright position. The breast is marked. In secondary reconstructions the breast borders are marked with regard to the contralateral breast. The upper border and the IMF are landmarks. For centring the volume, the midline should be marked too. If a mastopexy or reduction is planned with the contralateral breast, it should be also marked.

The leg should be flexible. Patient is wearing her underwear. She stands on the contralateral leg and mildly rotates the knee externally. The surgeon can palpate the origin of the adductor magnus and mark the muscle. The gracilis muscle is directly dorsal from that muscle. The dominant pedicle enters the gracilis about 7–10 cm distal to the origin from the lateral. Usually it is a branch from the medial circumflex femoral artery. Sometimes the dominant pedicles originate directly from the profunda femoris artery.

The greater saphenous vein is the ventral border of the flap (■ Fig. 10.61). It runs from medial distal to lateral proximal on the adductor longus. Dorsally the flap ends at the midline of the inferior gluteal fold (IGF, ■ Fig. 10.62). Proximally the upper incision starts on the thigh, about 1–2 cm, below the inguinal crease and crosses the

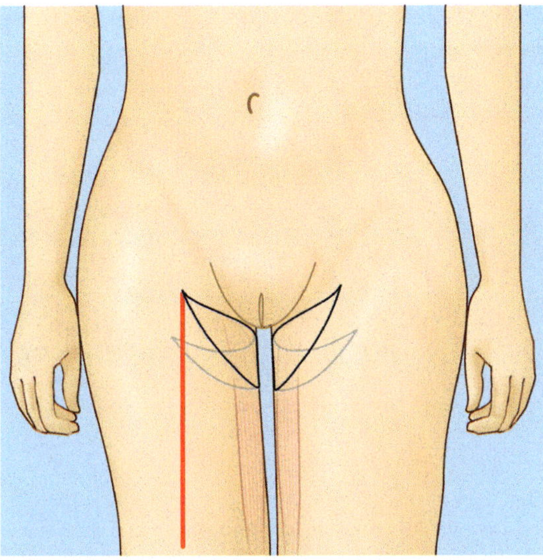

Fig. 10.61 The anterior border of the IT-flap is the greater saphenous vein. The proximal incision lies on the thigh, not in the inguinal crease, to avoid distortion of the labia. The incision runs with the relaxed skin tension lines

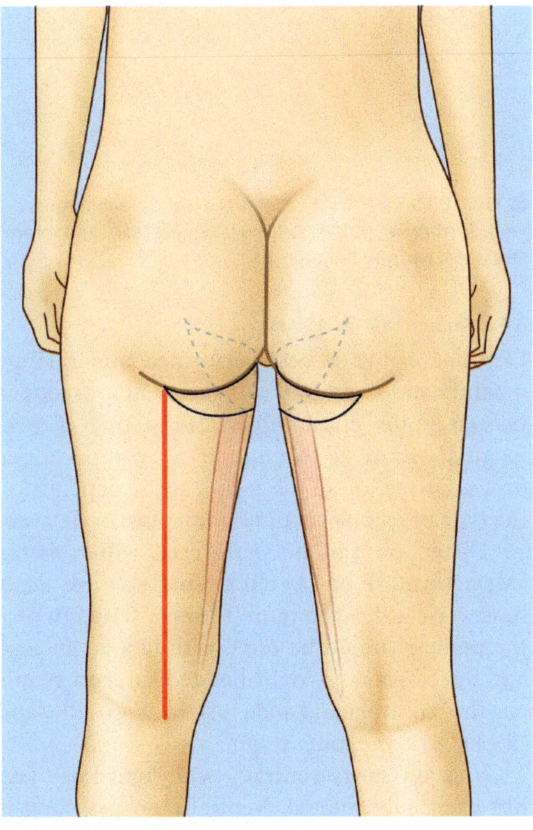

Fig. 10.62 The posterior border is the middle of the thigh at the inferior gluteal fold. The flap can also be harvested shorter

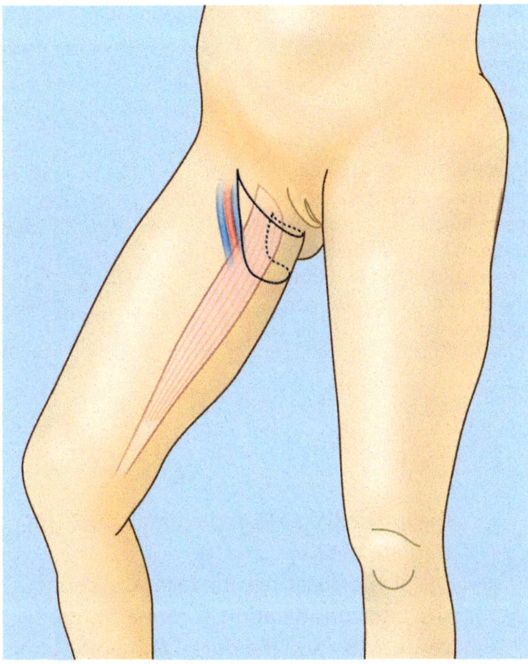

Fig. 10.63 The dominant vascular pedicle enters the gracilis muscle approx. 7–10 cm distally of its origin. The muscle is slightly dorsal to the adductor magnus, which is well palpable

inner thigh to the IGF (Fig. 10.63). The distal incision takes the flap size into consideration. Perfusion should be safe if flap height is at least 6 cm. However the height can be assessed by pinching and taking the reconstructive needs into account. Distally and dorsally additional tissue can be included into the flap by bevelling the tissue, leaving skin for closure at the thigh (Fig. 10.64). The level of bevelling should be marked on the skin.

If a vertical island is used, the skin island should be located above the proximal third of the gracilis muscle. Pinching the skin can assess the width. Bevelling can also increase the volume.

If the thigh has enough tissue and it is needed for the breast, island can be shaped in a fleur-de-lis design. Closure is then in T-shape like a thigh lift.

Anatomic landmarks of the IT-flap

- Ventral: greater saphenous vein.
- Dorsal: midline of IGF.
- Proximal: proximally the upper incision starts on the thigh, about 1–2 cm, below

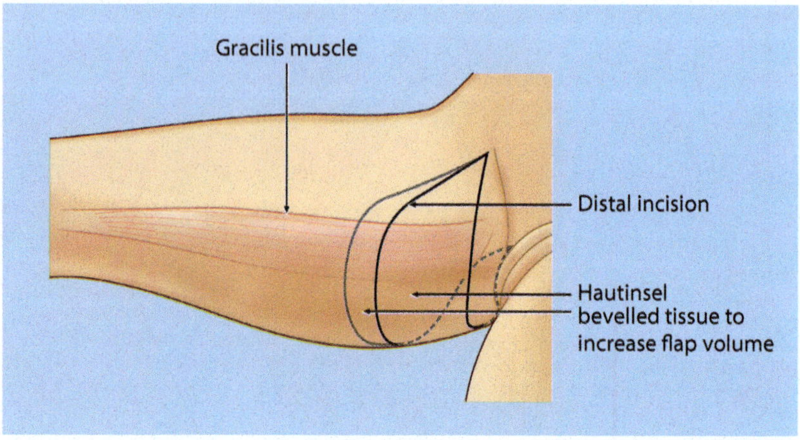

Fig. 10.64 The distal incision depends on the planned flap size. To ensure safe perfusion, the skin island should have a height of at least 5–6 cm. Distal and dorsal additional subcutaneous tissue without skin can be included into the flap by undermining and bevelling. The extent of this undermining should also be planned and marked

the inguinal crease and crosses the inner thigh to the IGF.

- Distal: the distal incision takes the flap size into consideration. It connects the ventral start and the dorsal end point so that an ellipse is formed. Perfusion should be safe if flap height is at least 6 cm.

10.2.6 Technique

10.2.6.1 Positioning on the Operation Table, IV Lines

Patient is placed supine. Arms are adducted by 45–30° in the shoulder. The elbows are placed on little arm pads and the hands are placed under the lumbar region. In a two-team approach, simultaneously two electrosurgery devices with two electrodes are required. A Foley catheter is recommended and directed under the thigh that is not used. The patient's body temperature can be managed with a convective warming device (e.g. Bair Hugger) on the non-operated leg. Two peripheral lines are sufficient, preferred at the ankle/feet or at the arm of the not operated side. In bilateral operations the IV lines are placed in both arms. The anaesthesiologist is located at the foot. Breast and thigh are prepared. The thigh is completely prepared to allow hip movement. The lower leg is sterile covered with a stockinette. The vulva/perineum is covered with a sponge. A U-shaped sterile sheet can cover the whole situs from caudal including the breast. A large sheet is used to cover the cranial part. One sheet can cover the abdomen to prevent loss of body temperature.

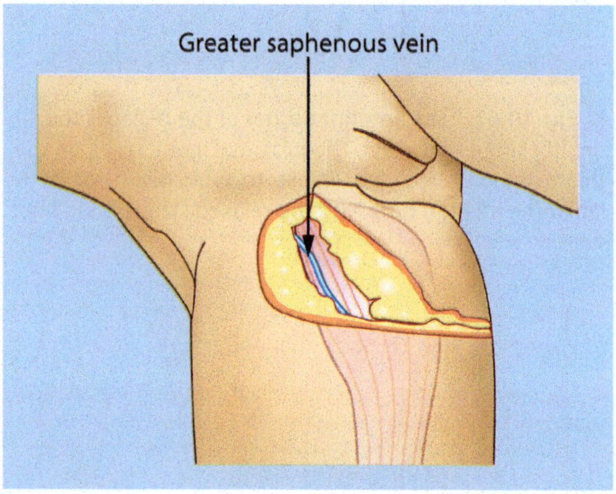

Fig. 10.65 Ventral border is the greater saphenous vein. Further ventral dissection is unnecessary and interferes with lymph drainage

10.2.6.2 Operation

Flap harvesting is best performed under loupe magnification with a headlight. A microscope is necessary for anastomosis. Harvesting is performed within 25–45 min if no complications occur. Dissection of the recipient site depends on the type of reconstruction, immediate or delayed.

Dissection can be performed with scissors (Metzenbaum) or by electrosurgery. The latter however can lead to more seroma. Dissection of the pedicle should be done with bipolar forceps and fine scissors. A right-handed surgeon stands on the contralateral side of the flap side and "looks" into the inner thigh.

Incision starts ventrally with bent knee and hip externally rotated. Ventrally no bevelling is recommended. The incision is made straight to the muscle fascia of the adductor longus muscle. The fascia is included in the flap (Fig. 10.65). Do not dissect laterally to the greater saphenous vein to keep the lymph nodes and the lymph collectors intact. Almost always a large subcutaneous vein from the flap enters the saphenous vein. The branch is clipped. The gracilis muscle is localized dorsally and medially from the adductor muscle. The dominant pedicle can be seen from here, how it enters from laterally underneath the adductor longus above the adductor magnus the gracilis muscle. The subcutaneous fat is left on the gracilis. The perforators run through the muscle and enter the fat. Then the distal dissection starts. If no bevelling is planned, the incision goes straight down to the muscle fascia. If a bevelling is planned, the superficial subcutaneous fascia should be left at the thigh if possible. The skin island should be about 5–7 cm high (from proximal to distal) directly over the gracilis muscle to include one or two sufficient perforators.

After the distal part is cut the dissection continues from the dorsal (◘ Fig. 10.66). The thigh is bent in the hip and externally rotated; the knee is bent. This allows to access the dorsal aspect without turning the patient. Bevelling is also dorsally possible. The incision goes down to the fascia and the fascia is included into the muscle. The flap is released from all muscles but the gracilis muscle. Now the incision is continued proximally. Proximally the incision is made straight down to the muscle without bevelling. Dorsal and medial several perforators arise from the muscles and enter the fatty tissue. They originate from the profunda femoris system. Strong perforators can be kept and temporarily clamped. If perfusion stays stable from the gracilis pedicle, they can be coagulated. Usually the gracilis perfusion is sufficient. If not the perforators that arise from dorsal of the gracilis muscle can be followed. These are the perforators of the *profunda artery perforator flap (PAP-flap)*.

The flap is now only based on the gracilis muscle. From the distal incision, the distal part of the muscle can be cut. The 2–3 vessels within the muscle have to be coagulated carefully because a bleeding from the stump is hard to control as the muscle contracts. If a long muscle is desired, a second distal incision may become necessary. We usually stop at the distal incision border and do not harvest a long muscle. Then the proximal gracilis is cut. The muscle is mobile now.

Then the pedicle is dissected staring with the entrance into the muscle and following the vessels

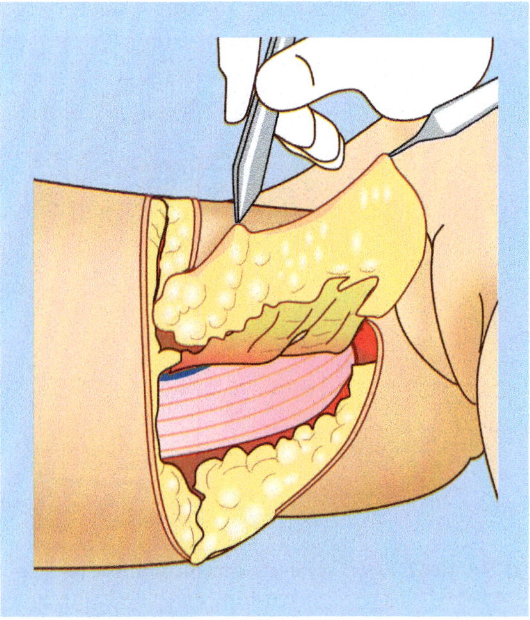

◘ Fig. 10.66 After the flap is incised ventrally, distally and proximally, the flap is elevated from dorsal to ventral up to the border of the gracilis muscle. The fascia around the muscles should be integrated into the flap

from periphery to central. A fine DeBakey forceps and a Stevens Tenotomy (or similar) are recommended. Small branches are clipped with small clips, larger ones with medium clips. The hip is in a straight position so that the muscle has no tension. A relaxation by the anaesthesiologist is helpful. The branch of the obturator nerve enters the muscle from proximal and lateral. The nerve can be left until the flap is completely harvested as it "holds" the flap in place (◘ Fig. 10.67).

It is evident in most cases which of the veins is the better one. Usually only one vein is sufficient. Some branches (artery and vein) enter the dorsal adductor. They can be clipped or coagulated. The first big branch runs ventrally into the adductor longus muscle. It should be isolated and clipped. The assistant can hold the adductor now away with a Langenbeck hook. Some more branches are clipped. Deep (medial) lies the medial circumflex femoris artery or the profunda femoris artery. If another branch runs from the gracilis pedicle to any adductor, it should be clipped close to the branching to avoid any intravascular turbulence, especially if these branches are bigger than the gracilis artery. Before the pedicle merges into the medial circumflex femoris or profunda femoris artery, the artery can be separated from the veins.

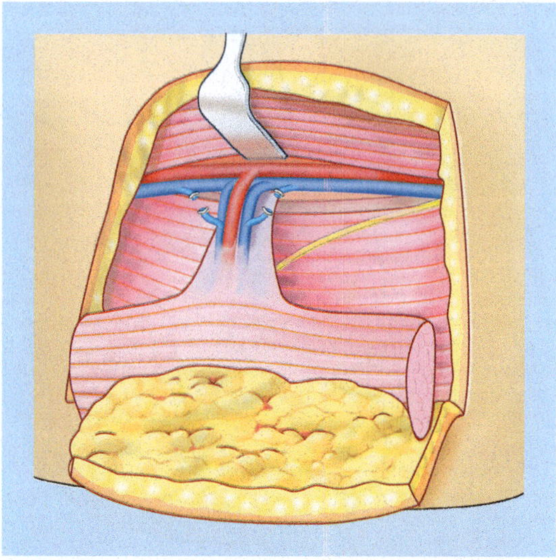

Fig. 10.67 After complete circumcision, the pedicle (arrow) is dissected from the muscle laterally to the origin of the vessels. The M. adductor magnus must be elevated with a Langenbeck hook. The patient should be relaxed. Branches from the pedicle usually go upwards into the adductor. These can be clipped with a fine Ligaclip. The pedicle can be harvested to a length of 5–7 cm. One only needs the artery and one, preferably, the stronger vein. The other vein can be clipped. If the nerve branch from the obturatorius nerve is initially left, it holds the flap without tension on the on the pedicle

We use a blunt dissector (fine Overholt forceps or similar). The smaller vein is clipped, leaving one artery and one vein (Fig. 10.68).

Others describe an access to the gracilis pedicle from the lateral passing the adductor longus muscle. The assistant has not to hold the strong muscle away and one approaches the vessels directly. However we do not use this approach, as the lateral mobilization can interfere with the lymphatics of the thigh.

Pedicle dissection has to be meticulous. The branches should be clipped close to the artery avoiding intravascular turbulences.

The flap is now based on the pedicle and the nerve and can be harvested now. We place a Redon drain in the inguinal area and a second one distal (watch the saphenous vein when placing the drain). If the skin island was large, the thigh has to be mobilized. A blunt manual dilation with the surgeons hand underneath the fascia can help. The subcutaneous fascia should be sutured with strong Vicryl. The closure should start dorsally.

10.2.6.3 Mastectomy and Flap Weight

For an adequate symmetry, the mastectomy specimen should be weighed. In a secondary recon-

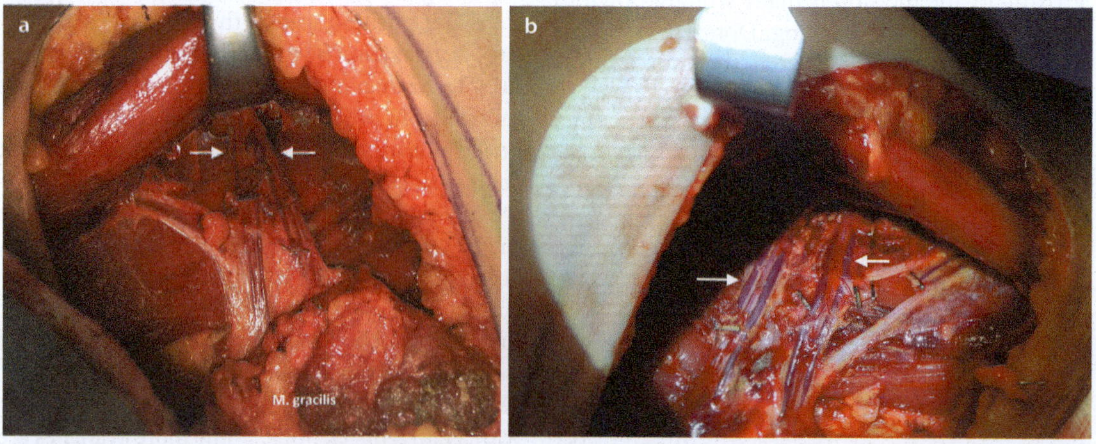

Fig. 10.68 Usually the pedicle is constant; this allows a quick harvest. In few cases there are variations like here: **a** a double pedicle from one central vessel. Both pedicles can be lifted without much effort. **b** Double pedicle with two origins from central. It is recommended to temporarily clamp the smaller vascular pedicle, or the one with more branches, with a clamp and then assess the circulation of the flap. For a good assessment, the clamp should be left at least 5 min, and the blood pressure should be normotonic. If the blood flow within the flap is poor, the clamp can be placed on the other pedicle to assess the blood flow over the other pedicle

struction, the mastectomy specimen weight is usually documented in the histopathology report. After the flap is resected, it can also be weighed. Normally the gland and the IT-flap have a similar volumic density. Only if the gland is very dense and heavy, the weight is not a real indicator because the gland is then heavier despite a small volume. However in most cases, weighing is a valuable tool to estimate symmetry. In a conversion from implants/expander, their weight can also give a rough estimate if the breasts were symmetrical before the operation.

10.2.6.4 Shaping and Inset of the Flap, Buried Flap

The IT-flap is oval-shaped; the gracilis runs perpendicular to the skin island (◘ Fig. 10.69). If the flap is large enough or a wide breast is desired, it can be put in transversely. However this can result in volume loss in the décolleté.

Mostly the flap should be sutured with itself using some 3-0 Vicryl. The flap then looks like an "anatomic implant" (◘ Figs. 10.70 and 10.71). If using the ipsilateral flap, the muscle runs from medial caudal to lateral cranial. The muscle can replace the axillary part of the gland. By this positioning the dorsal part of the flap lies caudal sternal, the ventral part cranial medial.

There are many concepts regarding the flap sutures. The part where the pedicle enters the muscle should be fixed after anastomosis to the pectoral muscle to avoid a twisting or kinking of the pedicle. We think that the flap should at least be fixed medially and in the IMF to avoid dents and malposition and allow smooth transitions. Cranially and laterally sutures should be applied if the flap is better positioned and shaped. To avoid fat necrosis, the flap side should only be fixed at Scarpa's fascia or the dermis.

We normally use drains which are not put next to the pedicle. If the mastectomy skin flap is not well perfused or cannot be assessed properly, the flap skin can be left on the flap. The mastectomy flap is placed over the flap. The flap is now buried. After some days viability of the mastectomy skin can be assessed. If the mastectomy skin has survived, the thigh skin is removed in a short second operation; if not the mastectomy skin can be replaced by flap skin.

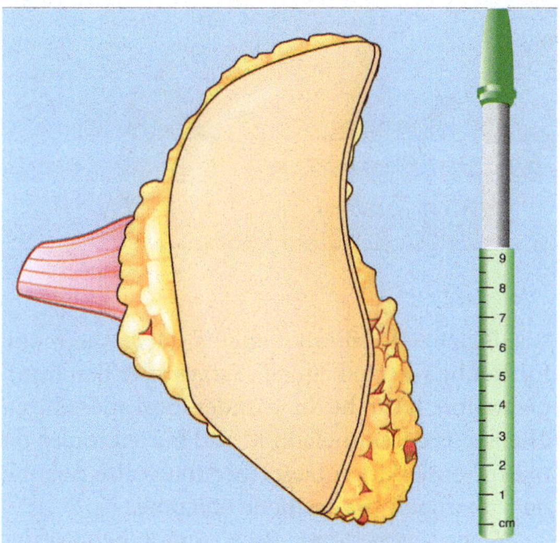

◘ Fig. 10.69 The ventral flap is thinner than dorsal. This must be taken into account when shaping the flap

10.2.6.5 Anastomoses

The general technique has been described in ► Sect. 8.3. For the IT-flap, the anastomoses should be done at the IMA or IMAP vessels. IMAP calibre resembles the gracilis vessel size and is therefore preferred. The calibre is matching and the positioning is easy.

The standard IMA approach is in the 3rd or 4th ICS. Perforator veins or the IMV can be coupled. The IMAP veins show more valves. At the anastomotic site, no valve should be present. IMAP veins are thinner than the IMV; thus gentle handling is required.

The arterial anastomosis to the IMA is not easy as mostly a calibre mismatch is present. To facilitate the anastomosis, the flap artery can be dilated with dilator or micro-needle holder. A dilation can also be made by flushing the artery: place a bulldog clamp on the artery near to the gracilis muscle and flush intraluminal. If the vessel is temporarily blocked at the lumen entrance, the vessel will dilate. Anastomosis can be done in the preferred technique. Short pedicles can be best sutured with the backhand technique. In a persistent calibre mismatch, the distance between the stiches on each side of the vessel should be proportional, thus wider at the larger side and narrower at the smaller sider. An 8-0 to 10-0 nylon with small needles should be adequate.

The anastomosis to the subscapular vessels requires interposition grafts and is not primarily recommended. Only if two IT-flaps are used for one breast, the lateral/cranial one is anastomosed to the axilla.

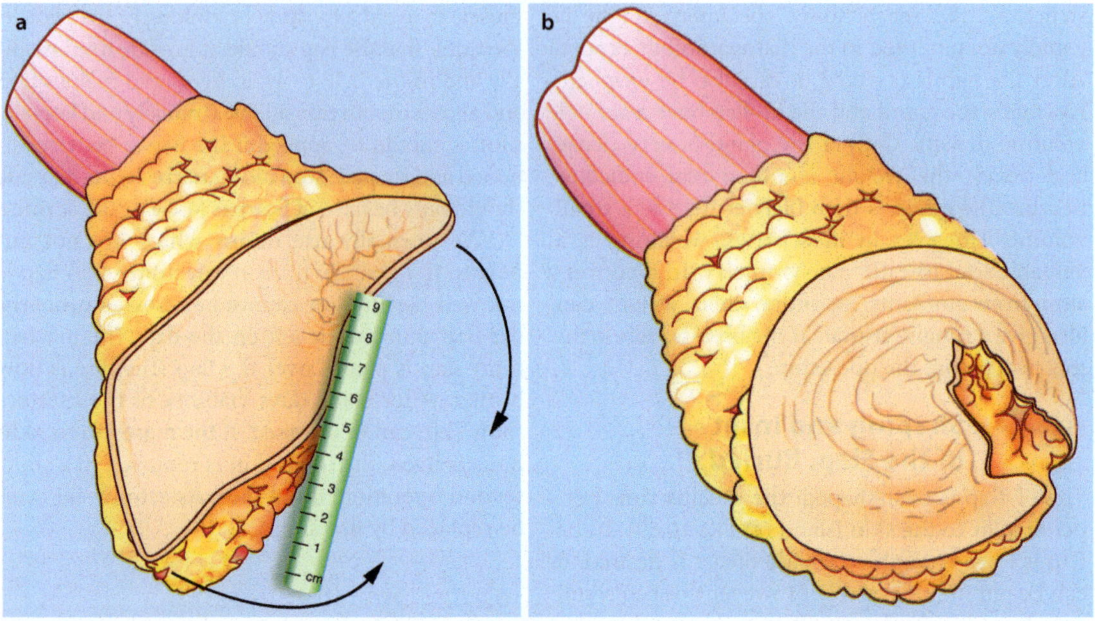

Fig. 10.70 **a** To imitate an "anatomical implant", the flap can be sutured together via its proximal side. This creates **b** a hemispherical shape. On the left, the subcutaneous fat content is visible from undermining/bevelling

Fig. 10.71 The flap is de-epithelialized in the areas that are placed under the breast skin. Flap skin is only left where it replaces the breast skin or is used for monitoring. The easiest way to de-epithelialize is using sharp scissors

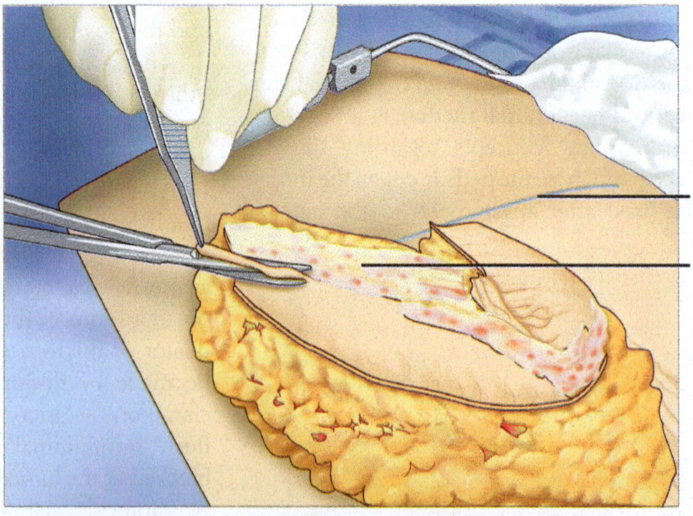

10.2.7 Monitoring

After mastectomy and immediate reconstruction or secondary reconstruction, the decision has to be made if skin from the flap has to be used. If so the skin can be used to monitor flap viability. If no skin island is required, one should consider placing a temporary monitor island at the incision line to assess flap viability. A small, representative part is sufficient. If viability remains stable, the monitor can be resected after 2–5 days after flap transplantation. It can be done under local anaesthesia. The flap is de-epithelialized and buried under the mastectomy skin. A later resection is also possible but can impair the aesthetic outcome.

If the mastectomy skin cannot be assessed intraoperatively regarding its viability, the flap skin can be left temporarily underneath the mastectomy skin for some days. The flap is kept buried until the viability is clear. If mastectomy skin has to be resected, the resulting defects can be replaced by flap skin in a second operation short after.

10.2.8 Aftercare

The patients are mobile as soon as they can get up. They should get up from the bed not sitting on the operated side. They should be supported and instructed by PT or nurses when getting up the first times. In the first days, they should avoid sitting on the operated side and prefer soft padded chairs. The Foley catheter can be removed at the first postoperative day. A raised WC seat can help the first days. The wound at the thigh is best covered with a spray-on liquid plaster. A bra that does not compress the pedicle can be used if necessary. A stocking can stabilize the leg in the first postoperative weeks. The stocking should not compress the scar and avoid mechanical irritation.

Thromboprophylaxis is recommended. Drains should be removed with regard to the fluid amount. Work and daily activities should be possible after 1 week and should not exceed the standard. Sporting, sauna and sun tanning should be avoided for at least 6 weeks.

A loss of sensitivity at the dorsal thigh and the breast is usual. Seromas at the donor site can be punctured if necessary.

10.2.9 Corrective and Additional Surgery

If additional surgery is necessary, it should be planned at least 3–6 months later then the flap surgery. If dents or irregularities occur in the transition zones between flap and original tissue, they can be mildend by lipofilling; a secondary augmentation can also be done by lipofilling. A contralateral operation, if not done together with the reconstruction, can be planned at that time too. A secondary augmentation can also be done with an implant with respect to the flap pedicle because the flap does not achieve full vascular autonomy in most cases. Usually the pedicle of the IT-flap is more caudal than the DIEP-flap pedicle; thus the dissection for an implant should be more careful.

If a contralateral donor site alignment is planned, it should take place at the earliest after 3–6 months after the flap reconstruction. If the patient desires a refinement, the contralateral thigh can be suctioned, and the aspirate can be used to undertake possible breast refinements. If the skin is not elastic, a thigh lifting can be considered, if necessary after harvesting the fat for lipofilling.

The reconstruction of the NAC is considered to be the last operation.

10.2.9.1 Results After IT-Flap Reconstructions

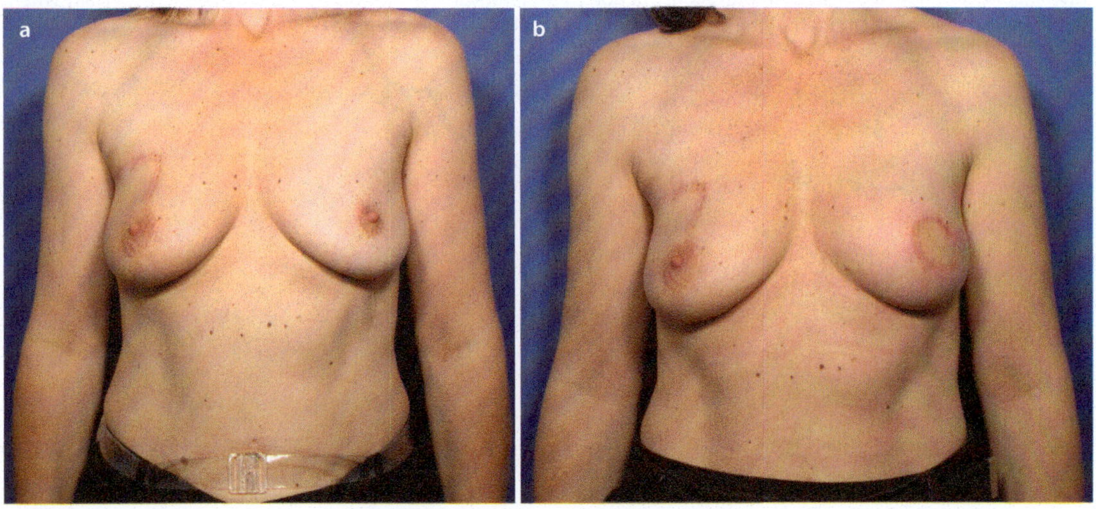

Fig. 10.72 **a, b** Periareolar SSM left; BCT due to breast cancer on the right side. The highly unusual BCT incision on the right side was made elsewhere (!). Primary reconstruction with IT-flap. Thigh skin replaces the areola. Result after 4 months

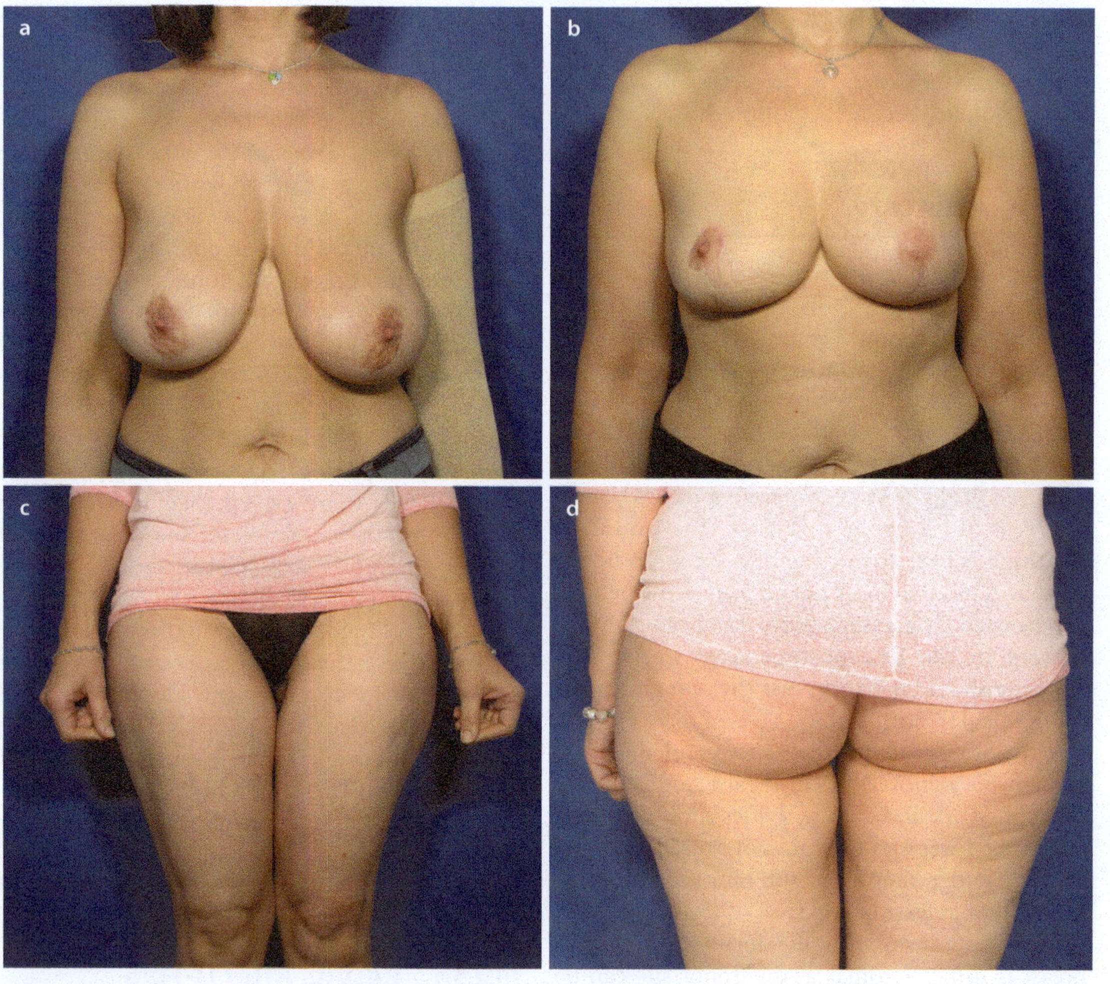

Fig. 10.73 **a–d** Cancer left breast. SSM and single-stage primary reconstruction with IT-flap and reduction mammaplasty of right side. Later nipple reconstruction with local flap and pigmentation of the areola. Result after 12 months. **c, d** Donor site on the left thigh. The scar runs dorsally in the infragluteal fold. Even with a single-sided removal, the asymmetry is hardly visible, especially when clothing is worn

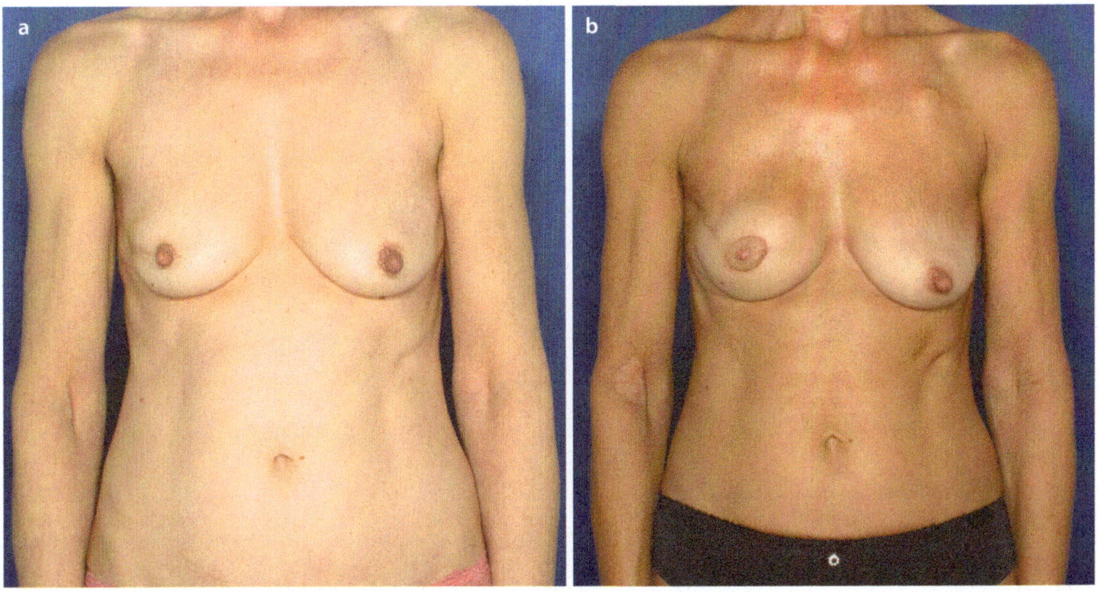

Fig. 10.74 **a, b** Right breast carcinoma with axillary infiltration. SSM and primary reconstruction with IT-flap. Irradiation of the flap. Results 18 months after primary surgery with nipple sharing. An adjustment of the opposite side was not desired

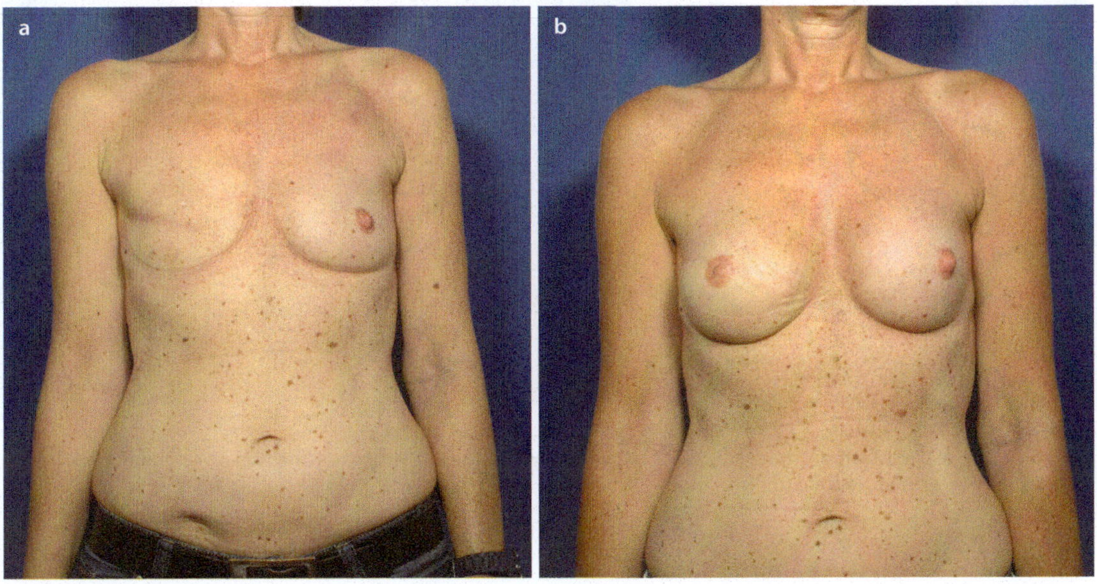

Fig. 10.75 **a, b** Mastectomy right and radiation therapy. Secondary reconstruction with right IT-flap and left augmentation with round implant in a single-stage operation. Later nipple reconstruction with local flap and pigmentation

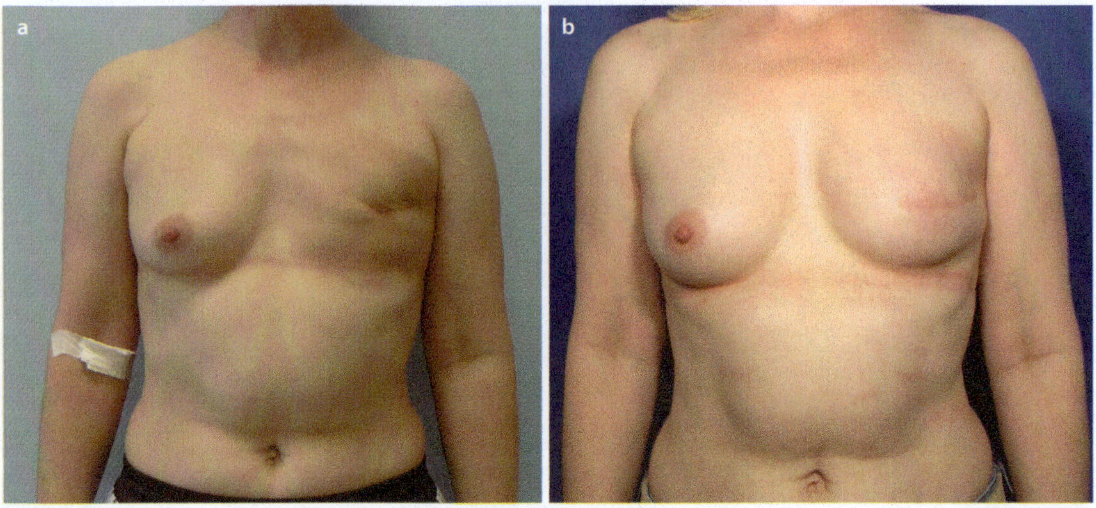

Fig. 10.76 **a** Mastectomy and radiation therapy left. First epipectoral expansion, then **b** secondary reconstruction with IT-flap. Result after 2 years

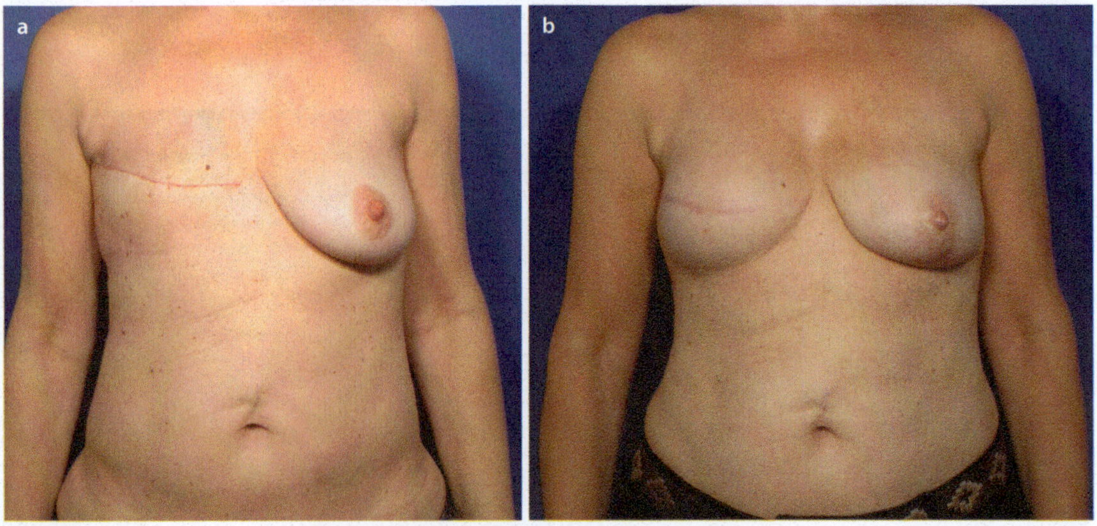

Fig. 10.77 **a, b** Mastectomy right with radiation; BRCA2 was detected later; reconstruction right with buried IT-flap. NSM left and also IT-flap. Result after 6 months

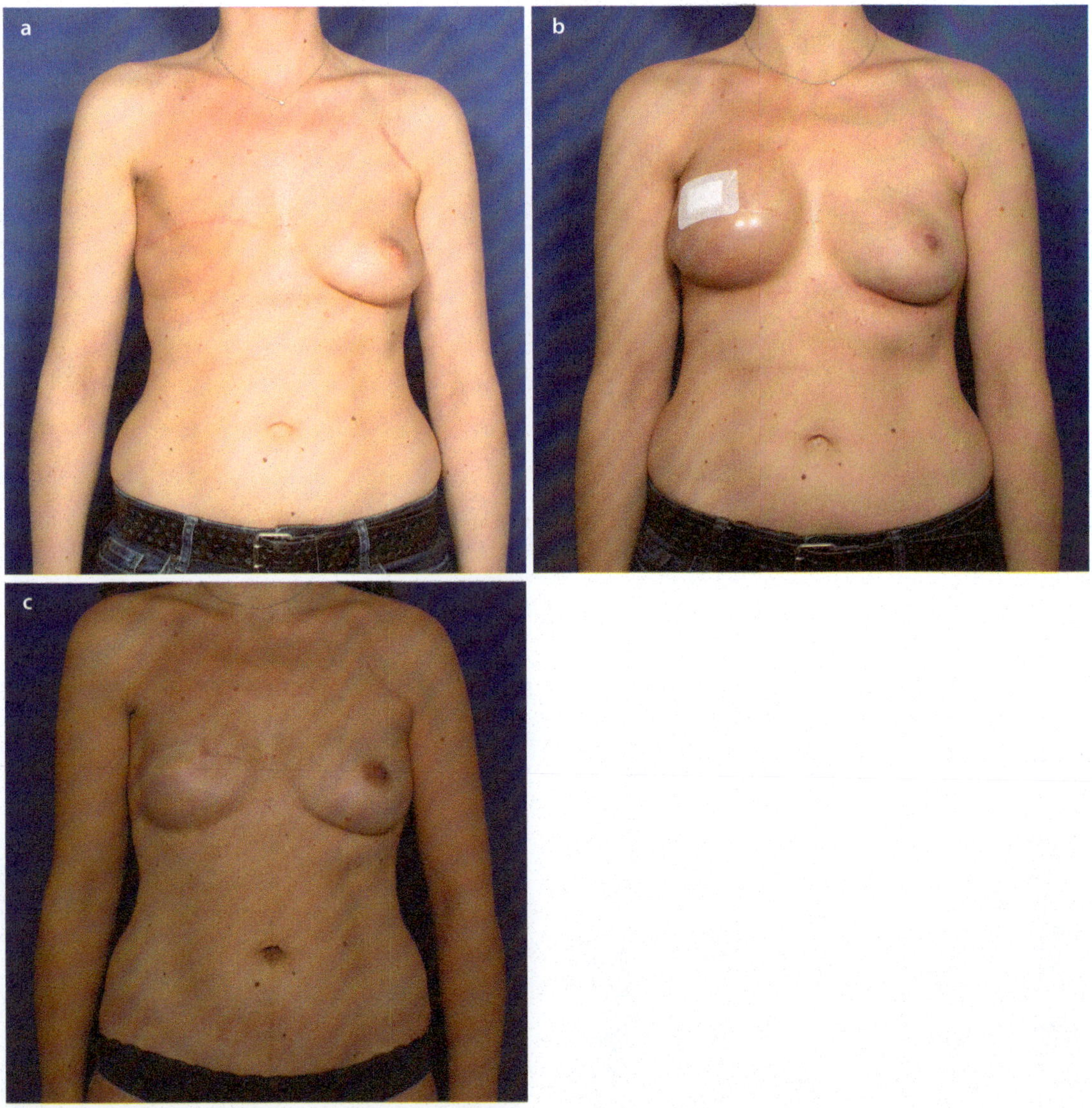

Fig. 10.78 **a** Mastectomy right with radiation therapy and planned NSM left. **b** First operation with expander right to use as little thigh skin as possible; NSM and IT-flap left side. **c** Second operation with expander removal and IT- flap right with small skin island

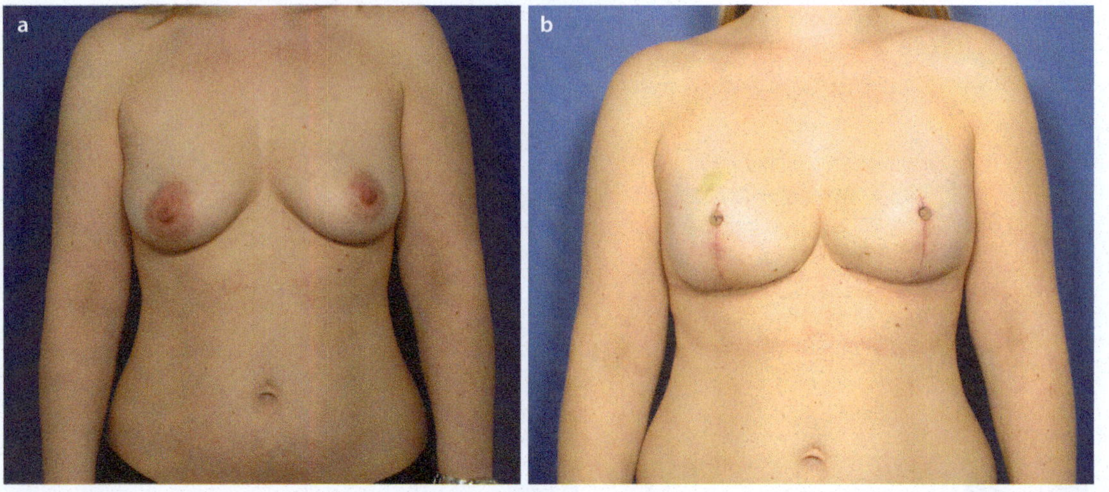

Fig. 10.79 **a** BRCA1 patient. **b** Bilateral SSM with Wise pattern and primary reconstruction with bilateral thigh flaps. The patient desired immediate nipple reconstruction, results after 6 weeks

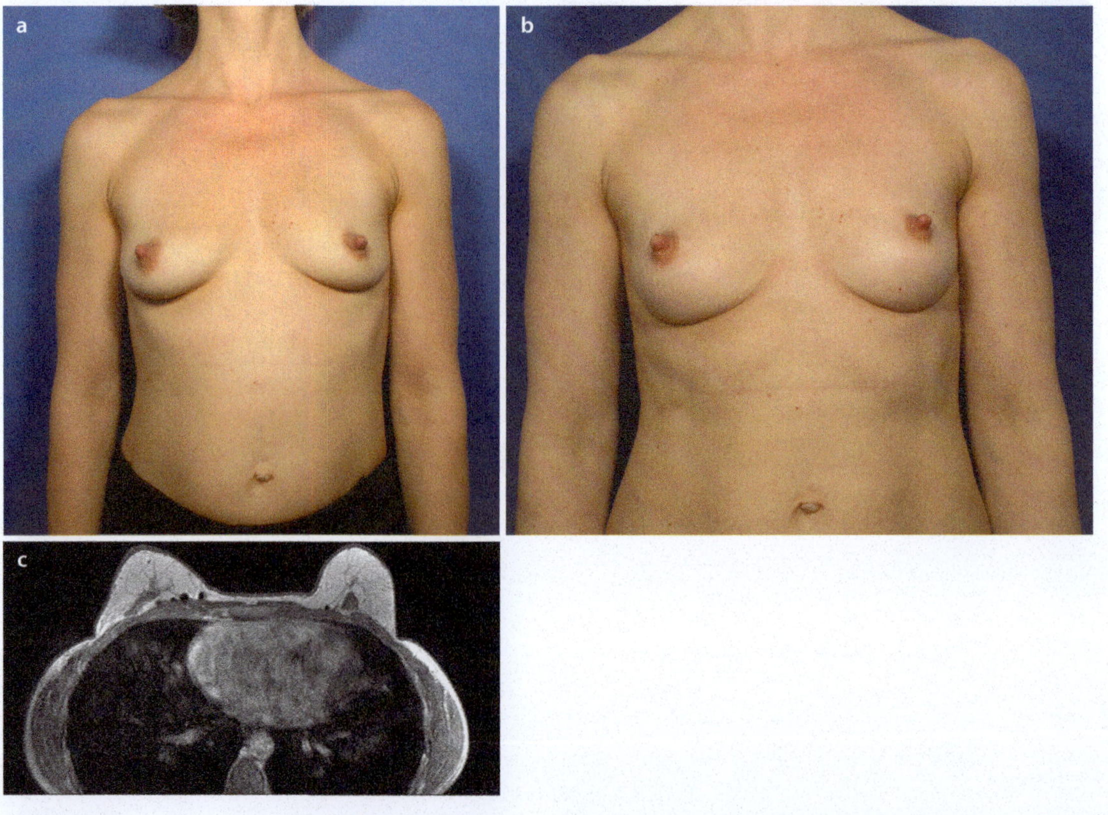

Fig. 10.80 **a** BRCA1 patient. **b** Bilateral SSM from an IMF incision and reconstruction with bilateral IT-flaps, result after 9 months. **c** MRI 6 months postoperatively for evaluation of mastectomy and further planning of intensified early detection. Glandular tissue is no longer visible; only fat and parts of the gracilis muscle can be seen

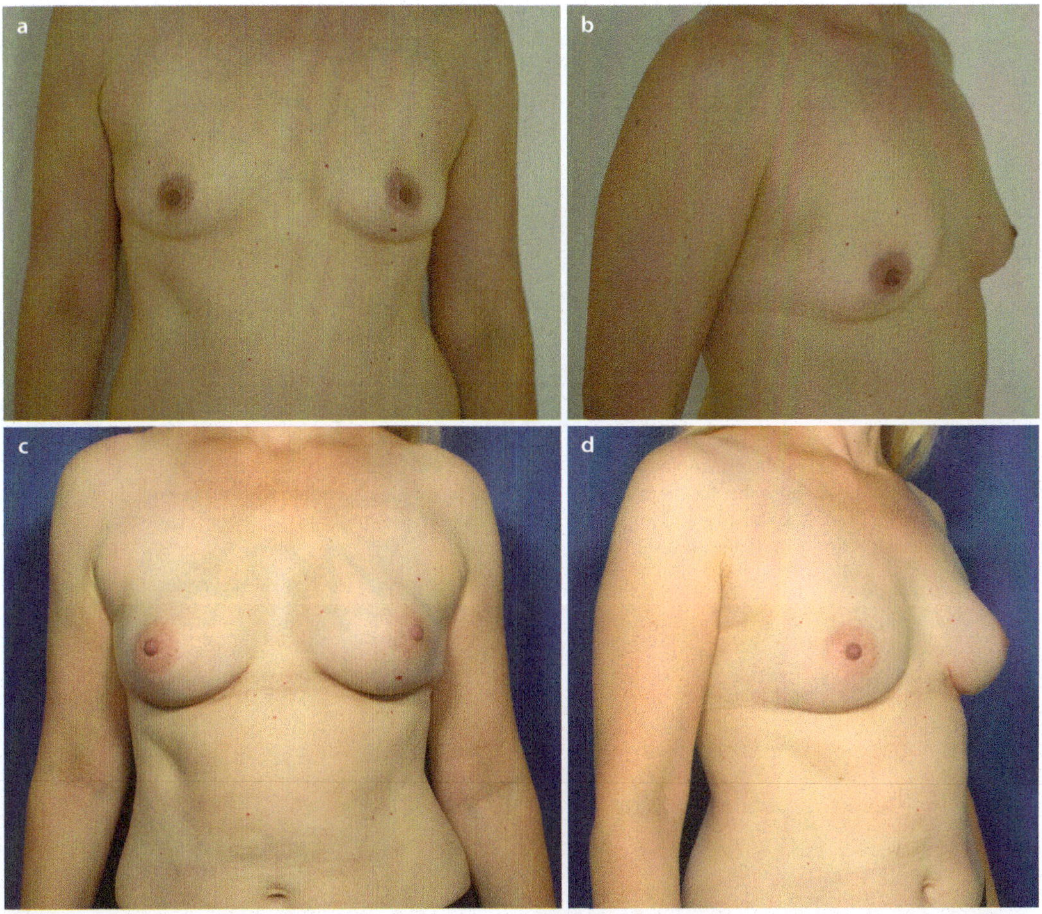

Fig. 10.81 **a, b** BRCA2 patient. **c, d** NSM from an IMF incision and reconstruction with IT-flap; result after 6 months. IT-flaps allow shaping an anatomical breast shape with good projection. Especially with a skin excess, a good volume can be achieved if the nipple-IMF distance is not greater than 8–9 cm

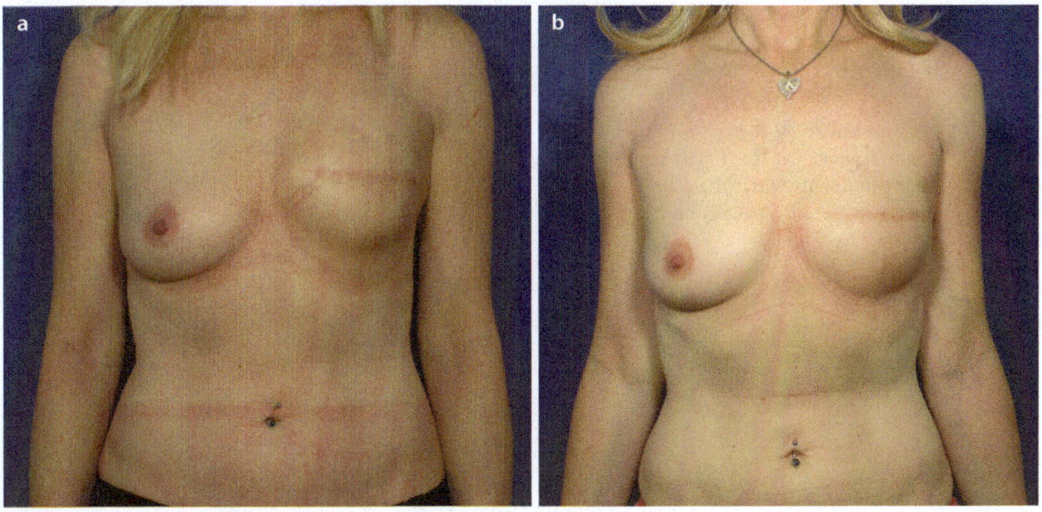

Fig. 10.82 **a** Patient with SSM left, implant reconstruction and radiation. Capsular contracture with cranial dislocation, asymmetry, hardening and pain. **b** Conversion to autologous tissue with capsule and implant removal and reconstruction with IT-flap

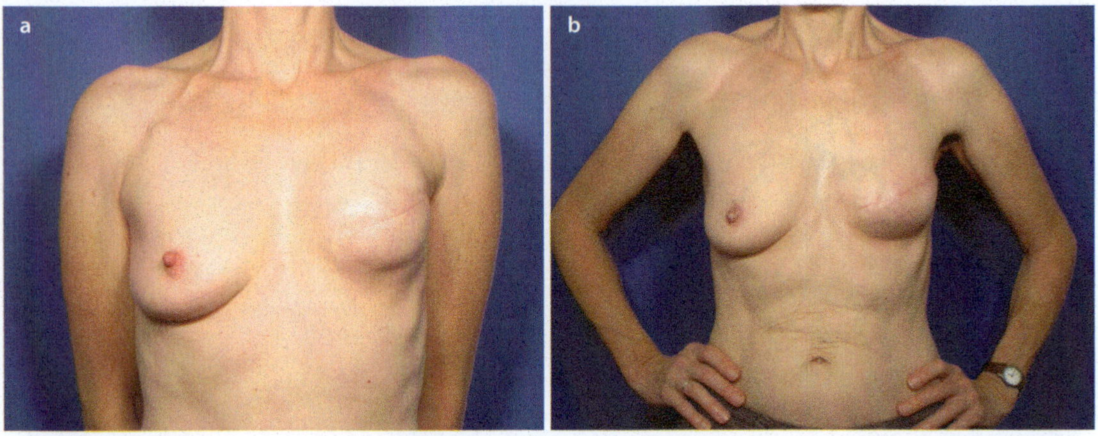

Fig. 10.83 **a** Patient with SSM left, implant reconstruction and radiation. Also here due to the radiation pronounced capsular fibrosis. **b** Capsule and implant removal and reconstruction with IT-flap. It is difficult to resect the rigid fibrosis in such a way that the breast skin can be caudalized again without the need to insert the skin from the thigh

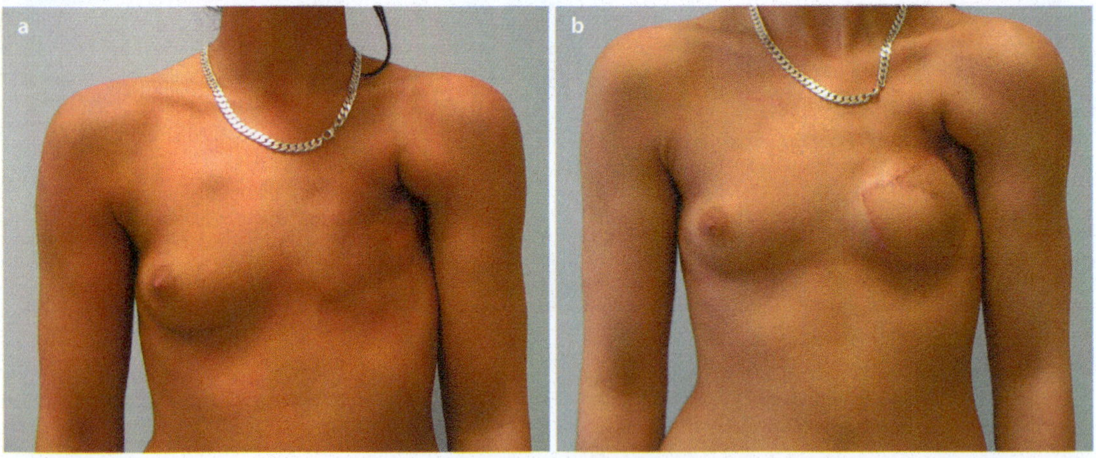

Fig. 10.84 **a** 18-year-old female patient with resection of the breast, the entire pectoralis musculature up to the ribs due to a sarcoma of the thoracic wall. Radiation. **b** Reconstruction with IT-flap with skin, since no local skin could be recruited; result after 3 months

Fig. 10.85 Donor site of left IT-flap from the frontal view, patient from Fig. 10.76. The scar is on the thigh, not in the inguinal crease. The asymmetry is noticeable to the patients, but is usually hardly visible wearing trousers

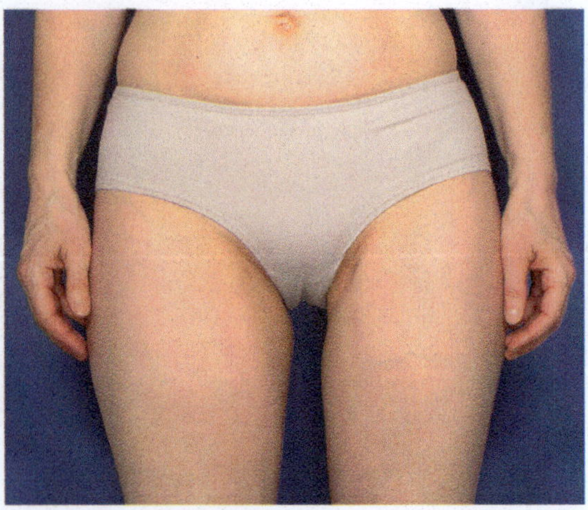

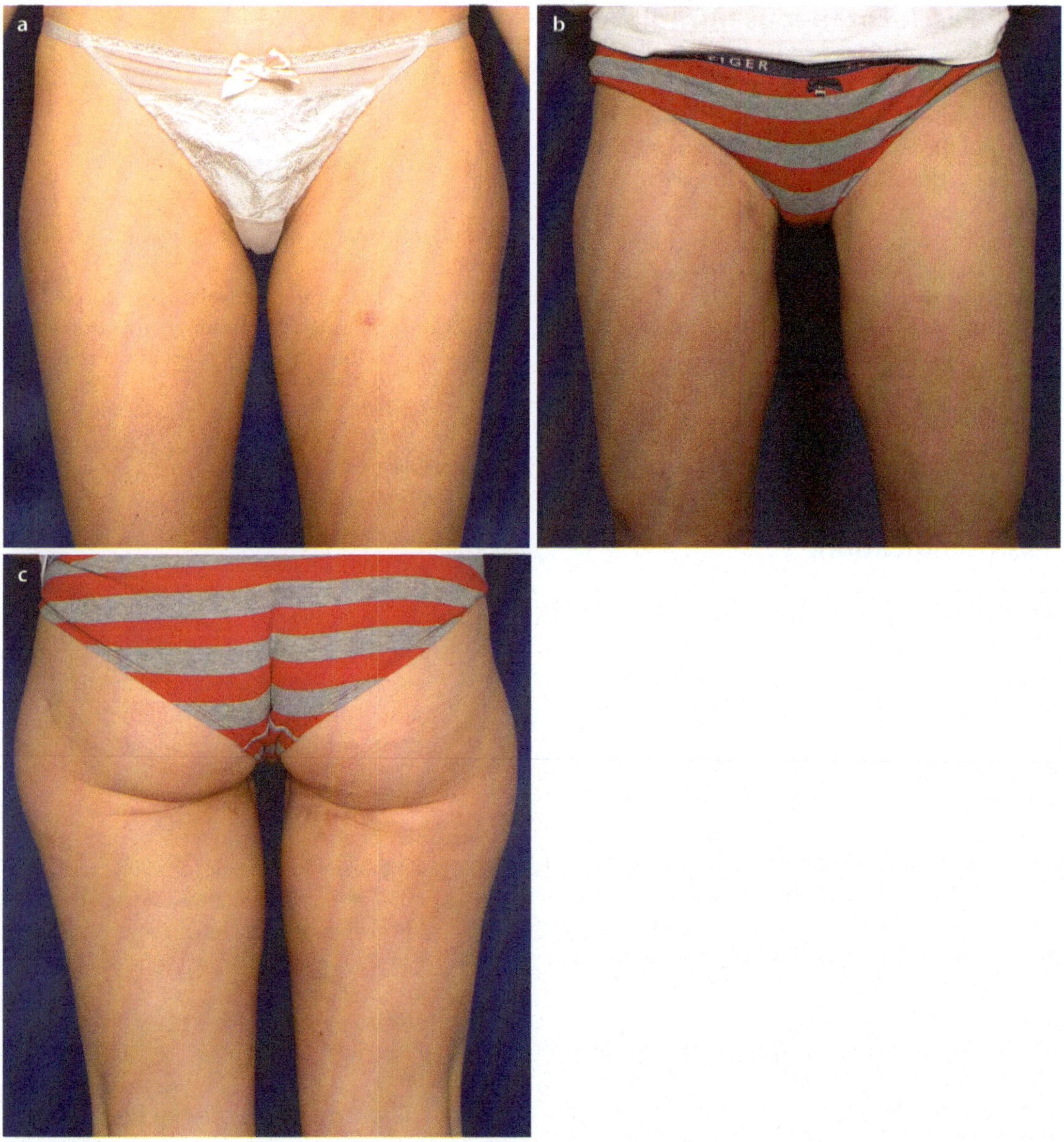

Fig. 10.86 **a** Donor site of IT-flaps on both sides, patient from Fig. 10.80. Preoperative. **b** Postoperative from frontal and dorsal view. **c** Dorsally the donor site runs into the lower gluteal fold. Flap weight was about 215 g

Conclusion

The inner thigh flap (IT-flap) is a discrete flap that is a significant alternative to the DIEP-flap. The volume is enough to reconstruct a small- to medium-sized breast with slender patients. In bilateral reconstructions, this technique does not have to respect the existing size as it creates two new symmetric breasts. It can be applied very well for prophylactic reconstructions. The tissue is harvested with a transverse island from the inner thigh and the IGF. Bevelling increases flap volume and leaves skin for tension-free closure at the thigh. The short pedicle is best anastomosed to the IMA or IMAP. The vessels are smaller than the epigastric vessels; thus the arterial anastomosis requires microsurgical expertise. However success rates are similar to the DIEP-flaps. The patients should know that in the beginning a loss of sensitivity and some tension are evident at the dorsal thigh.

10.3 Fasciocutaneous Infragluteal Flap (FCI-Flap)

Fasciocutaneous infragluteal flap (FCI-flap) is a fat flap from the lower gluteal fold. The same harvesting area is the infragluteal perforator flap (IGAP). Here, however, the pedicle comes from the descending branch of the inferior gluteal artery. The posterior femoral cutaneous nerve accompanies the pedicle. The FCI-flap is an alternative flap to the flaps described above. Disadvantages are the prone position for harvesting the flap and possible sensitivity and sitting problems in the donor site. But especially for very slim patients, it can be a possible donor region.

10.3.1 Indication

Breast

The FCI-flap is suitable for the reconstruction of patients with small- to medium-sized breasts, i.e. with rather smaller bra cups (A–C) and a narrower upper body. In the case of bilateral reconstructions, this flap can be used independently of the existing breast size, since symmetry can be achieved by surgery on both sides.

Primary reconstructions with SSM and NSM are best suited for this flap, as they keep the breast skin intact. In secondary reconstructions, skin smaller from the lower gluteal fold must usually be inserted in the form of a spindle in order to shape the breast accordingly.

The FCI-flap can also be used in the case of defects after a BCT to replace the volume deficit. If such a visible skin spindle is not desired, the local skin can be stretched by means of a previous expander surgery. In this case, it is sufficient to place the expander epipectorally, since the flap is inserted in this position.

Donor site

If the lower abdomen and inner thigh can be used as a donor site, we recommend to use a DIEP-flap or IT-flap; however the preferences of the patient and the surgeon should be taken into account. In the case of previous operations on the lower abdomen smaller that have affected the deep and/or superficial epigastric blood circulation system, or on the thigh, or insufficient volume at these points, the FCI is an ideal donor site. The possible harvesting volume can be estimated by a pinch test and compared with the breast volume.

10.3.2 Contraindication

Patients who had liposuction or operations on the lower gluteal fold should be carefully examined to determine whether the previous operations (scars, retractions, missing fatty tissue) are a contraindication. A previous thigh lift is usually a contraindication.

Overview FCI (Fig. 10.87)
Indication: small- to medium-sized breasts

Skin island:
- Transversal in the lower gluteal fold.
- Size: up to 20 cm wide and 6–10 cm high, depending on buttocks.
- By subcutaneous bevelling of the flap, the skin on the buttocks and thighs can be left for better closure, and the volume of the flap can be increased.

Vascular pedicle:
- Skin branch from the descending branch of the inferior gluteal artery or from the medial or lateral circumflex femoris artery
- Accompanied by the posterior femoral cutaneous nerve
- Pedicle length: about 5–15 cm

10.3.3 Tissue Characteristics

The tissue of the inferior gluteal fold is usually soft but has septa. It therefore cannot be sutured to itself and shaped well as the inner thigh flap. However, it can be inserted en bloc into the breast. The sense of touch is firmer than with a DIEP- or IT-flap. The tissue does not "sag" with gravity like other flaps. Therefore, the flap must be formed carefully in situ.

The colour of the skin on the buttocks is lighter than the breast skin. Some patients may have hairy donor site. Since most of the flap is de-epithelialized, this is not very important. If hair-bearing parts remain, these can later be removed by laser hair removal or other permanent techniques.

As a rule, the volume of the flap remains stable. If radiation therapy becomes necessary after the reconstruction, our experience has shown that the entire flap can be included in the radiation field.

Single-sided removal results in a slight asymmetry of the lower gluteal fold. This is visible to the patients in front of the mirror but is hardly noticeable when the leg is clothed. Usually no further surgery is necessary. If necessary, however, an adjustment should only be made later. In the case of elastic skin, the contralateral side can undergo a liposuction, and the lipoaspirate can be used for lipofilling possible dents or for increasing the volume. If the skin is inelastic, a contralateral lifting should be performed, if necessary after suction for lipofilling.

10.3.4 Informed Consent

The disclosure of general and special risks should be documented with standardized and evaluated forms. Infection, haematoma and wound-healing complications can occur. The risk of complete and partial flap loss should be mentioned, as well as wound-healing complications at the donor site. Seroma formation and visible scars can result. In mastectomy cases loss of sensitivity to the breast skin and the NAC is often. Loss of sensitivity can also occur at the donor site (lower gluteal fold, perineal and dorsal thigh). Especially in FCI-flaps, sitting can be painful in the first weeks, and in rare cases, a neuropathic pain can result from the nerve. A skin necrosis and NAC necrosis can occur and may require a reoperation. Smaller wound-healing problems can remain conservatively treated.

A lymph oedema of the breast and thoracic wall is possible in rare cases. The patient should be aware that breast shape, colour and symmetry are altered. Aesthetic change can result in psychological problems which may require psycho-oncologic consultation.

The incisions should be visualized in a drawing. The indication for a SSM or NSM should be discussed carefully. Scarring can distort the NAC in an NSM. Fat necrosis can occur. In most cases it shows no symptoms but can be detected by ultrasound. Second operations should be mentioned if histopathology is unclear or wound-healing problems occur or a contralateral mastopexy/reduction is required. A significant change after radiation is not likely to occur if the flap is well perfused; however it should be mentioned. If the patient does refuse recommended surgery or parts, this should also be documented.

If a bra and compression garments are recommended, the patients should be informed prior to surgery. Also the after treatment should be explained.

10.3.5 Preoperative Markings and Measures

In single-sided procedures, the flap can first be harvested in the prone position, and the flap is then prepared on an operating table. The patient is then placed in a supine position, the breast is operated on according to the plan, the recipient vessels are dissected, and the flap is anastomosed. With this technique, the ischemia time is extended, but only one a position change is necessary. Alternatively, one can start in supine position, then repositioning to prone position for harvesting and then again back to supine position.

First, the inferior gluteal fold is marked with the patient in an upright position (◘ Fig. 10.88). The skin island is then marked centred on the crease. The tissue that is to be taken along cranially and caudally is also marked. The skin island should be selected so that the lifting area can be closed without tension. Overresection should be avoided at all costs. The pedicle usually enters in the middle third of the gluteal fold, rather medially. The vessel can be marked by Doppler examination.

Anatomic landmarks of FCI-flap
- Central: inferior gluteal fold.
- Medial: ischium.
- Lateral: end of inferior gluteal fold.
- For volume augmentation the flap is bevelled, and subcutaneous tissue is integrated cranially and caudally into the flap.

10.3.6 Technique

10.3.6.1 Positioning on the Operation Table, IV Lines

For flap harvesting the patient is placed in a prone position. When the flap is anastomosed, the patient is in supine position. Arms are adducted by 45–30° in the shoulder. The elbows are placed on little arm pads and the hands are placed under the lumbar region. In a two-team approach, simultaneously two electrosurgery devices with two electrodes are required. A Foley catheter is recommended and directed under the thigh that is not used. The patient's body temperature can be managed with a convective warming device (e.g. Bair Hugger) on the non-operated leg. Two peripheral lines are sufficient, preferred at the ankle/feet or at the arm of the not operated side. The anaesthesiologist is located at the foot. The lower leg is sterile covered with a stockinette. The vulva/perineum is covered. A U-shaped sterile sheet can cover the whole situs.

10.3.6.2 Operation

Flap harvesting is best performed under loupe magnification with a headlight. A microscope is necessary for anastomosis. Harvesting is performed within 45–60 min if no complications occur. Dissection of the recipient site depends on the type of reconstruction, immediate or delayed.

Dissection can be performed with scissors (Metzenbaum) or by electrosurgery. The latter however can lead to more seroma. Dissection of the pedicle should be done with bipolar forceps and fine scissors. A surgeon stands on the ipsilateral side.

The incision is made around the flap and includes the subcutaneous tissue cranially, caudally and laterally. In this case, care must be taken to gently bevel the flap in order to avoid subsequent step formation, especially on the cranial breast (◘ Fig. 10.89). The fat and the bursa above the ischium are always spared. One can now dissect from cranial on the muscle to the caudal muscle border or as in the original description of Papp et al. [21] from lateral. In a cranial preparation, the perforator vessels from the gluteal muscle can be left in place until the pedicle is visible. The pedicle runs with the posterior cutaneous femoral nerve. The medial and lateral branch of the nerve should be preserved and protected by microsurgery to avoid dysesthesia and sitting problems (◘ Fig. 10.90). Nerve branches running through the vascular bifurcation must be severed. After the flap has been harvested, they can be coapted again if necessary (◘ Figs. 10.89 and 10.91).

Once the pedicle has been identified and secured, the gluteus maximus can be elevated cranially, the ischiocrural muscles can be held laterally and medially with self-retaining hooks, and the pedicle can be further prepared centrally. The pedicle runs in a fatty fascia. The dissection should be done very carefully until the infrapiriform foramen, where the inferior gluteal artery usually arises. The pedicle can be lengthened by ligating some branches but keeping the inferior gluteal nerve intact. The arteries and the accompanying veins should be carefully separated. The flap now only hangs on the pedicle and can then be harvested. After the pedicle is cut with Ligaclips, a Redon drain is placed. If there is enough subcutaneous fascia, it should be closed with absorbable sutures (e.g. Vicryl or Monocryl).

! Medially the fat above the ischium must be retained. The medial and lateral nerve branches must also be protected.

10.3.6.3 Mastectomy and Flap Weight

For an adequate symmetry, the mastectomy specimen should be weighed. In a secondary reconstruction, the mastectomy specimen weight is usually documented in the histopathology report. After the flap is resected, it can also be weighed. Normally the gland and the FCI-flap have a similar volumic density. Only if the gland is very dense and heavy, the weight is not a real indicator because the gland is then heavier despite a small volume. However in most cases weighing is a valuable tool to estimate symmetry. In a conversion from implants/expander, their weight can also give a rough estimate if the breasts were symmetrical before the operation.

10.3.6.4 Shaping and Inset of the Flap, Buried Flap

The FCI-flap is oval-shaped and inserted en bloc. Coning sutures or other shaping attempts are difficult due to the septa within the flap. We prefer to suture the flap in the IMF. A medial fixation can avoid "dents" towards the décolleté. Cranially, an attempt can be made to smooth the transition with sutures between the flap and the subcutaneous fascia.

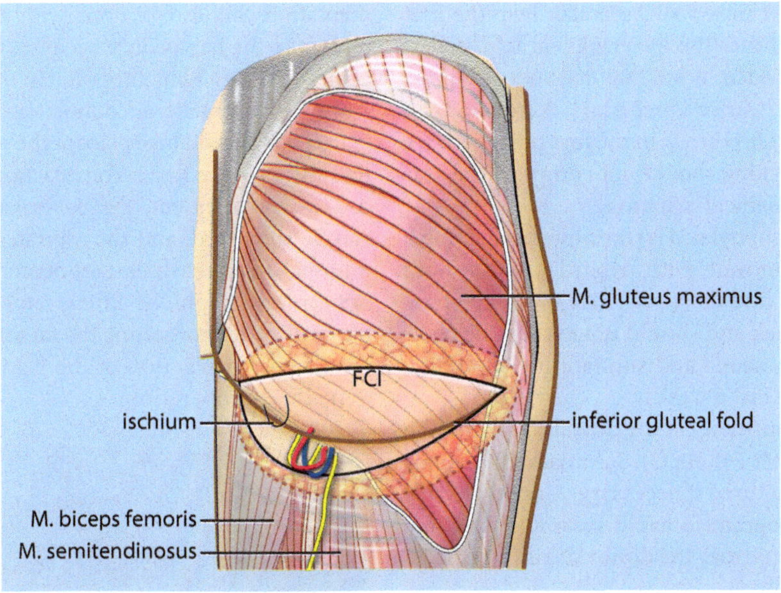

Fig. 10.87 The skin island of the FCI is placed over the inferior gluteal fold. The subcutaneous tissue cranial, caudal and lateral can be integrated into the flap. The fat and the bursa above the ischium are always spared. The pedicle enters the flap in the middle third of the fold. It runs posteriorly with the posterior femoral cutaneous nerve. The medial and lateral branch of the nerve should be preserved and protected to avoid sensibility/dysesthesia and sitting problems. Once pedicle has been identified and secured, the gluteus maximus can be elevated cranially, and the ischiocrural muscles can be held laterally and medially, and the pedicle can be further prepared centrally. The dissection should be done very carefully until the infrapiriform foramen (sciatic nerve)

We normally use drains which are not put next to the pedicle. If the mastectomy skin flap is not well perfused or cannot be assessed properly, the flap skin can be left on the flap. The mastectomy flap is placed over the flap. The flap is now buried. After some days viability of the mastectomy skin can be assessed. If the mastectomy skin has survived, the thigh skin is removed in a short second operation; if not the mastectomy skin can be replaced by flap skin.

10.3.6.5 Anastomoses

The basic details are described in ▶ Sect. 8.3. The anastomosis itself can be performed using the technique preferred by the surgeon.

10.3.7 Monitoring

After mastectomy and immediate reconstruction or secondary reconstruction, the decision has to be made if skin from the flap has to be used. If so the skin can be used to monitor flap viability. If no skin island is required, one should consider placing a temporary monitor island at the incision line to assess flap viability. A small, representative part is sufficient. If viability remains stable, the monitor can be resected after 2–5 days after flap transplantation. It can be done under local anaesthesia. The flap is de-epithelialized and buried under the mastectomy skin. A later resection is also possible but can impair the aesthetic outcome.

If the mastectomy skin cannot be assessed intraoperatively regarding its viability, the flap skin can be left temporarily underneath the mastectomy skin for some days. The flap is kept buried until the viability is clear. If mastectomy skin has to be resected, the resulting defects can be replaced by flap skin in a second operation short after.

10.3.8 Aftercare

The patients are mobile as soon as they can get up. They should get up from the bed not sitting on the operated side. They should be supported and instructed by PT or nurses when getting up the first times. In the first days, they should avoid sitting on the operated side and prefer soft padded chairs. The Foley catheter can be removed at the first postoperative day. A raised WC seat can help the first days. The wound at the lower gluteal fold is best covered and padded. A bra that does not compress the pedicle can be used if necessary. A stocking can stabilize the thigh/buttock in the first postoperative weeks. The stocking should not compress the scar and avoid mechanical irritation.

Thromboprophylaxis is recommended. Drains should be removed with regard to the fluid amount. Work and daily activities should be possible after 1 week and should not exceed the standard. Sporting, sauna and sun tanning should be avoided for at least 6 weeks.

A loss of sensitivity at the dorsal thigh and the breast is usual (◘ Fig. 10.92). Seromas at the donor site can be punctured if necessary. A good physiotherapeutic program to avoid permanent neuropathic irritations from the donor site is important.

10.3.9 Corrective and Additional Surgery

If additional surgery is necessary, it should be planned at least 3–6 months later then the flap surgery. If dents or irregularities occur in the transition zones between flap and original tissue, they can be mildend by lipofilling; a secondary augmentation can also be done by lipofilling. A contralateral operation, if not done together with the reconstruction, can be planned at that time too. A secondary augmentation can also be done with an implant with respect to the flap pedicle because the flap does not achieve full vascular autonomy in most cases.

If a contralateral donor site alignment is planned, it should take place at the earliest after 3–6 months after the flap reconstruction. If the patient desires a refinement, the contralateral thigh/IGF can be suctioned, and the aspirate can be used to undertake possible breast refinements. If the skin is not elastic, a thigh/IGF lifting can be considered, if necessary after harvesting the fat for lipofilling.

The reconstruction of the NAC is considered to be the last operation.

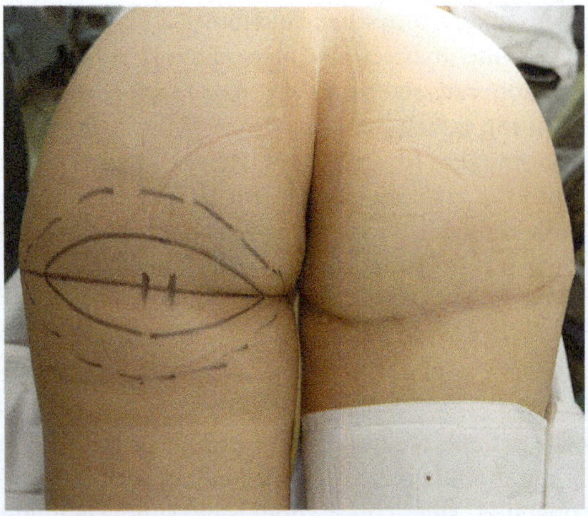

◘ **Fig. 10.88** Prone position for harvesting the FCI on the left side. FCI-flap was previously harvested on the right side. Transverse marking if the IGF. The vertical markings show the Dopplered pedicle. The first marking around the IGF is the incision; the second is the bevelled area

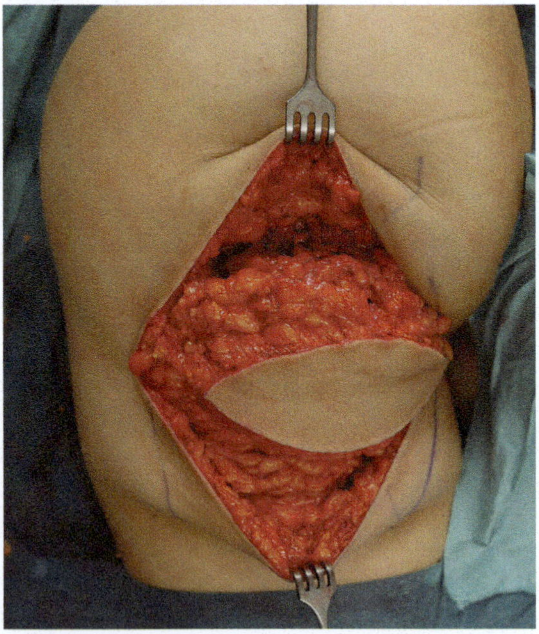

◘ **Fig. 10.89** Harvested flap with cranial and caudal subcutaneous tissue from bevelling

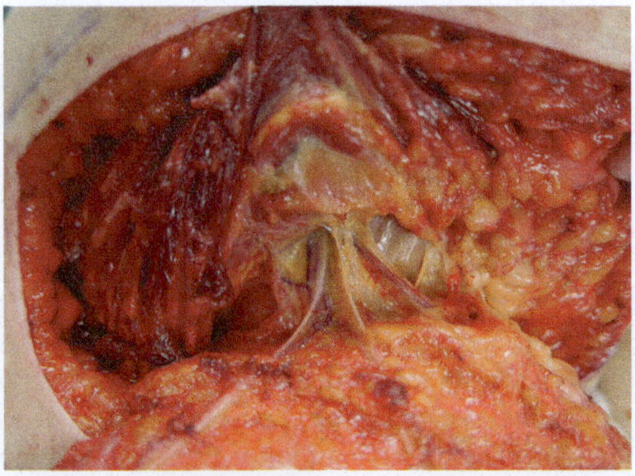

◘ **Fig. 10.90** Pedicle directly under the gluteus maximus muscle border. Note the branches of the nerve

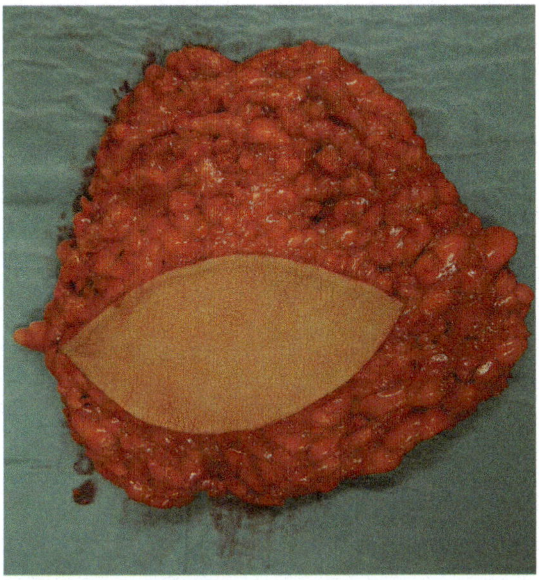

Fig. 10.91 FCI-flap before anastomosis. Cranially enough tissue can be harvested. It is important to shape the cranial transition to the thoracic tissue to avoid an edge towards the décolleté

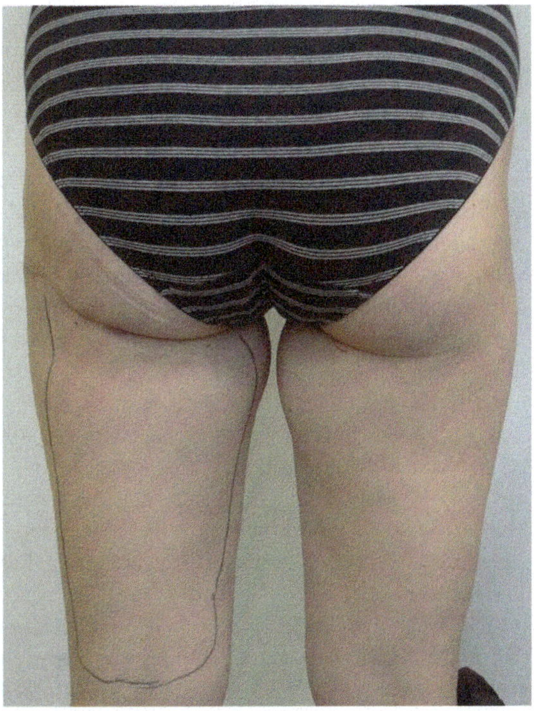

Fig. 10.92 Donor site left after 6 weeks. Hardly visible asymmetry to the right. Black markings on the thigh show the initial numbness dorsally

10.3.9.1 Results After FCI-Flap Reconstructions

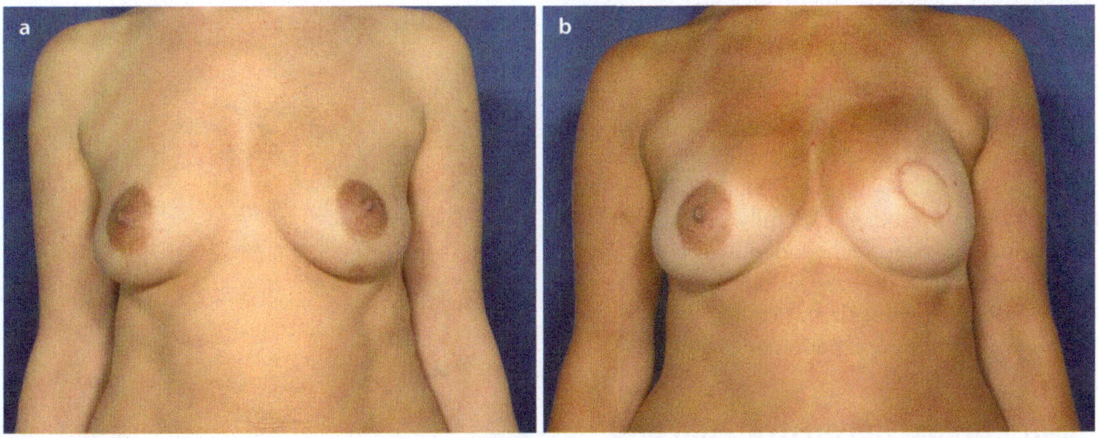

Fig. 10.93 **a**, **b** Large DCIS on the left side. SSM left with a periareolar incision and primary reconstruction with FCI- flap. The reconstructed breast is slightly larger than the right one. If desired, this can be adjusted by augmentation of the right breast or liposuction of the left breast

Conclusion

FCI-flap surgery is an alternative to DIEP or TMG flap surgery. In our hands it is not the first choice flap if the first mentioned can be carried out. It is suitable for slim and normal weight patients with small- to medium-sized breasts. The tissue is resected transversely from the lower gluteal fold. Subcutaneous bevelling increases the flap volume and facilitates skin closure in the donor site. The flap is soft, but less pliable than tissue from the lower abdomen or thigh due to the septa. The donor site and the dorsal thigh may initially be irritated by the nerve involvement after removal from the ischium.

10.4 Lymph Node Transplantation

Lymph oedema of the arm is a complication of the resection of sentinel lymph nodes and axillary lymphadenectomy. Many factors, some of which are not yet clear, can trigger lymph oedema. If the sentinel lymph nodes or the lymph nodes in axillary adenectomy are located close to the axillary vein, direct damage to the lymph drainage of the arm is possible. Furthermore, chemotherapy or radiation therapy can increase postoperative fibrosis in the axilla so that lymphatic flow obstruction with lymph oedema can occur.

The standard therapy of lymph oedema is still conservative. Complex physical decongestion therapy, a combination of lymph drainage, skin care, compression and physiotherapy, is the cornerstone. In recent years, however, microsurgical therapy has developed further. Three basic forms of therapy are available: (1) the transplantation of lymph collectors (formerly, lymph vessels). Collectors are removed from the leg and then microsurgically transplanted as a bypass between arm lymph collectors and the neck. (2) The transplantation of lymph node packages from the groin, contralateral axilla or neck. After careful adhesiolysis of the affected axilla, the lymph node package is microvascularly connected. (3) Anastomoses between the lymph collectors and veins/venules on the affected arm. Two to three lymphovenous anastomoses at different levels of the arm should create an "unphysiological" bypass.

All procedures are used with different successes. The study situation is not sufficient to place one procedure above the other. Carefully planned studies are required to evaluate the individual procedures.

In our hands axillary adhesiolysis followed by lymph node transplantation has been shown to improve arm lymph oedema (Fig. 10.94).

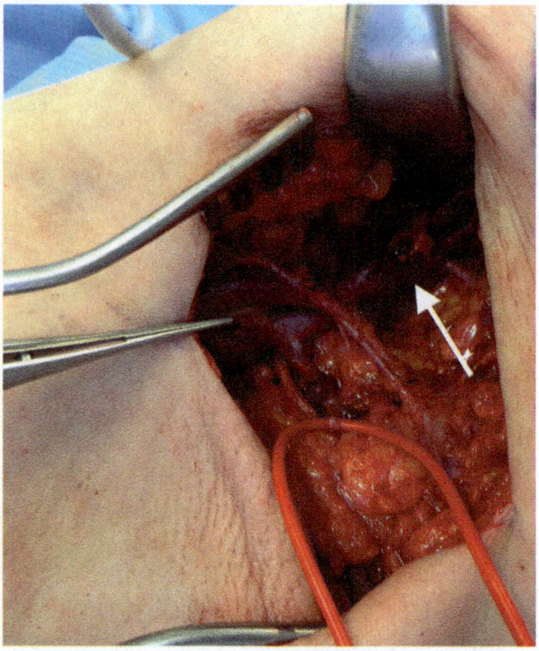

Fig. 10.94 In lymph oedema after axillary dissection, the axilla is scarred. The anatomic structures in the axilla must be exposed before a lymph node transplantation, and the adhesions must be resected. At the same time, the vessels can be dissected for lymph node transfer. The lead structure is the axillary vein (arrow). Looped with the red loop is a venous vessel for later anastomosis

10.4.1 Breast Reconstruction and Lymph Node Transplantation in a Single Flap

If indicated, usually after mastectomy and existing lymph oedema, breast reconstruction can be performed with a DIEP-flap. Together with the DIEP-flap, lymph nodes that are located either at the superficial inferior epigastric vessels (SIEA/V) or at the superficial circumflex iliac vessels (SCIA/V) can be harvested. The DIEP portion is connected to the IMA/V or its perforators, adhesiolysis takes place simultaneously in the axilla, and the lymph nodes are connected via the SIEA/V or SCIA/V to vessels in the axilla (Figs. 10.95, 10.96, 10.97, 10.98, and 10.99). The indications are

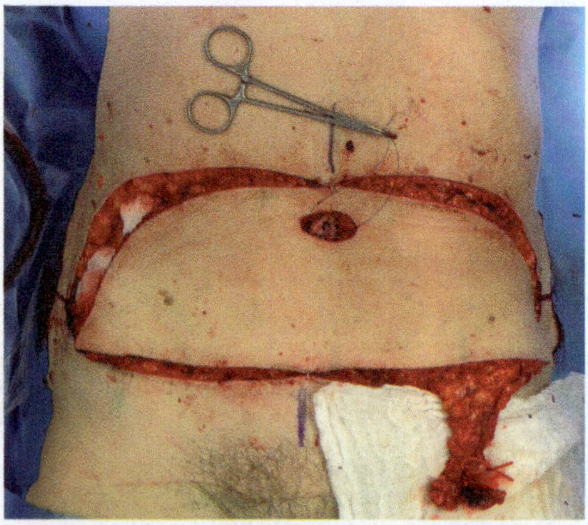

Fig. 10.95 DIEP-flap with DIEP pedicle from the right and lymph nodes around the left SIEA/V. A reconstruction of the right breast and lymph node transplantation to the right axilla are planned. The flap is rotated by 180°. The DIEP is connected to the IMA and the SIEA is placed in the axilla

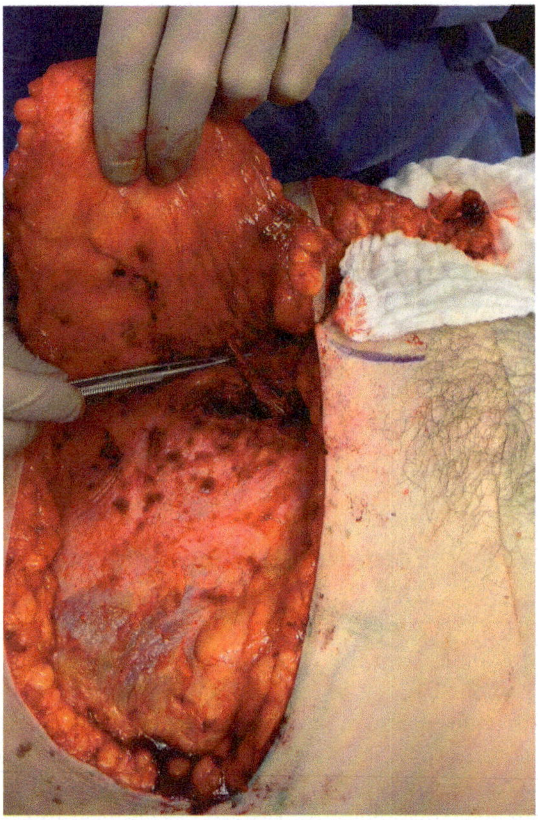

Fig. 10.96 The DIEP-flap is harvested at a medial caudal perforator on the right side

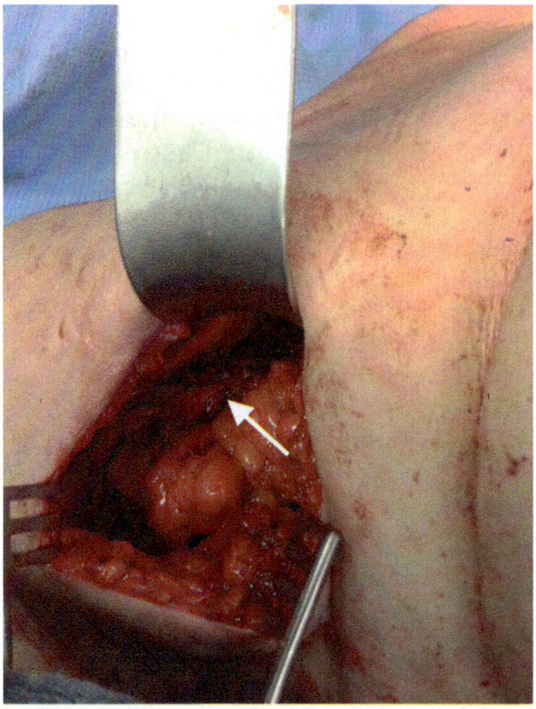

Fig. 10.98 The flap is placed. The SIEA vessels are placed in the axilla. It is connected to the vessels in the axilla. The lymph node package is placed on the axillary vein. Blind ending lymph collectors can also be connected to the lymph nodes by microsurgery

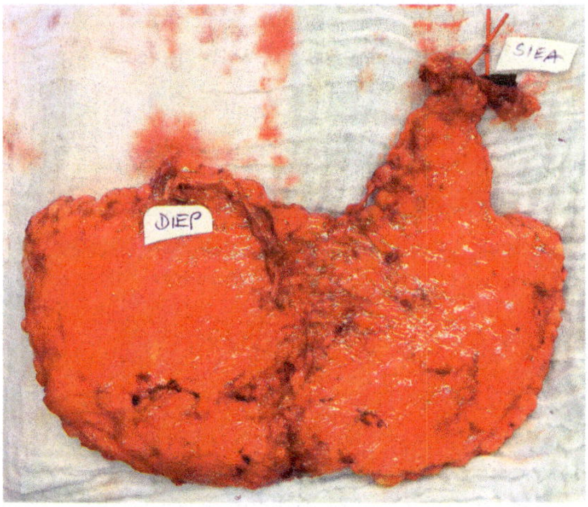

Fig. 10.97 Flap seen from dorsal with the two pedicles and the lymph node flap around the SIEA

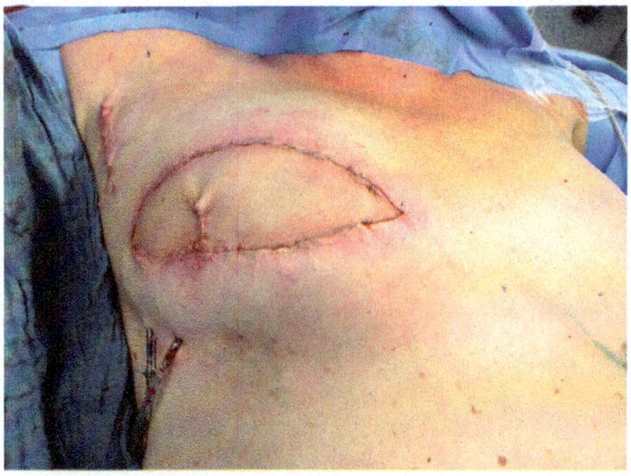

Fig. 10.99 At the end of the operation, the breast has been reconstructed and the lymph nodes transferred into the axilla

rare, but with this chimeric flap, a good result can be achieved with regard to breast reconstruction and lymph drainage. In our opinion, the prerequisite is an arterial and venous anastomosis in the axilla, or at least a venous anastomosis.

10.5 Special Indications

10.5.1 Failure of Implants, ADM and Meshes; Conversion to Autologous Tissue

With increasing numbers of primary reconstructions using expanders and implants in combination with ADM (acellular dermal matrices) and meshes, the number of complications has increased. The complications are additionally increased if the patients require radiation therapy. There are complications that require additional surgery for medical reasons but also due to a poor aesthetic result. The best way to deal with complications from implant and ADM/mesh surgery is to convert to autologous tissue.

While the conversions were demonstrated for each flap in this short chapter, we present some intraoperative details that highlight the problems of implant/ADM reconstruction in conversion surgery (◘ Figs. 10.100, 10.101, 10.102, 10.103, 10.104, 10.105, 10.106 and 10.107).

10.5.2 Bilateral Surgery

If bilateral procedures are planned, the same flaps should always be used for symmetry reasons. While DIEP-flap surgery can usually be performed in one operation on both sides and should also be performed for logistical reasons, IT-flap and FCI-flap surgery can always be performed separately. While IT-flap surgery can also be performed bilaterally in one operation, FCI-flap surgery consumes time and energy because the repositioning of the patient has to be taken into account. In principle, the surgeon in charge should decide with the patient whether the procedure is a single stage or not.

In some patients, there is a later indication for a second flap surgery if, for example, a contralateral or second carcinoma occurs or implant problems become evident only later. Here the common flaps can then be combined with each other. Patients should be made aware of the primary asymmetry that usually occurs (◘ Figs. 10.108, 10.109 and 10.110). Alignment measures can then be secondary.

10.5.3 Extended Defect Coverage and Palliative Interventions

In some cases the cancer has progressed due to tumour biology or lack of therapy in such a way that the goal is not breast reconstruction, but defect coverage of the thoracic wall. Depending on the extent and tumour, this can be done with curative or palliative intent (◘ Figs. 10.111, 10.112, 10.113 and 10.114). Such extensive resections and defect detections should always be discussed in the breast centre in order to jointly develop the most gentle and effective therapy approach and to initiate adjuvant therapies pre- and postoperatively. Patients should always be involved with their wishes and expectations.

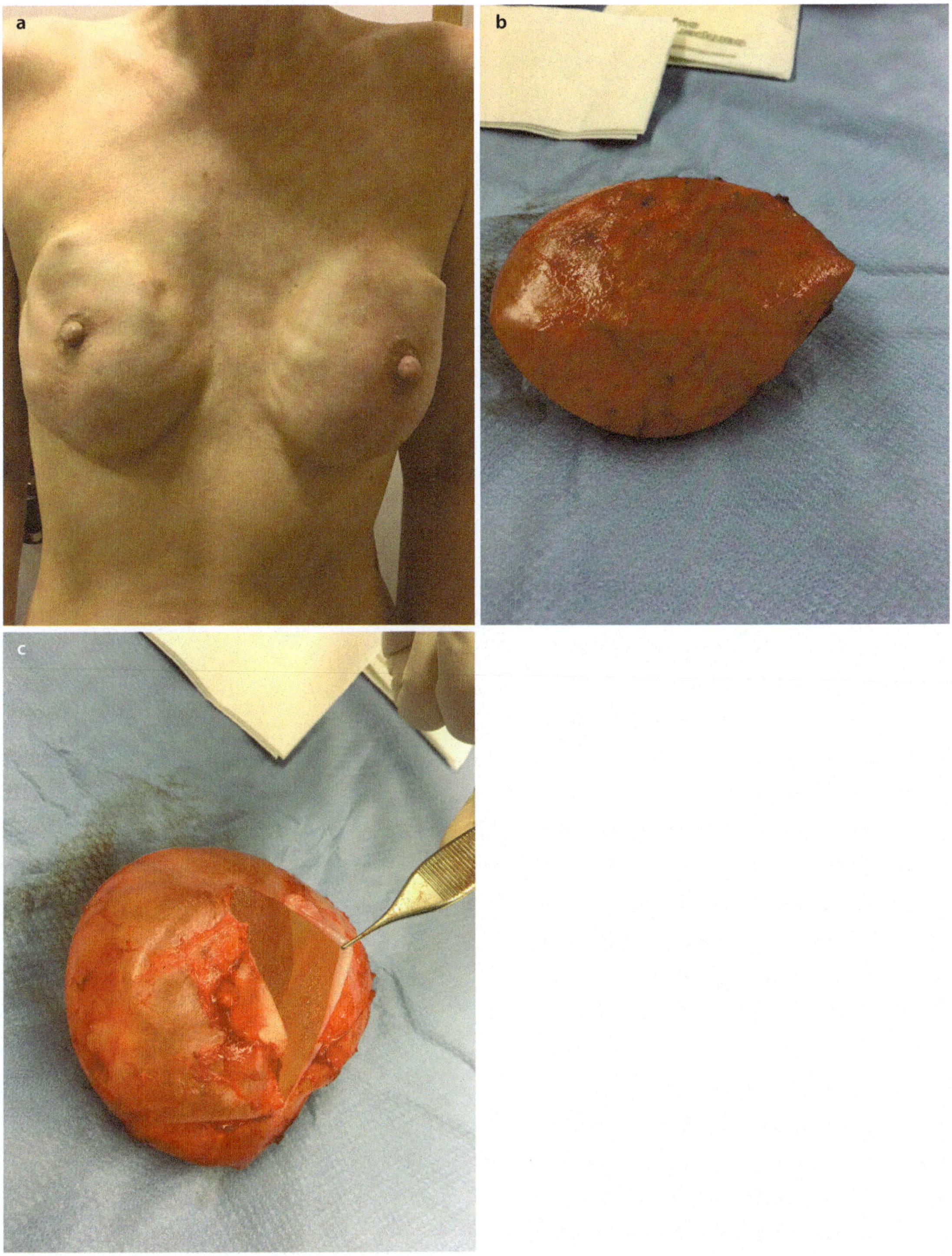

Fig. 10.100 **a** Epipectoral implant reconstruction causing pain due to severe capsular contracture. **b, c** Removal of implants and capsule. The implant is deformed. Reconstruction is better done with autologous tissue

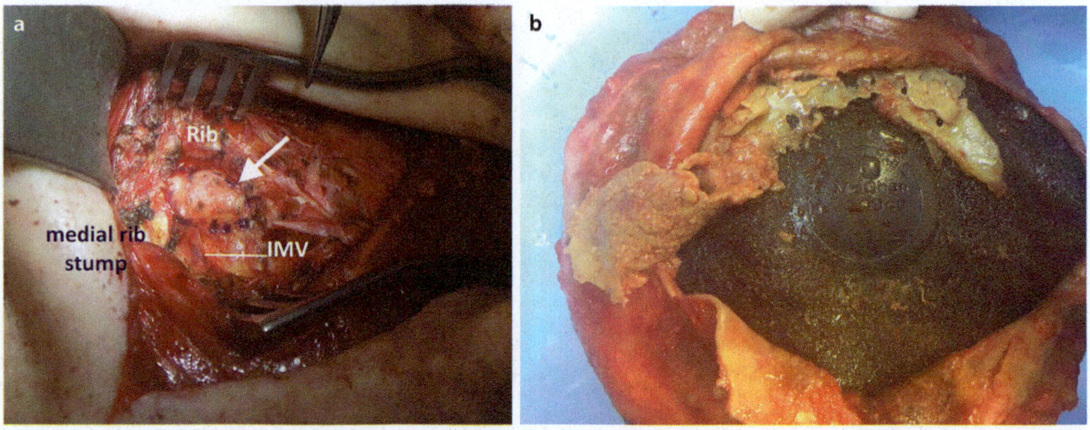

Fig. 10.101 **a** Patient with implant reconstruction (elsewhere). Nodules in the axilla were noted. Siliconomas were seen in the MRI. Implant and capsule resection, lymph nodes thickened along the IMA (dotted intraoperatively with ink, arrow) were found during IMA exposure for autologous tissue reconstruction in the ICS. Silicone took the entire vessel tract. Axillary vessel was used for anastomosis. **b** The capsule shows unclear deposits (possibly old haematoma) and a defective implant. The removed lymph nodes showed silicone deposits

Fig. 10.102 **a** Exposed implant on the left with mesh (elsewhere). Conservative therapy was not successful. A single-stage change to autologous tissue was performed. Afterwards complication-free healing. **b** Exposed implant cranial (elsewhere) after the calcified capsule has perforated the skin. The implants were removed. **c** Exposed implant on the right after SSM and reconstruction with mesh and implant (elsewhere). The skin is thinned out by mechanical irritation and a cortisone treatment. Autologous tissue reconstruction was performed. In all these cases, conservative therapy is not indicated. If an implant is exposed, a surgical revision with a change of procedure should be initiated. **d**, **e** Exposed implant and mesh left side after NSM. Patient was treated with intermittent antibiotics for more than 1 year. Single-stage implant and mesh removal and conversion to IT-flap

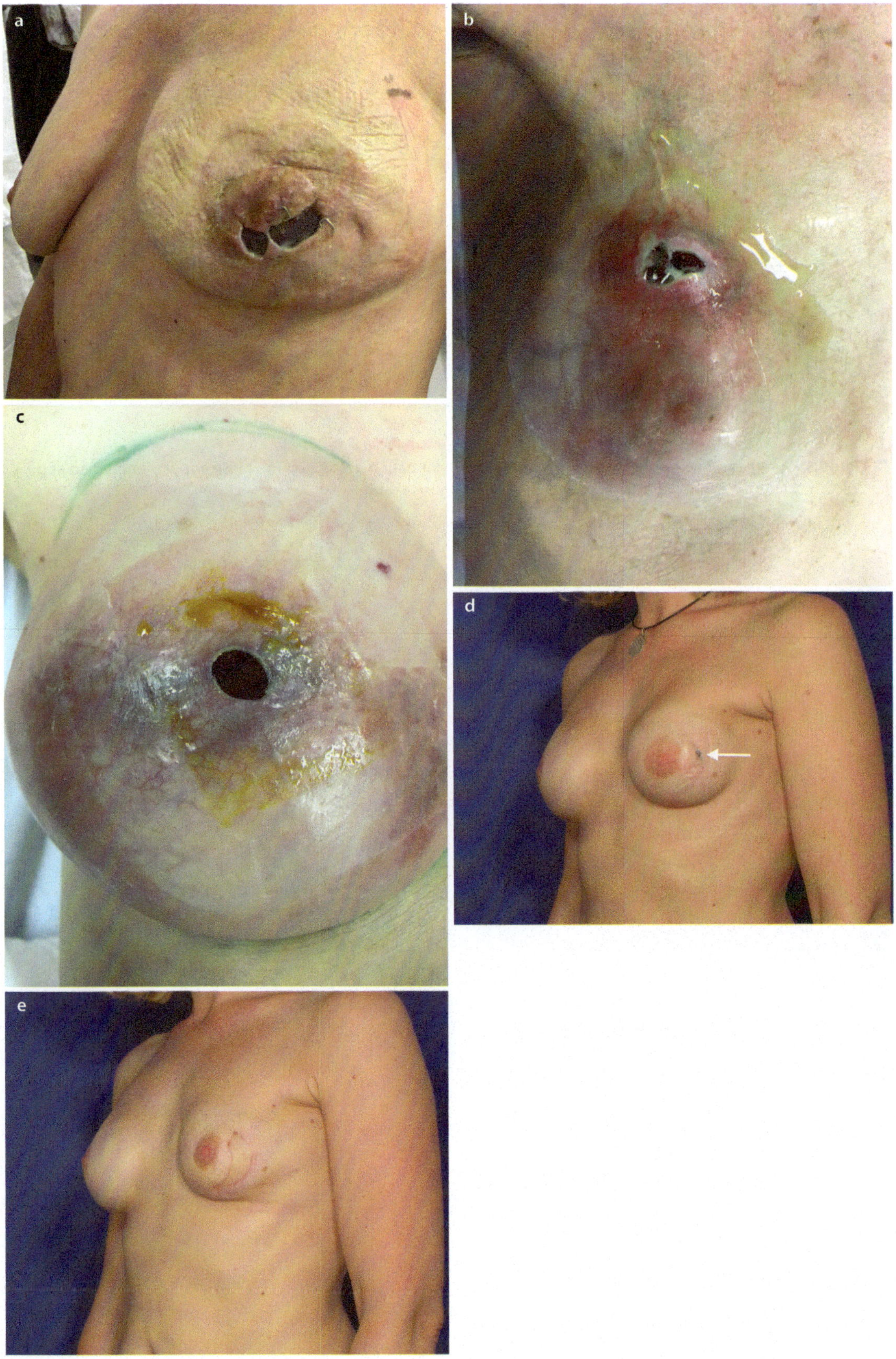
a
b
c
d
e

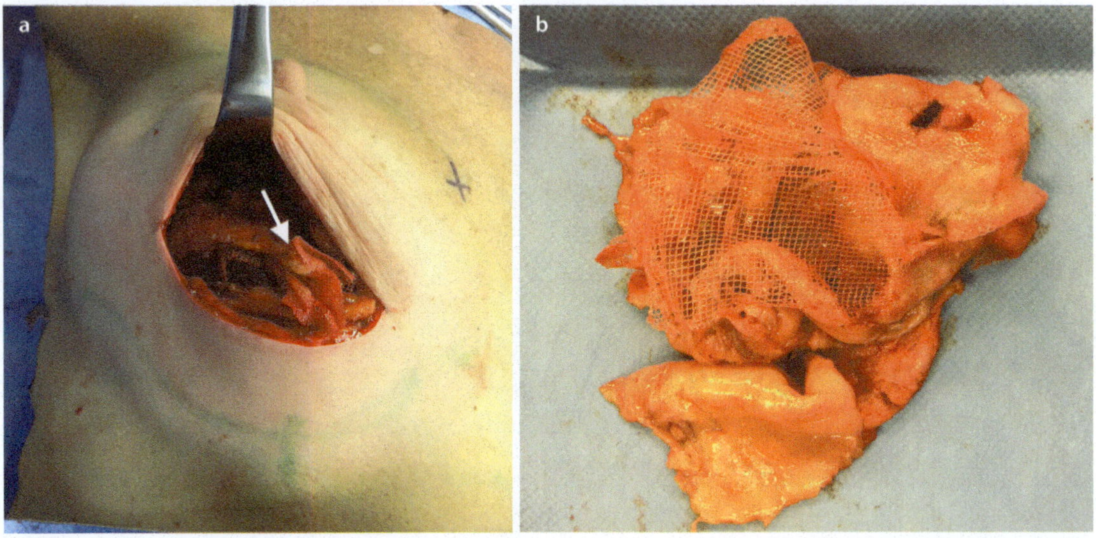

Fig. 10.103 **a** Revision of a 4° capsular contracture with animation deformity. The mesh appears entangled and completely scarred. **b** Removed mesh. Conversion to autologous tissue

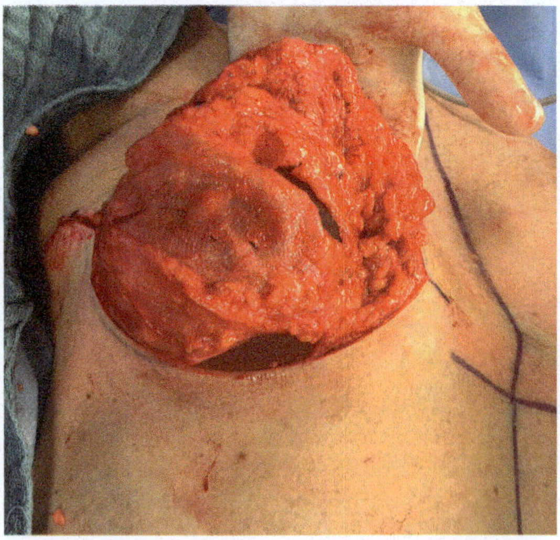

Fig. 10.104 Patient with skin retractions and chronic pain from mesh. In these kinds of revisions, it is difficult to loosen and maintain the continuity of skin. Conversion to autologous tissue here

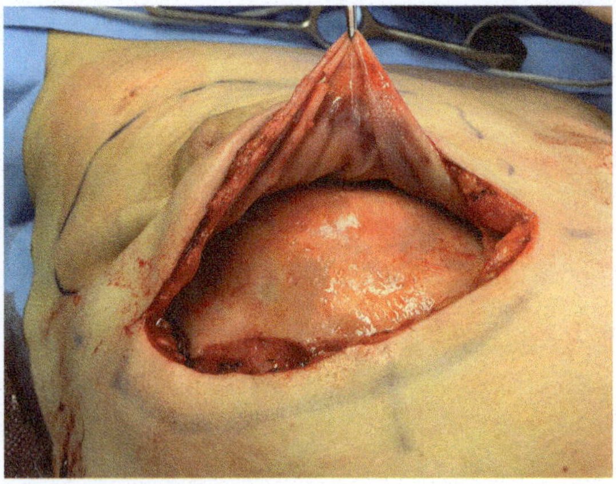

Fig. 10.105 Capsular contracture. The mesh is healed. However, the strong capsule and the pain make removal necessary. Conversion to autologous tissue

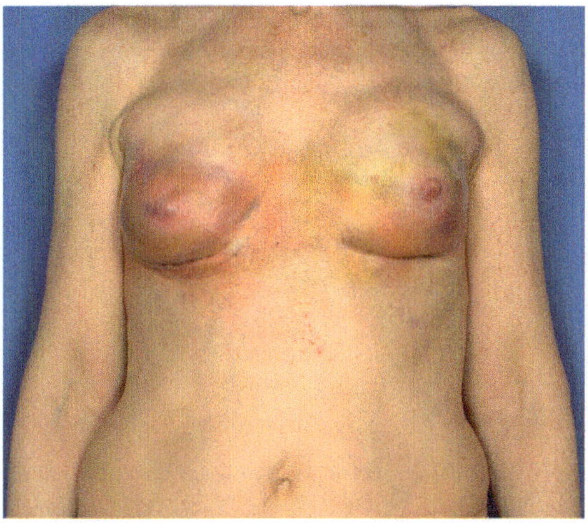

Fig. 10.106 "Red breast syndrome" in response to the ADM. This is not a bacterial infection, but an inflammatory reaction to the matrix. In some cases cortisone therapy is recommended. We prefer the removal of the triggering matrix and the conversion to another technique

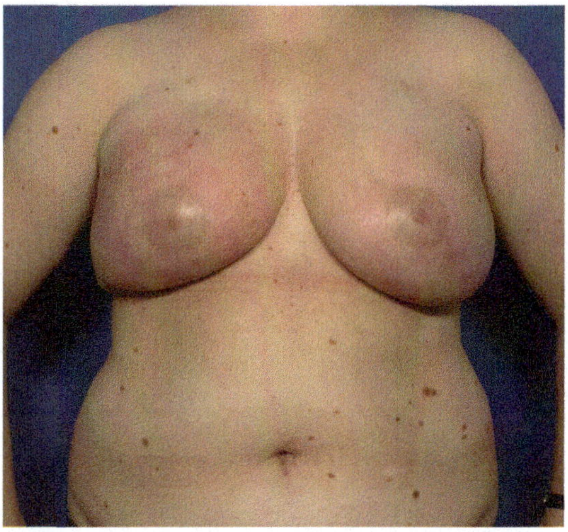

Fig. 10.107 Chronic inflammation with redness and oedema of the skin after bilateral ADM and implant reconstruction in prophylactic mastectomy. After 6 months of cortisone therapy (elsewhere), resection was performed, and conversion to autologous tissue was done

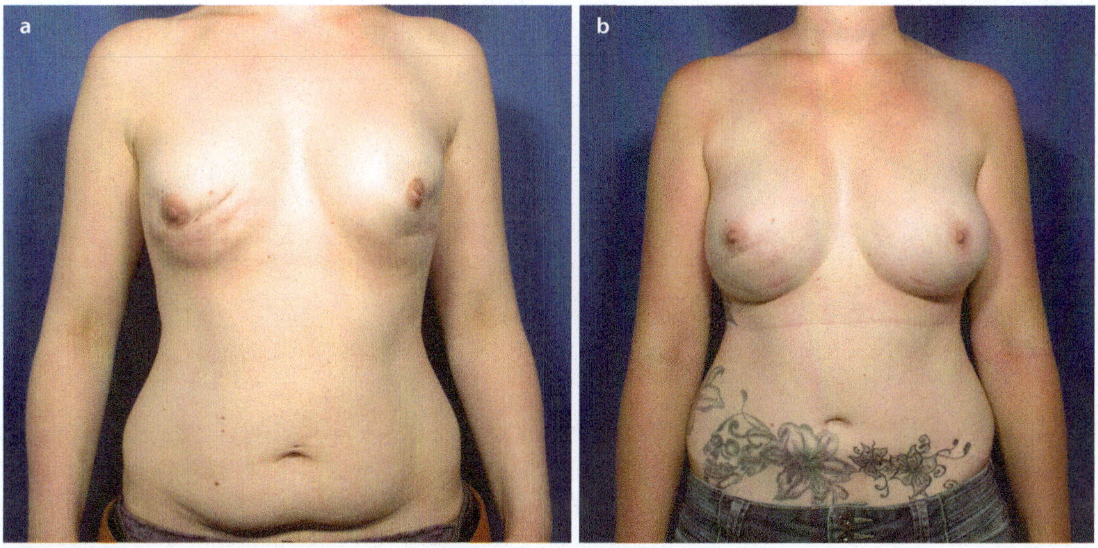

Fig. 10.108 **a** Patient with extensive capsular contracture after implant placement after bilateral mastectomy and right breast cancer with radiation therapy. **b** On the right, a DIEP-flap was performed. Due to the rigid skin, a skin island was inserted; a IT-flap was performed on the left

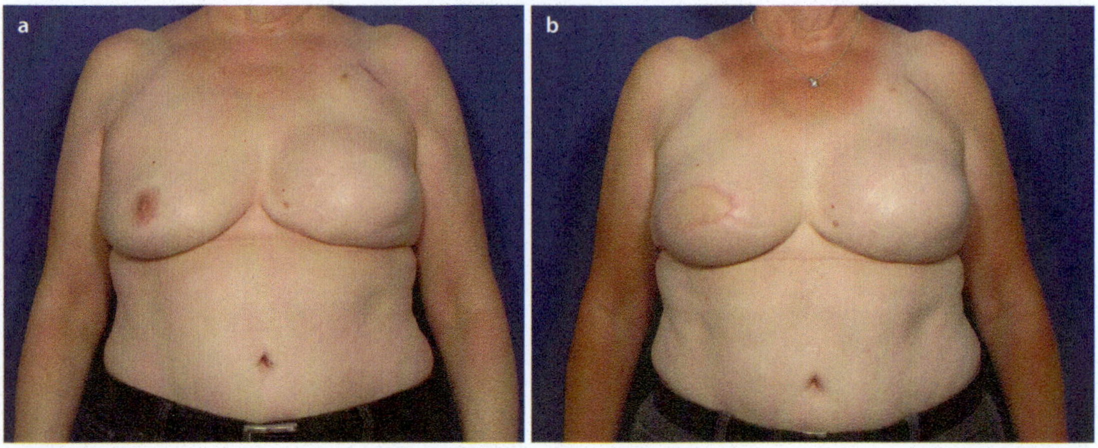

Fig. 10.109 **a, b** Patient with DIEP-flap after left cancer. Five years later, right mastectomy was performed due to a contralateral carcinoma, and the reconstruction was done with a IT-flap

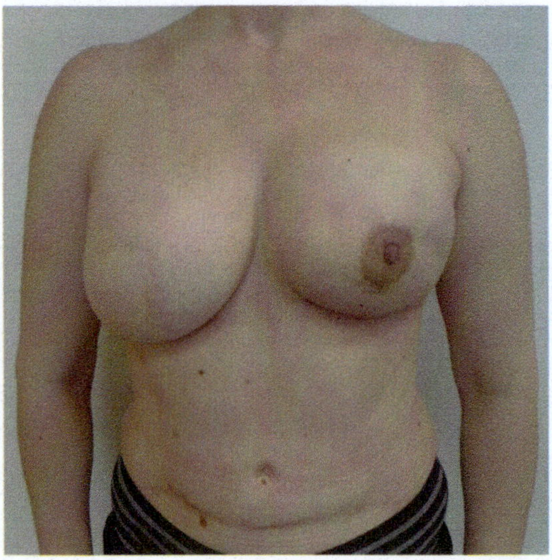

Fig. 10.110 DIEP-flap right in a breast cancer; 3 years later a FCI-flap on the left side was done due to an extensive DCIS

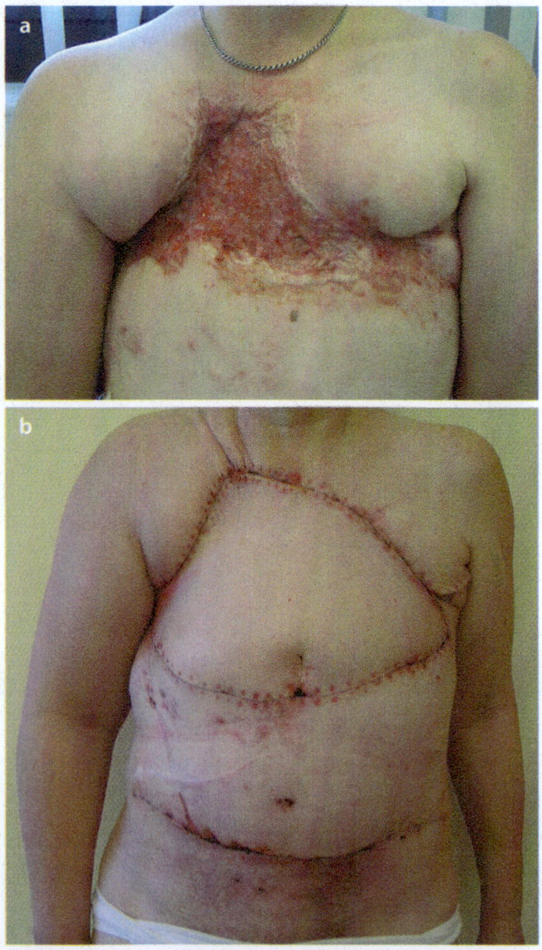

Fig. 10.111 **a, b** Patient with local recurrence of bilateral cancer. First, resection and defect coverage was performed with a bilateral DIEP-flap plastic with anastomosis to both IMA/V. This was followed by irradiation

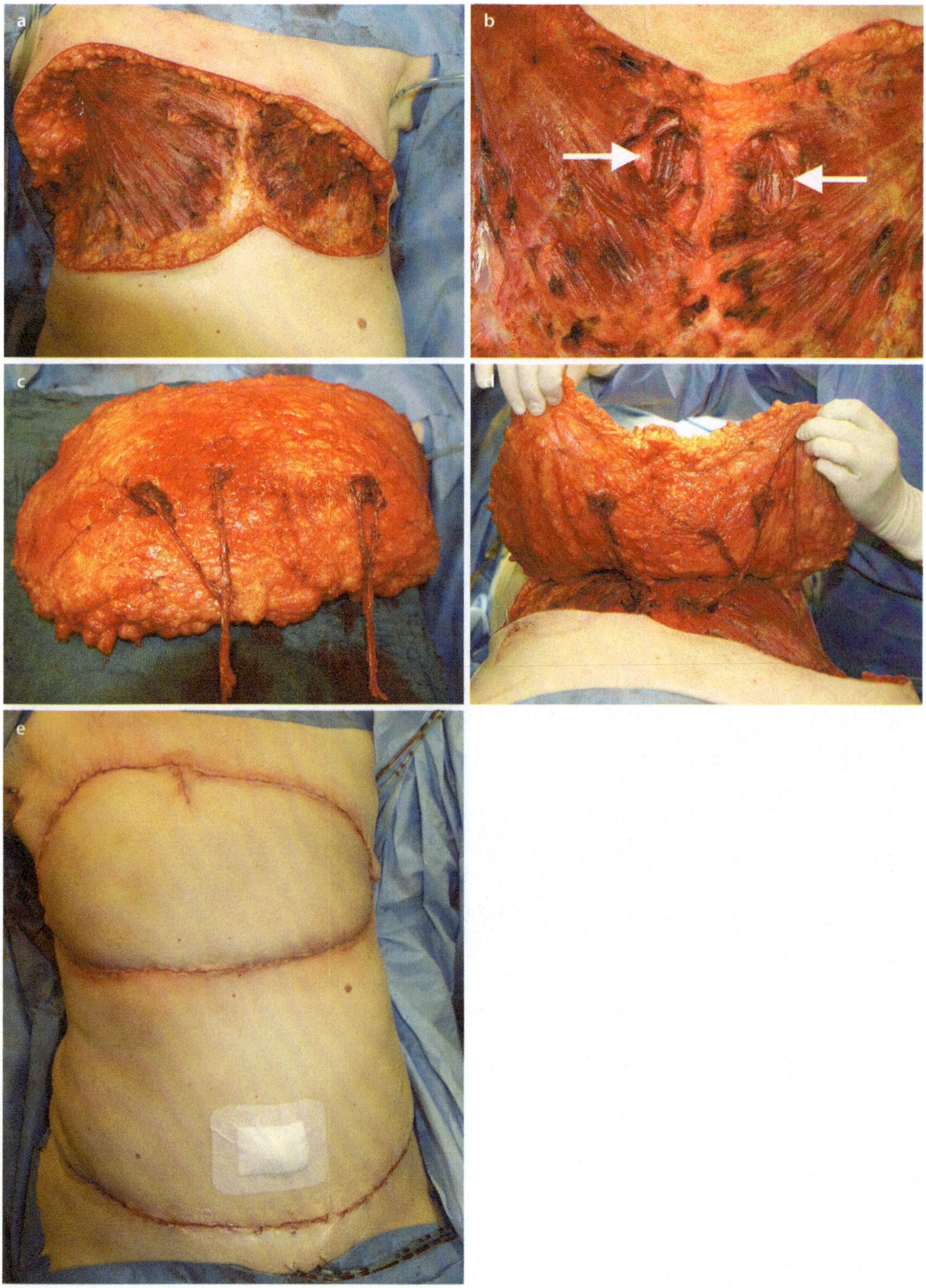

Fig. 10.112 **a** Similar resection in a bilateral cancer. **b** The two IMA/V are shown in detail (arrows). **c** A DIEP-flap on both sides was harvested with two perforators each. **d** The epigastric vessels were then anastomosed to the IMA vessels. **e** Final result in the OR

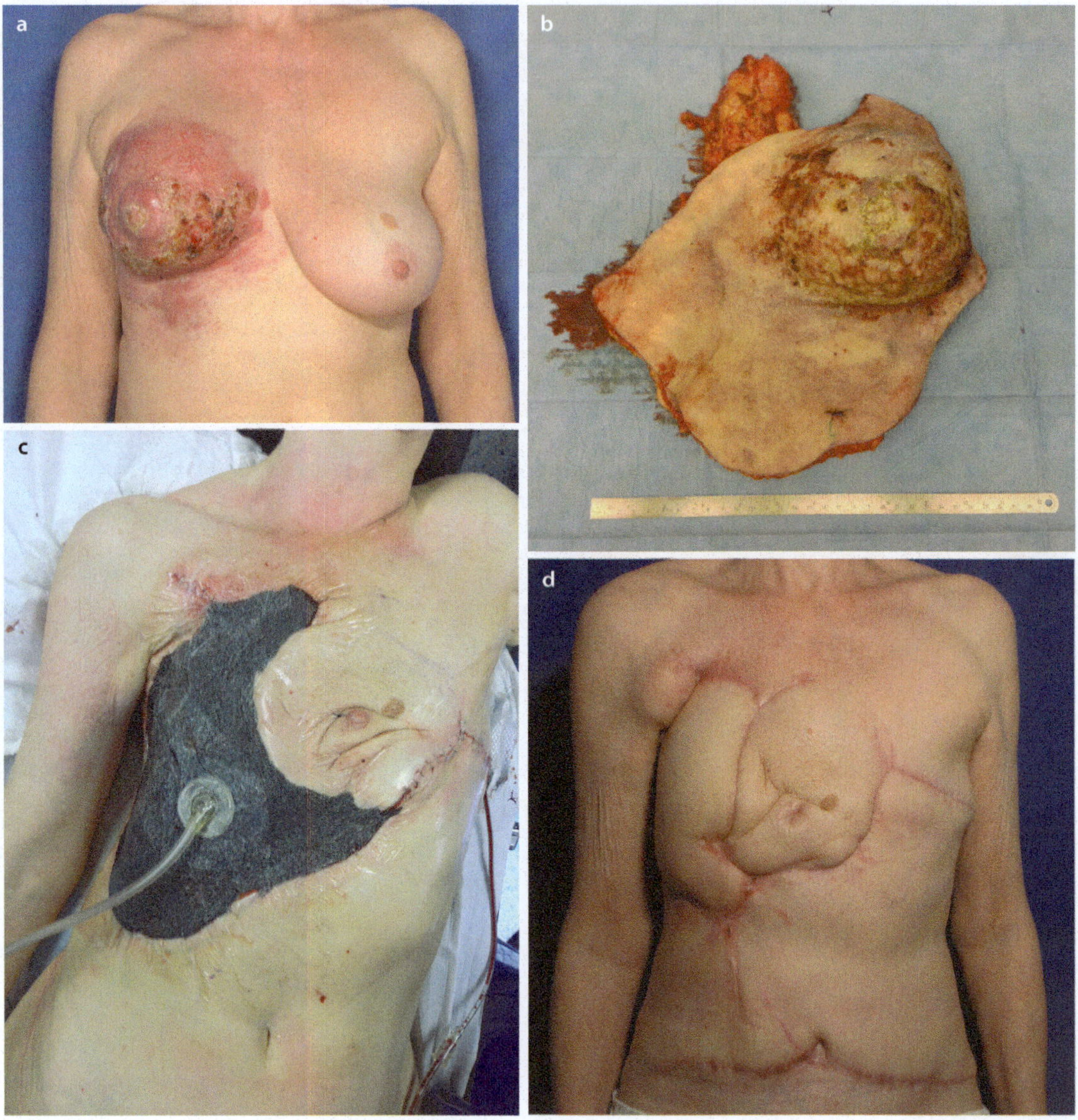

Fig. 10.113 **a** Patient with ulcerated breast cancer on the right and extensive carcinoma on the left that does not infiltrate the skin. **b** Specimen right and SSM left preserving the skin and its circulation. **c** Temporary defect coverage until final histology with NPWT dressing. **d** The defect was covered by a DIEP-flap and skin from the left breast pedicled on the IMA perforators from the left side

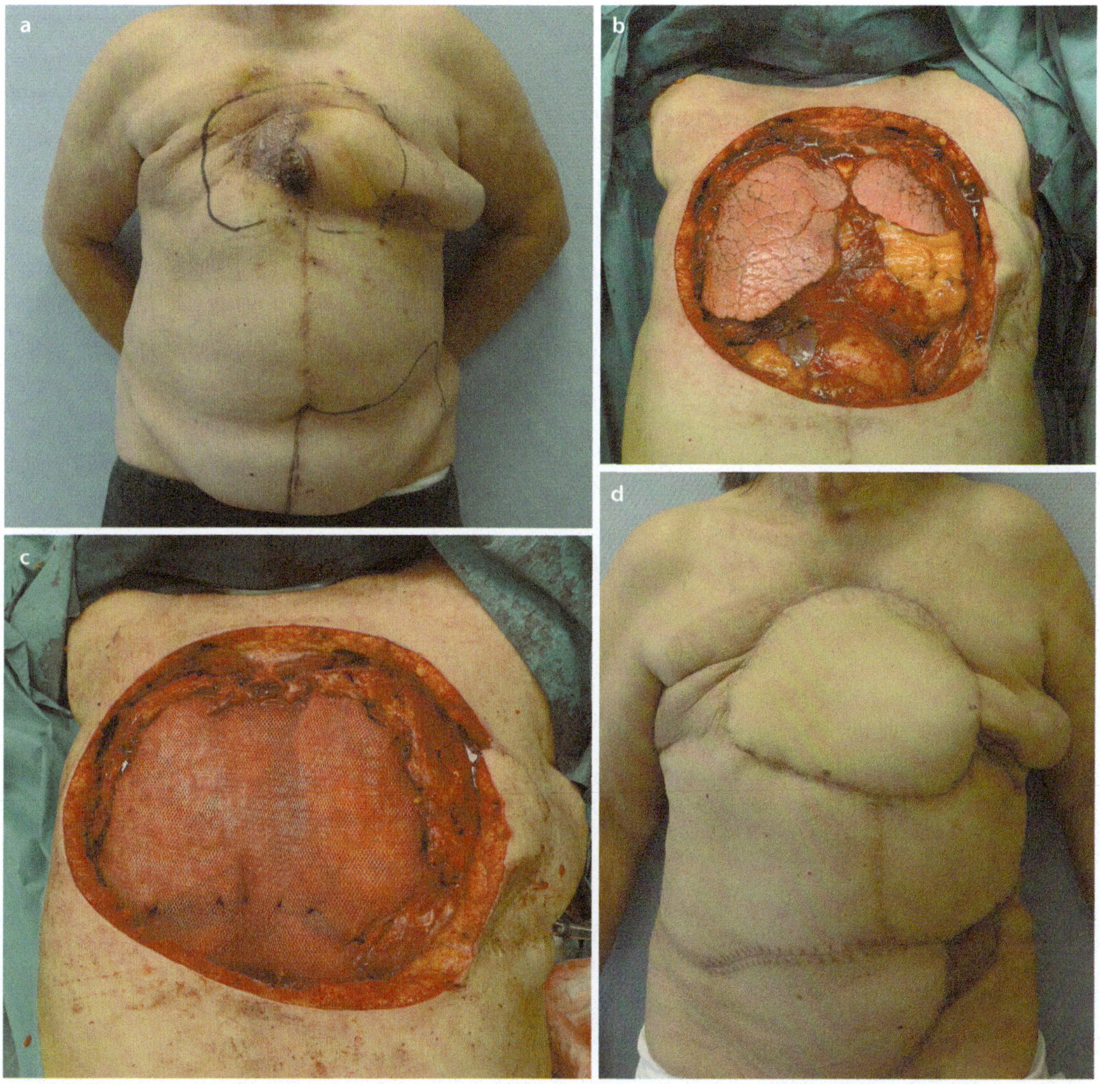

Fig. 10.114 **a** Patient with angiosarcoma 7 years after radiation therapy of breast cancer. **b** All layered thoracic wall resection with opening of the thorax, abdominal cavity and parts of the diaphragm. **c** Stabilization with a mesh; insertion bilateral chest tubes. **d** Defect coverage by single-sided, extended DIEP from the left side; the right epigastric artery could not be used due to previous injuries. Result after the operation. Patient is free of recurrence 8 years after the procedure (The procedure was performed together with thoracic surgeon Dr. J. Stapenhorst, Bielefeld)

Literature

DIEP-Flaps, ms-TRAM Flaps and SIEA-Flaps

1. Chen L, Hartrampf CR Jr, Bennett GK. Successful pregnancies following TRAM flap surgery. Plast Reconstr Surg. 1993;91:69–71.
2. Eom JS, Kim DY, Kim EK, Lee TJ. The low DIEP flap: an enhancement to the abdominal donor site. Plast Reconstr Surg. 2016;137:7e–13e.
3. Figus A, Wade RG, Gorton L, Rubino C, Griffiths MG, Ramakrishnan VV. Venous perforators in DIEAP flaps: an observational anatomical study using duplex ultrasonography. J Plast Reconstr Aesthet Surg. 2012;65:1051–9.
4. Gravvanis A, Tsoutsos D, Papanikolaou G, Diab A, Lambropoulou P, Karakitsos D. Refining perforator selection for deep inferior epigastric perforator flap: the impact of the dominant venous perforator. Microsurgery. 2014;34:169–76.
5. Mohan AT, Zhu L, Wang Z, Vijayasekaran A, Saint-Cyr M. Techniques and perforator selection in single, dominant DIEP flap breast reconstruction: algorithmic approach to maximize efficiency and safety. Plast Reconstr Surg. 2016;138:790–803.
6. Moon HK, Taylor GI. The vascular anatomy of rectus abdominis musculocutaneous flaps based on the deep superior epigastric system. Plast Reconstr Surg. 1988;82:815–32.
7. Munhoz AM, Pellarin L, Montag E, Filassi JR, Tachibana A, Gebrim H, Gemperli R, Ferreira MC. Superficial Inferior Epigastric Artery (SIEA) free flap using perforator vessels as a recipient site: clinical implications in autologous breast reconstruction. Am J Surg. 2011;202:612–7.
8. Pülzl P, Schoeller T, Wechselberger G. Respecting the aesthetic unit in autologous breast reconstruction improves the outcome. Plast Reconstr Surg. 2006;117:1685–91.
9. Sarik JR, Bank J, Wu LC, Serletti JM. Superficial inferior epigastric artery: learning curve versus reality. Plast Reconstr Surg. 2016;137:1e–6e.
10. Walle L, Fansa H, Frerichs O. Smartphone-based thermography for perforator localization in microvascular breast reconstruction. Handchir Mikrochir Plast Chir. 2018;50:111–7.

Inner Thigh Flaps (IT-Flap)

11. Allen RJ, Haddock NT, Ahn CY, Sadeghi A. Breast reconstruction with the profunda artery perforator flap. Plast Reconstr Surg. 2012;129:16e–23e.
12. Arnez ZM, Pogorelec D, Planinsek F, Ahcan U. Breast reconstruction by the free transverse gracilis (TUG) flap. Br J Plast Surg. 2004;57:20–6.
13. Fansa H, Schirmer S, Warnecke IC, Cervelli A, Frerichs O. The transverse myocutaneous gracilis muscle flap: a fast and reliable method for breast reconstruction. Plast Reconstr Surg. 2008;122:1326–33.
14. Fansa H, Schirmer S, Cervelli A, Gehl HB. Computed tomographic angiography imaging and clinical implications of internal mammary artery perforator vessels as recipient vessels in autologous breast reconstruction. Ann Plast Surg. 2013;71:533–7.
15. Fattah A, Figus A, Mathur B, Ramakrishnan VV. The transverse myocutaneous gracilis flap: technical refinements. J Plast Reconstr Aesthet Surg. 2010;63:305–13.
16. Hunter JE, Lardi AM, Dower DR, Farhadi J. Evolution from the TUG to PAP flap for breast reconstruction: comparison and refinements of technique. J Plast Reconstr Aesthet Surg. 2015;68:960–5.
17. Park JE, Alkureishi LW, Song DH. TUGs into VUGs and friendly BUGs: transforming the gracilis territory into the best secondary breast reconstructive option. Plast Reconstr Surg. 2015;136:447–54.
18. Schoeller T, Huemer GM, Wechselberger G. The transverse musculocutaneous gracilis flap for breast reconstruction: guidelines for flap and patient selection. Plast Reconstr Surg. 2008;122:29–38.
19. Whitaker IS, Karavias M, Shayan R, et al. The gracilis myocutaneous free flap: a quantitative analysis of the fasciocutaneous blood supply and implications for autologous breast reconstruction. PLoS ONE. 2012;7(5):e36367. https://doi.org/10.1371/journal.pone.0036367. Lin SJ, ed.
20. Yousif NJ, Matloub HS, Kolachalam R, Grunert BK, Sanger JR. The transverse gracilis musculocutaneous flap. Ann Plast Surg. 1992;29:482–90.

Fasciocutaneous Infragluteal Flap (FCI-Flap)

21. Papp C, Windhofer C, Gruber S. Breast reconstruction with the Fasciocutaneous Infragluteal free flap (FCI). Ann Plast Surg. 2007;58:131–6.
22. Struckmann V, Peek A, Wingenbach O, Harhaus L, Kneser U, Holle G. The free Fasciocutaneous Infragluteal (FCI) flap: outcome and patient satisfaction after 142 breast reconstructions. J Plast Reconstr Aesthet Surg. 2016;69:461–9.

Lymph Node Transplantation

23. Becker C. Autologous lymph node transfers. J Reconstr Microsurg. 2016;32:28–33.
24. Saaristo AM, Niemi TS, Viitanen TP, Tervala TV, Hartiala P, Suominen EA. Microvascular breast reconstruction and lymph node transfer for postmastectomy lymphedema patients. Ann Surg. 2012;255:468–73.

Special Indications

Lateral Thigh Flap

25. Tuinder SMH, Beugels J, Lataster A, de Haan MW, Piatkowski A, Saint-Cyr M, van der Hulst RRWJ, Allen RJ. The lateral thigh perforator (LTP) flap for autologous breast reconstruction: a prospective analysis of 138 flaps. Plast Reconstr Surg. 2017. https://doi.org/10.1097/PRS.0000000000004072.

SGAP and IGAP Flaps

26. Feller AM, Richter-Heine I, Rudolf KD. The Superior Gluteal Artery Perforator flap (S-GAP-flap). Handchir Mikrochir Plast Chir. 2002;34:257–61.
27. LoTempio MM, Allen RJ. Breast reconstruction with SGAP and IGAP flaps. Plast Reconstr Surg. 2010;126:393–401.

Lumbar Flap

28. Hamdi M, Craggs B, Brussaard C, Seidenstueker K, Hendrickx B, Zeltzer A. Lumbar artery perforator flap: an anatomical study using multidetector computed tomographic scan and surgical pearls for breast reconstruction. Plast Reconstr Surg. 2016;138:343–52.

Autologous Reconstruction: Pedicled Flaps

H. Fansa, C. Heitmann, *Breast Reconstruction with Autologous Tissue*,
https://doi.org/10.1007/978-3-319-95468-4_11

11.1 Latissimus Dorsi Flap

The latissimus dorsi muscle runs from the thoracolumbar fascia of the lumbar and lower thoracic spine directly under the skin to its base on the upper arm (crista tuberculi minoris). The latissimus dorsi flap, first described by Tansini in 1906, quickly became the standard flap after its rediscovery by Olivari in 1976 due to its very constant anatomy. It can be used as a free flap or as a pedicled flap. In breast surgery it is used almost exclusively pedicled. Even today, the pedicled latissimus is a good procedure if free flaps are not indicated or have failed. The latissimus is an internal rotator and adductor in the shoulder. If the shoulder is intact and the remaining muscles are present, muscle harvesting is usually well tolerated.

11.1.1 Indication

11

The latissimus is suitable to cover defects after extensive resections in the ventral thorax or can be used to reconstruct the breast but then usually together with an implant. Usually the flap is not thicker than 2–3 cm, so that an implant is needed to form the breast. The latissimus can also be used as an extended latissimus without an additional implant in (rather rare) patients with a thick subcutaneous fat layer and rather small breasts.

However, since breast reconstruction with a latissimus usually requires an additional implant and thus combines the disadvantages of autologous (scar) and alloplastic procedures (capsule formation/implant exchange), latissimus has today become more of a backup procedure in breast reconstruction. In addition, some patients describe movement restrictions on the arm or long healing phases with seromas. When used to cover defects, the latissimus is still a suitable procedure, even in the palliative situation. However, the disadvantage is that the harvesting must always take place in a lateral position. Intraoperative positioning change is therefore a factor to be calculated.

Removal from the back is almost always possible. Only very slim, mostly young patients with a firm skin texture are less suitable for this technique. The possible harvesting volume can be estimated by a pinch test.

> The latissimus muscle flap is suitable for covering defects in the ventral thorax or for reconstructing the breast together with an implant. Today, the latissimus flap has become more of a backup procedure in breast reconstruction. When used to cover defects, it is still a suitable method, even in the palliative situation. Removal from the back is almost always possible. However, the disadvantage is that the harvesting must always take place in a lateral position.

11.1.2 Contraindications

Patients who are to undergo bilateral surgery are less suitable, as they often complain postoperatively about a constricted chest. This is understandable inasmuch as a bilateral latissimus removal results in an almost circular thoracic scar for both breasts. However, there is no absolute contraindication. An alternative should be considered for patients using wheelchairs or for diseases of neurodegenerative origin. An alternative should also be considered for patients who are very sporty.

In patients who have received a previous axillary dissection and, if necessary, additional radiation therapy of the axillary lymphatics, the lifting of the harvesting may be difficult, and the perfusion of the flap may be impaired. If a DIEP-flap has previously been anastomosed to the thoracodorsal vessels, the latissimus can only be used in exceptional cases.

> **Overview Latissimus Dorsi Flap**
> Indication: Defect coverage on the ventral thorax or breast reconstruction usually together with an implant
> Muscle:
> - 25–35 cm length and 15–20 cm width
>
> Skin island:
> - Mostly transverse or perpendicular to the fibre course.
> - Size: up to 25 cm long and 7 cm high, depending on pinch test.
> - By subcutaneously bevelling, a little more fat can be taken along with the flap without endangering the primary closure at the back.

Vascular pedicle:
- Thoracodorsal vessels from the subscapular vessels in the axilla. The thoracodorsal nerve runs along with the vessels.
- Length: 7–12 cm

11.1.3 Characteristics

The muscle itself is about 1–1.5 cm thick. It allows only a defect coverage if it is harvested with a skin island or is covered by an additional split skin transplantation. The latter should not be discussed in this context, as it has only a very limited indication in breast surgery. Reference is made to the textbooks of plastic surgery. The muscle tissue can also be used to cover an implant. However, it is better to use the skin island. This can be de-epithelialized and also be used in a NSM or SSM. Breast reconstruction only with the volume of the skin island is only possible in patients with a thick subcutaneous fat layer and small breasts. For all others, sufficient projection is not possible.

The flap usually remains volume stable despite the high muscle content. If radiation becomes necessary after the defect has been covered, our experience has shown that the entire flap can be included in the radiation field. In a reconstruction with an implant, the problem of capsular contracture after radiation also exists here.

A single-sided removal hardly results in asymmetry of the back but leaves a scar.

11.1.4 Informed Consent

The disclosure of general and special risks should be documented with standardized and evaluated forms. Infection, haematoma and wound-healing complications can occur. The risk of complete and partial flap loss should be mentioned, as well as wound-healing complications at the donor site. Seroma formation, visible scars and restricted movement of the arm can result. In mastectomy cases loss of sensitivity to the breast skin and the NAC is often. Loss of sensitivity can also occur at the donor site. A skin necrosis and NAC necrosis can occur and may require a reoperation. Smaller wound-healing problems can remain conservatively treated.

A lymph oedema of the breast and thoracic wall is possible in rare cases. The patient should be aware that breast shape, colour and symmetry are altered. Aesthetic change can result in psychological problems which may require psycho-oncologic consultation.

The incisions should be visualized in a drawing. The indication for a SSM or NSM should be discussed carefully. Scarring can distort the NAC in an NSM. Fat necrosis can occur. In most cases it shows no symptoms but can be detected by ultrasound. Second operations should be mentioned if histopathology is unclear or wound-healing problems occur or a contralateral mastopexy/reduction is required. A significant change after radiation is not likely to occur if the flap is well perfused; however ,it should be mentioned. If the patient does refuse recommended surgery or parts, this should also be documented.

If a bra and compression garments are recommended, the patients should be informed prior to surgery. Also the after treatment should be explained.

11.1.5 Preoperative Markings and Measures

Tip

The skin island on the back should either be concealed by the bra, i.e. it should run transversely, or be placed perpendicular to the course of the muscle fibres. The scar lies in the relaxed tension lines of the skin and is least conspicuous (◘ Fig. 11.1). The entire muscle flap can be dissected from the edge of the skin island without the need for a further incision in the axilla or at the front edge of the muscle. The smaller the skin island, the more precisely it has to be planned, since no perforator vessel may leave the muscle and enter the skin. A Doppler examination is then appropriate.

When marking, the patient should abduct the arm to 90°. The muscle runs from the spine and the upper dorsal pelvis via the caudal scapula tip to the axilla. Its tendon forms together with the teres major muscle tendon the posterior border of

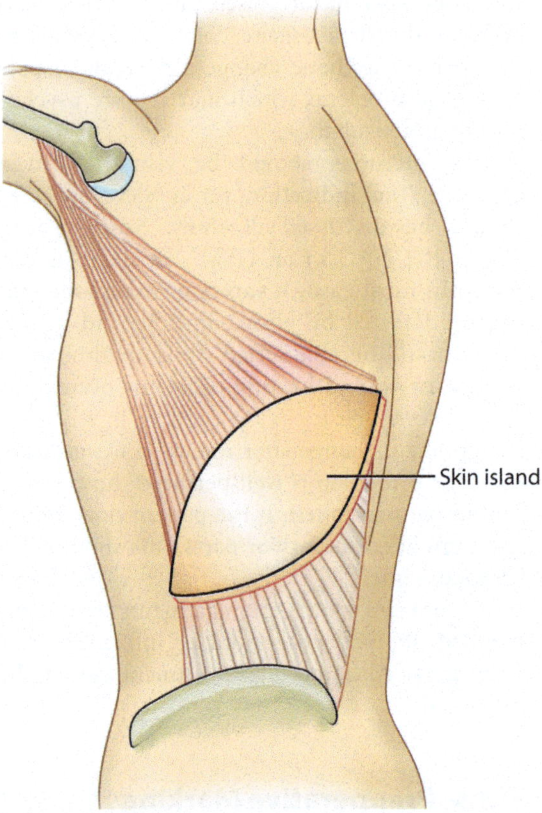

◘ **Fig. 11.1** In this example, the skin island on the back is placed at perpendicular to the course of the muscle fibres. The scar is located in the relaxed tension lines of the skin and is the least conspicuous. This looks quite rough at the beginning but usually leads to better scars. The extended latissimus can also be harvested via this incision. If only a small skin island is required, it can also be placed in the bra line. Basically, the skin island must be laid in such a way that it can be used after putting the latissimus at the recipient site. The pivot point is the axilla. The entire muscle flap can be dissected from the edge of the skin island

the axilla and can be well felt here. The anterior edge of the muscle runs in the posterior axillary line on the thorax. The pedicle enters the muscle centrally from the anterior third of the muscle about 9–12 cm caudally of the axilla. The position of the skin island depends on the requirements of the breast and should allow a primary closure on the back. When marking, the skin can be pinched to determine the width of the skin island. Usually a width of 7–8 cm can be closed easily. The length of the skin island can be up to 25 cm. It can then be drawn in as an ellipse.

11.1.6 Technique

11.1.6.1 Positioning on the Operation Table: IV Lines

The harvesting of the latissimus is an operation that must be performed in a lateral position. Either the breast operations are performed in supine position and the patient is repositioned or the surgeon is also able to operate on the breast in lateral position. If a reconstruction is planned together with an implant, the final fitting of flap and implant in symmetry to the opposite side has to be made in supine position.

The patient is placed on the unaffected side (◘ Fig. 11.2). The upper arm is bent 90° in the elbow and abducted 90° in the shoulder. It is best to fix it well padded to a right-angled bow at the operating table so that you have free access to the axilla. In a two-team approach simultaneously two electrosurgery devices with two electrodes are required. A Foley catheter is recommended. The patients' body temperature can be managed with a convective warming device (e.g. Bair Hugger). One to two peripheral lines are sufficient, preferred at the ankle/feet or at the arm of the not operated side.

The chest, back and axilla as well as the proximal upper arm are completely prepared. The easiest way is to cover the entire site with the breast using a U-shaped sterile sheet coming from below. A larger sheet is first fixed cranially around the arm and then down.

11.1.6.2 Operation

Flap harvesting is best performed under loupe magnification with a headlight. Harvesting is performed within 30–60 min if no complications occur. Dissection of the recipient site depends on type of reconstruction.

Dissection can be performed with scissors (Metzenbaum) or by electrosurgery. The latter however can lead to more seroma. Dissection of the pedicle should be done with bipolar forceps and fine scissors. The surgeon starts on the backside of the patient. The pedicle can also be dissected from ventrally.

The incision begins on the skin island. If bevelling is planned, this should be done below the subcutaneous fascia. When you are on the muscle, leave the muscle fascia intact and dissect the muscle as much as required. Separate the skin from the muscle, dissecting away from the skin island.

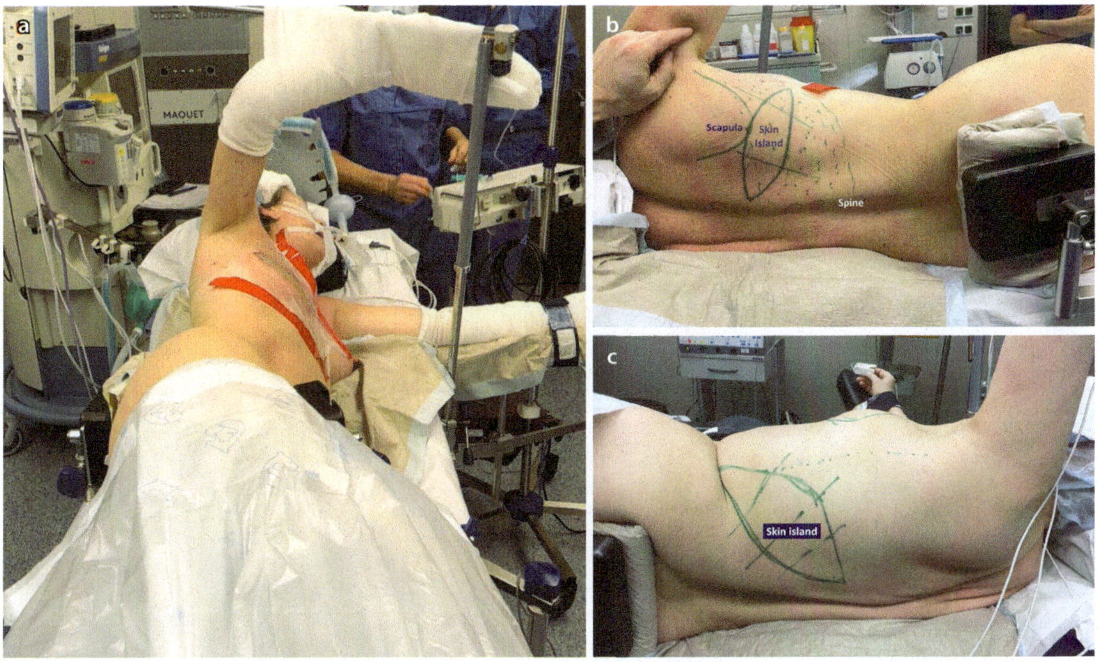

◻ Fig. 11.2 **a** Positioning on the healthy side. Arm abducted to 90° and bent in the elbow. Fixing to a transverse support which is attached ventrally to the operating table. This makes it easy to get into the axilla and allows the pedicle to be dissected safely. Preparation of the muscle and tunnelling can also be done in this way. **b** Positioning seen dorsally. The scapula edge, the planned skin island (here horizontally in the course of the bra) and the muscle coat to be lifted. **c** Different design with distal skin island in the relaxed tension lines (see ◻ Fig. 11.1). The scar is more visible than a horizontal design, but the scar is less conspicuous and you can take a lot of volume out of the flank. This design is particularly suitable for defect coverage

At the front edge of the muscle in the posterior axillary line, one can then dissect underneath the muscle. The pedicle enters the front third of the muscle, about 9–12 cm caudal of the dorsal axilla. It usually runs 2–3 cm dorsally of the anterior muscle margin. Stepping on the ventral side of the patient can now facilitate dissection. The pedicle should be carefully dissected. It runs on the anterior serratus muscle and from there enters the latissimus muscle dorsally. Usually the pedicle is well visible in the fat between the muscles. Now the latissimus is carefully separated from the serratus. The pedicle is carefully protected. If it is certain that the cranial thoracodorsal bundle is good, the branch usually going from the thoracodorsal bundle into the serratus can be ligated with a Ligaclip. This makes the latissimus more mobile. The vessels can now be dissected cranially. Smaller branches are removed with bipolar forceps, larger ones with clips. At the level of the caudal axilla, dorsal branches run to the teres major muscle and the scapula. These must also be clipped carefully. Occasionally there is a branch from the thoracodorsal bundle into the latissimus at this point. If this is the case, this branch should be spared. The muscle must then be separated from the scapula and the teres major muscle. The tendinous attachment to the arm is initially left in place to avoid tension on the pedicle. In some cases, the teres muscle and the latissimus muscle have a common tendon. It can be difficult to separate the two.

If the pedicle is secured, the muscle can now be detached caudally and spinally by diathermy. The muscle has strong perforators from the thorax. These must be carefully coagulated or clipped. These perforators allow harvesting the latissimus muscle as a free flap if the thoracodorsal vessels are not suitable due to a previous operation. The latissimus is now caudal and spinal and detached from the surrounding skin and thorax. The dissection at the caudal scapula tip and the teres major muscle should be approached a little more carefully, as the pedicle runs here.

Once the muscle is detached, a tunnel can be prepared ventrally to the breast. This should start

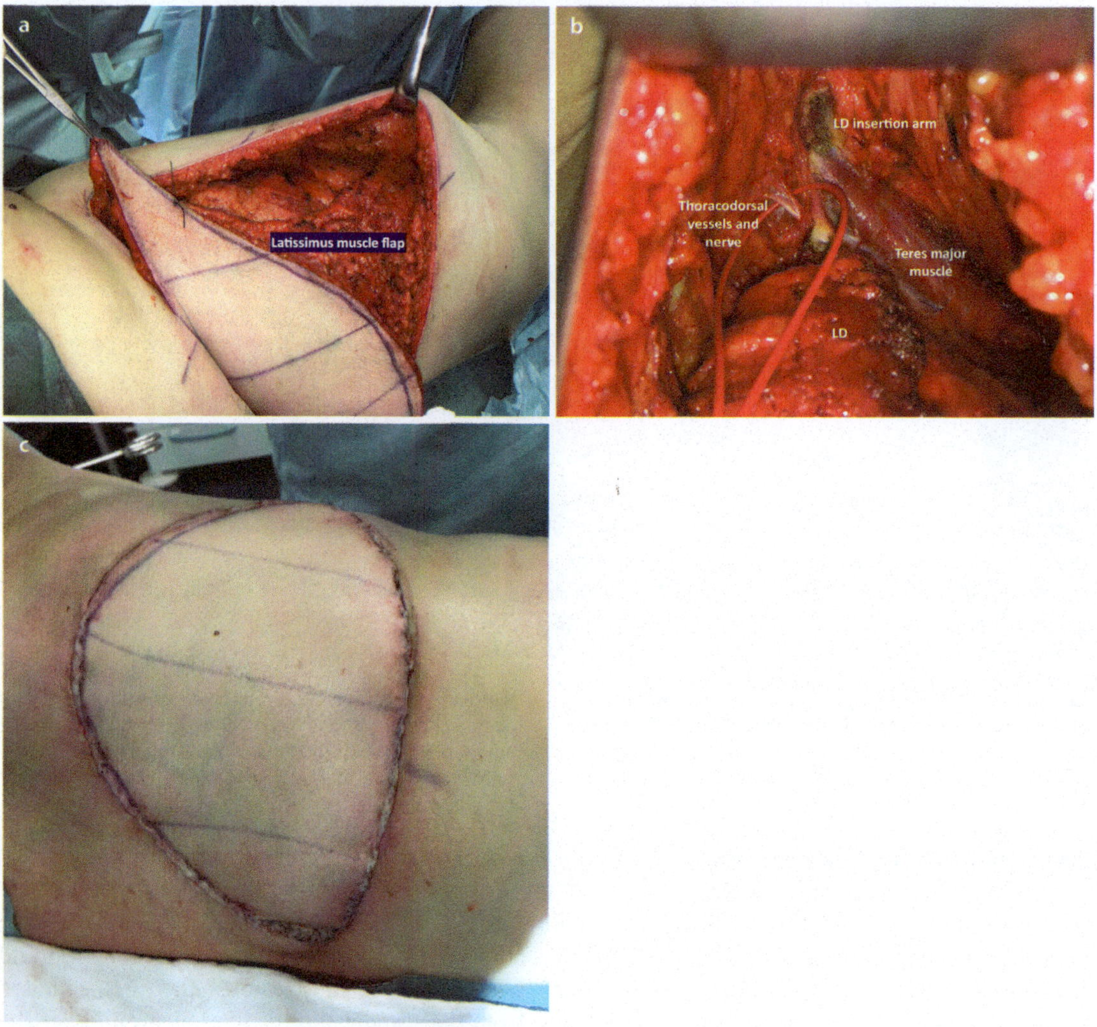

◘ **Fig. 11.3** **a**. Incision around skin island (25 × 12 cm) and dissection of the muscle up to the axilla. View from caudal to cranial. **b** View from ventral into the axilla. The muscle is tunnelled from dorsal to ventral. The thoracodorsal pedicle is looped. In the background the cut insertion of the latissimus muscle at the upper arm and the teres major muscle separated from the latissimus. **c** The skin island closes a ventral defect after extensive tumour resection

at the ventral axilla on the major pectoral muscle. If the mastectomy has already been performed, the tunnel can be prepared into the operating area. It is important not to make the tunnel too wide but to prepare it from the axilla towards the breast. The lateral breast should remain adherent so that the latissimus does not slip back into its former position.

If the muscle is completely dissected and well perfused, the thoracodorsal nerve can now be exposed. The easiest way to do this is at the pedicle. If the patient is not relaxed, a gentle pressure on the pedicle can cause the muscle to twitch and identify the nerve well. The nerve can be prepared bluntly with a fine forceps (e.g. Overholt dissector). It should be dissected to a length of a few centimetres. Then a section of the nerve should be excised. Denervating the muscle reduces the subsequent movement of the muscle. After the segmental excision of the nerve, the insertion of the tendon can be cut. This manoeuvre also reduces a possible joint movement, since the muscle is no longer stretched. Here too, a strong vascular branch runs in the muscle, which must be carefully coagulated (◘ Fig. 11.3).

The tendinous insertion of the muscle can now be temporarily fixed to the front edge of the pectoralis muscle with a strong suture while positioning the pedicle gently. This prevents any traction on the pedicle during transfer. The muscle can now be placed in the tunnel. Once the breast is dissected, the latissimus can be pulled through to the front and fitted in. If only a defect coverage is planned, the suture of the muscle and the skin island can be closed by a second surgeon after drain insertion. It is important that the pedicle is free of tension and that no tension is exerted later. If the breast has not yet been prepared, the muscle remains in the tunnel.

The donor site can be primarily closed after drainage has been inserted. If possible, the tension should be applied to the subcutaneous fascia with strong resorbable suture (Vicryl 2–0). Since the wound has a large surface that tends to form seromas, quilting sutures between the thorax and the subcutaneous fascia can reduce the dead space and thus reduce seroma formation, e.g. with Vicryl 2–0. The skin is then closed with running intracutaneous sutures.

▪▪ Using the Flap for Breast Reconstruction

If a repositioning is now planned, the wounds can be sterilely draped. The breast can be closed with a sterile surgical film. A repositioning to the supine position is carried out. If implant placement is planned, the arms should be placed on the elbow pads in 30–45° adduction. It should be possible to put the patient in a sitting position.

After positioning, the surgical film is removed and everything prepared again. The flap can now exposed. First it should be checked that the perfusion is sufficient and the pedicle is not twisted or under tension. For safety, the flap can be fixed towards the axilla with resorbable sutures.

If breast reconstruction with implants is planned, the pocket is now prepared subpectorally. After mastectomy, the pectoralis is horizontally detached from the caudal ribs or briefly cranial of the IMF. Proactive haemostasis also facilitates the preparation here. The sternal origins of the pectoralis muscle should only be cut caudally up to about the level of the medial IMF but maximally up to the 4th ICS. Only firmer tendinous structures of the pectoralis visible as white ligaments should be severed, if present. A further detachment of the muscle tissue medially can expose the implant medially or lead to a medial dislocation. It is important to harvest only the major pectoral muscle. All other muscles remain on the thorax. The preparation initially extends laterally to the height of the lateral pectoral minor margin.

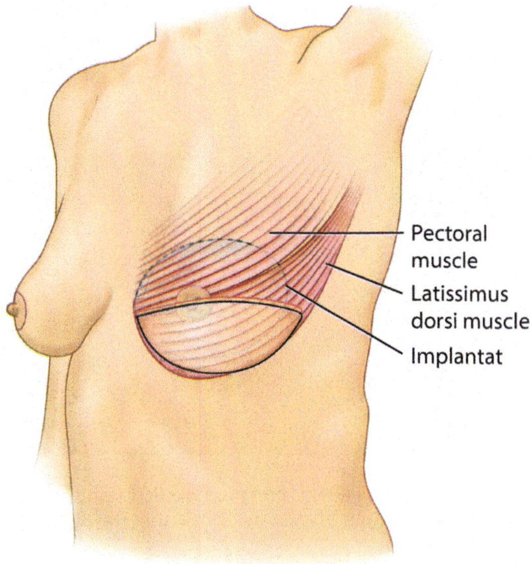

Fig. 11.4 Fitting of the latissimus at the breast with an implant. After insertion of the implant below the pectoral muscle, the latissimus is used as a caudal cover. If breast skin has to be replaced by latissimus skin, e.g. after removal of the MAK or skin over the tumour, this can now also be planned by fitting in the skin with temporary staples ("tailor tacking"). The skin of the latissimus that is not required is de-epithelialized. If no skin is needed from the latissimus, then the entire skin island can be de-epithelialized. In this case, the entire skin island can be used to stabilize the lower breast pole. The flap is then fixed cranially to the pectoral muscle and caudally to the IMF/Scarpa's fascia after insertion of the final implant. Absorbable sutures (Vicryl 3–0) are sufficient. Lateral fixation can also be used to prevent the implant from sliding laterally

The implant sizer can now be inserted. The latissimus is now sutured temporarily against the pectoralis and to the IMF, and the lower cover of the implant is estimated. The patient is now temporarily put in a sitting position to check the symmetry. If breast skin has to be replaced by latissimus skin, e.g. after removal of the MAK or skin over the tumour, this can now also be planned by fitting in the skin with temporary staples ("tailor tacking"). The excess skin is invaginated and temporarily fixed with the stapling device. The "stapled" lines are marked with the pen, the brackets removed, and the lines drawn exactly. The unneeded skin of the latissimus is de-epithelialized. If no skin is needed from the latissimus, the entire skin island can be de-epithelialized. In this case the entire skin island can be used to stabilize the lower breast pole (Figs. 11.4, 11.5, 11.6, 11.7, 11.8 and 11.9).

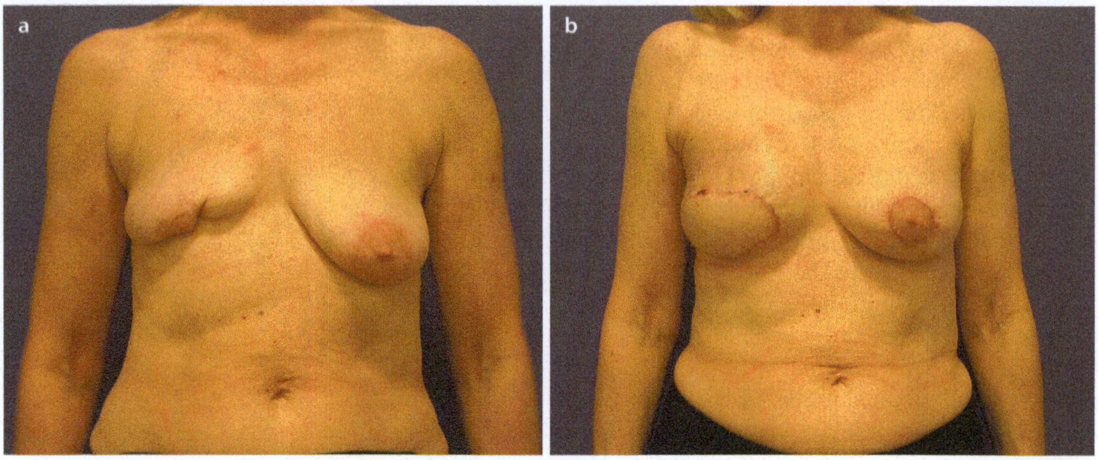

Fig. 11.5 **a, b** Patient after multiple BCT right side; no radiation. Reconstruction with a latissimus flap and a submuscular implant (about 200 cc). Adjustment of the opposite side with periareolar mastopexy. Result 21d after surgery

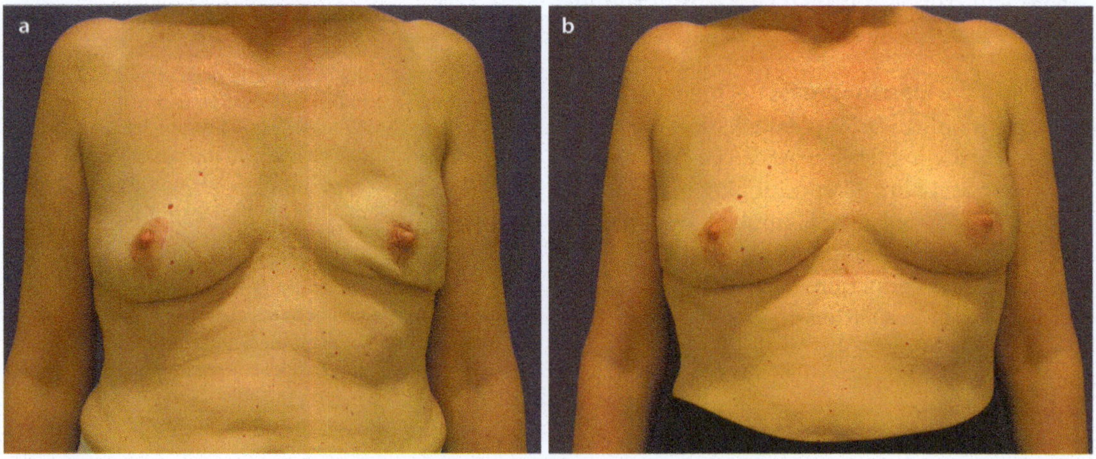

Fig. 11.6 **a, b** Patient with implant failure after subcutaneous mastectomy left. Alignment right. Reconstruction with latissimus flap and submuscular implant (175 cc). Result after 3 months

The flap is then fixed cranially to the pectoral muscle and caudally to the IMF after insertion of the final implant. Absorbable sutures (Vicryl 3–0) are sufficient. Lateral fixation can also be used to prevent the implant from sliding laterally. As with all implants, it is important that the pocket fits the implant so that it does not rotate or dislocate.

After the drains have been inserted, the sutures are made in the usual form.

! The dissection and subsequent transposition of the pedicle must be precise so that no tension or twisting is applied to pedicle and perfusion is reduced. The segmental resection of the thoracodorsal nerve and the discontinuation of the tendinous attachment of the muscle reduce the risk of breast co-movements (animation deformity).

11.1.6.3 Thoracodorsal Artery Perforator Flap (TDAP-Flap)

When harvesting as TDAP, the muscle is largely left in place. The skin island is planned as the normal flap. It is harvested at the intramuscular vessels and transposed with the thoracodorsal bundle. With this technique, the donor site morbidity is somewhat lower, but the muscle is not always functional afterwards.

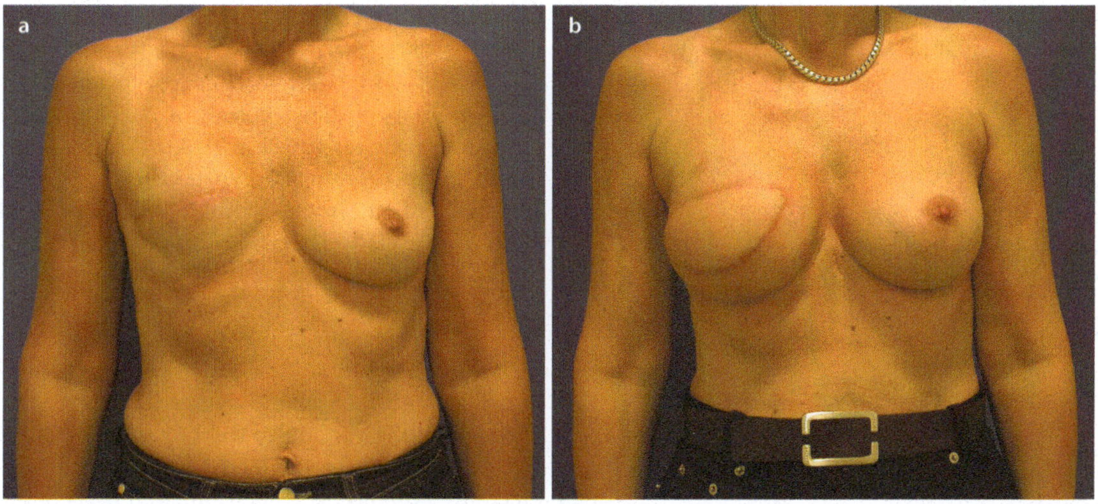

Fig. 11.7 **a, b** Patient with mastectomy right. Reconstruction with latissimus flaps and submuscular anatomical implant (370 cc); adjustment with implant augmentation (200 cc) left. Result after 6 months

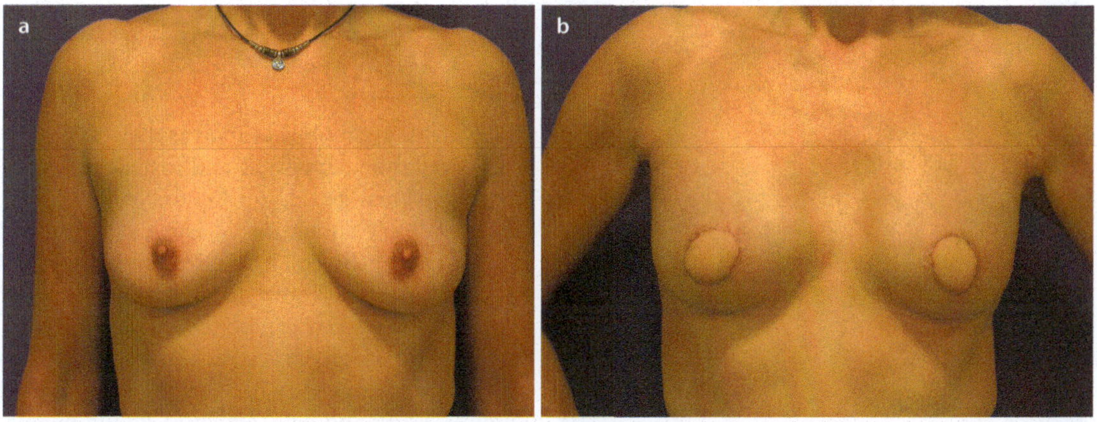

Fig. 11.8 **a, b** DCIS right and prophylactic mastectomy left. SSM on both sides and immediate reconstruction with bilateral latissimus flaps and 225 cc anatomical implants

The skin island is located in the upper medial part of the muscle via a strong perforator, which is previously identified by Doppler. These perforators lie within a radius of 8–10 cm around the entry of the thoracodorsal vascular bundle into the latissimus muscle. In some cases, a strong perforator may also originate from the thoracodorsal vessel on the frontal border of the muscle. After incision of the skin island, the skin island is removed from the muscle up to the perforator. The passage of the perforator through the muscle is spared, and then the muscle is cut caudally and dorsally of the entry of the perforator into the skin island. As a rule, the latissimus has a branching of its main perfusion from the entry of the thoracodorsal vascular bundle into four branches; one supplies the muscle cranially of the entry, and the three others branch out with the fibre course in a fan-shaped manner. These branches can now be followed until the thoracodorsal vascular bundle enters the muscle. This preparation is relatively simple because the latissimus is a thin muscle. But it becomes difficult if you want to maintain the nerve. This requires complete exposure and separation of the vascular pedicle and nerve.

Overall, the TDAP is an elegant procedure with low lifting morbidity when only parts of the skin are required.

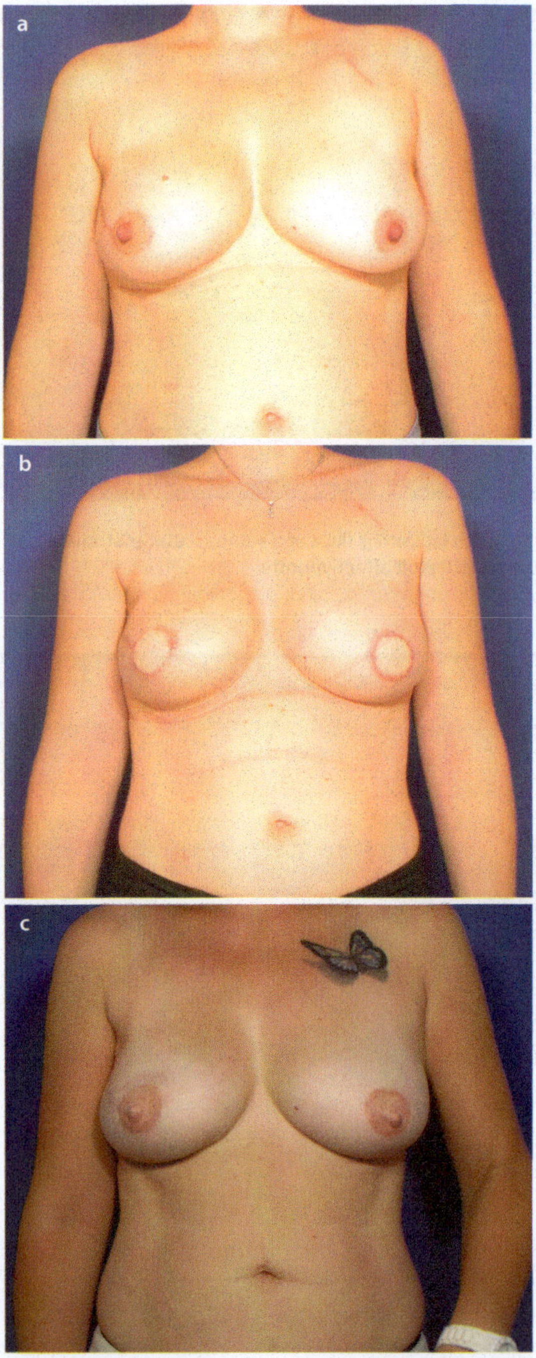

Fig. 11.9 **a–c** Patient with BET right and recurrence. Bilateral SSM and reconstruction with submuscular anatomical implant (395 cc) and latissimus flaps. Nipple reconstruction and pigmentation of the areola. Tattooing of the port scar by the patient

11.1.7 Monitoring

In the case of complication-free mastectomy or secondary reconstruction, a decision must be made whether to use flap skin. If this is the case, a flap monitoring can be carried out via this skin island. If you do not need a skin island and the flap is well perfused during the operation, you do not need to plan for a temporary monitor island.

If the perfusion of the mastectomy skin in a SSM or NSM cannot be clearly assessed intraoperatively, the skin can be completely left on the flap. With this buried flap technique, it is possible to wait up to 5 days until the status of the mastectomy skin has been determined. If parts of the mastectomy skin still have to be removed because it is not well perfused, the resulting defect can be replaced in a second operation with the skin of the flap.

11.1.8 Aftercare

The patients are mobile as soon as they can get up. They should be supported and instructed by PT or nurses when getting up the first times. In the first days, they should avoid using the operated arm to get up. The Foley catheter can be removed at the first post-operative day. A bra that does not compress the pedicle can be used if necessary.

Thromboprophylaxis is recommended. Drains should be removed with regard to the fluid amount. Work and daily activities should be possible after 1 week and should not exceed the standard. Sporting, sauna and sun tanning should be avoided for at least 6 weeks. Seromas at the donor site can be punctured if necessary.

11.1.9 Corrective and Additional Surgery

If additional surgery is necessary, it should be planned at least 3–6- months later than the flap surgery. If dents or irregularities occur in the transition zones between flap and original tissue they can be mildend by lipofilling; a secondary augmentation can also be done by lipofilling. A contralateral operation, if not done together with the reconstruction, can be planned at that time too.

The reconstruction of the NAC is considered to be the last operation.

Conclusion

The latissimus flap is now the second choice for breast reconstruction. However, it is suitable for patients in whom only defect coverage is planned or breast reconstruction with free autologous tissue is not possible, e.g. in the case of coagulation disorders. Intraoperative repositioning and possible axillary pre-operations make the operation somewhat lengthier. The combination with an implant may combine the negative aspects of autologous tissue and implant reconstruction. Nevertheless, latissimus flap surgery is a valuable technique that can provide good results for the correct indication.

11.2 Pedicled Transverse and Vertical Rectus Abdominis Muscle Flap (TRAM/VRAM-Flap)

For a long time, the pedicled TRAM-flap, transversal rectus abdominis muscle flap, was the procedure of choice for breast reconstruction. The rectus muscle is transposed cranially into the chest with a transverse skin island. If the skin island is used vertically, it is the VRAM flap. Flap perfusion comes from the superior epigastric artery. The disadvantage is that the transverse island of the lower abdominal skin, which is supposed to provide the volume in breast reconstruction, is actually dominantly supplied from the deep inferior epigastric artery, and the anastomoses between the superior and inferior epigastric artery are not always sufficient to completely supply the lower abdomen. The removal of the entire muscle and fascia sometimes leads to problems of the abdominal wall, such as abdominal wall weaknesses or even hernias, consecutive mesh inserts or pain.

Free, muscle-sparing TRAM-flap or DIEP-flaps are now the standard procedure. In our opinion, a pedicled TRAM-flap is more of a backup procedure if a free flap is not possible or useful.

11.2.1 Indication

Free flap from the lower abdomen is preferred: see ► Sect. 10.1. The inability to operate on a free flap is not an indication for a pedicled flap. If a free flap is not possible because of coagulation disorders or because the abdomen has been operated on in such a way that harvesting of the deep inferior epigastric vessels seems impossible, a pedicled TRAM-flap can be performed. It should be noted that in the case of a pedicled TRAM-flap, the perfusion is poor because it comes from the superior vascular system. As a result, the harvested volumes are usually limited to zones 1 and 2 for TRAM-flap. A vertical design is rather untypical in breast reconstruction because it does not provide sufficient volume. In the case of defects in the sternum, e.g. after metastasis resection, a vertical design can, however, provide a good closure of the defect. In our experience, a Caesarean section is not a contraindication for TRAM-flap; appendectomy scars, rectus muscle diastases or small umbilical hernias do not exclude the reconstruction.

11.2.2 Contraindication

In general, patients who had liposuction of the lower abdomen should be carefully examined to determine whether the previous operations (scars, retractions, missing fatty tissue) are a contraindication. A previous complete abdominoplasty is usually a contraindication. Median laparotomies can be a contraindication if the tissue on one side of the abdomen is not sufficient. Here, however, an alignment of the contralateral breast or the transplantation of both parts of the lower abdomen on two pedicles can be considered. Existing or operated abdominal wall hernias are a contraindication. Reconstruction on both sides is only possible if the abdominal wall is supported with a mesh after flap harvesting. The risks must be carefully weighed up here.

CT or MR angiography (▸ Sect. 10.1.5.1) allows a preoperative assessment of the donor site in case of possible doubts.

Overview Pedicled TRAM-Flap

Indication: all breasts form, if a free flap plastic is not possible.

Skin island:

- Mostly transversal, rarely vertical
- Size: maximum 30 cm width possible and 10–20 cm high, depending on abdomen

Vascular pedicle:

- Superior epigastric artery and vein; origin from the IMA/V
- Pedicle length: up to 20 cm possible

Side:

- The easiest way is to use the contralateral rectus muscle for the breast.

11.2.3 Characteristics

11.2.3.1 Perfusion

The pedicled TRAM-flap receives its perfusion through the superior epigastric artery which originates from the IMA. It branches cranially of the umbilicus in the rectus muscle and releases perforators there. The significant perfusion system for the lower abdomen is the deep inferior epigastric artery. The anastomoses between the two systems are not always optimally formed, so that the TRAM-flap usually has a less optimal perfusion than the DIEP. Usually, therefore, less volume can be harvested. Zones 3 and 4 are almost always less perfect (▸ Sect. 10.1.3.1). Venous drainage is also not optimal.

As with a DIEP-flap, a preoperative CTA can provide information on the structure of the perfusion.

11.2.3.2 Tissue Characteristics

The tissue of the pedicled TRAM-flap corresponds to the DIEP. As a rule, the volume of the flap remains stable. However, fat necrosis is more common than with DIEP. Shrinkage of the reconstructed breasts could not be seen in our patients with a stable body weight, so that the size achieved during the reconstruction should remain constant. If radiation therapy should become necessary after the reconstruction, shrinkage may occur more frequently with pedicled TRAM-flaps than with DIEP-flaps due to different perfusion. Unfortunately, the fibrosis caused by insufficient perfusion and irradiation in pedicled TRAM-flaps was mistakenly transferred to DIEP-flaps, which usually survive irradiation better due to their better perfusion. Recent studies confirm this.

11.2.4 Informed Consent

The disclosure of general and special risks should be documented with standardized and evaluated forms. They are basically the same as for DIEP-flaps. Infection, haematoma and wound-healing complications can occur. The risk of complete and partial flap loss should be mentioned, as well as wound-healing complications at the donor site like abdominal wall weakness and hernia which are increased compared to the DIEP-flap harvesting because the abdominal wall has to be dissected wider. Wide mobilization can result in more wound-healing problems, especially in heavy smokers. It may be necessary to use a mesh for rectus sheath closure. The use may cause weakness, hernias and adherence-related pain. By removing the rectus sheath on one side of the abdomen, the umbilicus can be pulled out of the midline. In rare cases a partial or complete necrosis of the umbilicus can occur.

The rectus muscle is pedicled cranially. At the pivot point at the level of the costal arch, a visible and palpable bulge often occurs. This can disturb some patients. Seroma formation and visible scars can result. In mastectomy cases loss of sensitivity to the breast skin and the NAC is often. Loss of sensitivity can also occur at the donor site. A skin necrosis and NAC necrosis can occur and may require a reoperation. Smaller wound-healing problems can remain conservatively treated.

A lymph oedema of the breast and thoracic wall is possible in rare cases. The patient should be aware that breast shape, colour and symmetry are altered. Aesthetic change can result in psychological problems which may require psycho-oncologic consultation.

The incisions should be visualized in a drawing. The indication for a SSM or NSM should be discussed carefully. Scarring can distort the NAC in an NSM. Fat necrosis can occur (more often than in DIEP-flaps). In most cases it shows no symptoms but can be detected by ultrasound. Second operations should be mentioned if histopathology is unclear or wound-healing problems occur or a contralateral mastopexy/reduction is required. A significant change after radiation can occur if the flap is not well perfused. If the patient does refuse recommended surgery or parts, this should also be documented.

If a bra and compression garments are recommended, the patients should be informed prior to surgery. Also the after treatment should be explained.

11.2.5 Planning and Preoperative Markings

11.2.5.1 CT Angiography (CTA) and Other Preoperative Imaging Techniques

As with the DIEP-flap (see ▶ Sect. 10.1), the CTA can provide important information on perfusion in advance. In this CTA, the examination should be extended to the upper abdomen and caudal thorax in order to visualize the IMA and its terminal branch, the superior epigastric artery. Thus, the course of the superior and deep inferior epigastric arteries and their anastomoses in the muscle can be visualized. In the coronary plane, the epigastrica branches out in the muscle. With a single-sided TRAM-flap, it can also be determined in advance whether one sticks to the planned muscle or uses the contralateral one.

11.2.5.2 Preoperative Markings and Measures

The markings and measures correspond to those for the DIEP-flap. Since cranial perforators are used, the cranial incision is usually slightly higher than with DIEP. This causes the resulting scar on the abdomen to run slightly higher than in DIEP-flaps or abdominoplasty. The easiest way to fit the flap is to use the contralateral rectus muscle as a pedicle.

11.2.6 Technique

11.2.6.1 Positioning on the Operation Table: IV Lines

Positioning and IV lines are the same as for the DIEP-flap.

11.2.6.2 Pedicled Flap

Flap harvesting is best performed under loupe magnification with a headlight. Harvesting is performed within 45–60 min if no complications occur. Dissection of the recipient site depends on type of reconstruction, immediate or delayed.

Dissection can be performed with scissors (Metzenbaum) or by electrosurgery. The latter however can lead to more seroma. Dissection of the pedicle should be done with bipolar forceps and fine scissors. A right-handed surgeon stands on the right side of the patient. The operation corresponds to the DIEP-flap surgery; harvesting is somewhat easier and is shown below.

▪▪ Common Technique

The incision is made along the markings. The umbilicus can already be cut and looped with the stay suture. Cranial abdominal wall preparation is now performed somewhat more generously than with DIEP-flaps. Dissection of the adhesions medially over the linea alba to the xiphoid and on both sides somewhat laterally of it to the costal arches. On the breast side that is to be reconstructed, the medial IMF can be dissected, and an epifascial tunnel can be made to the breast site. It should be at least 4–5 cm wide; for larger flap volumes, it must be enlarged.

The caudal veins at the lower incision margin and SIEA/V are coagulated or clipped. Once you have reached the abdominal fascia/rectus sheath, you can dissect from caudal to cranial or from lateral to medial. The midline is the line of adherence on the linea alba. As a rule, no perforators run here. Smaller perforators can usually be coagulated caudally and continue to be dissected cranially. The TRAM-flap does not have to be harvested with the complete fascia. Here, too, a muscle- and fascia-saving approach or the inclusion of perforators in a cranial position is sufficient. The perforators should be located at the level of the umbilicus or slightly cranially. If the perforators for the flap are cranial to the arcuate line, the risk of abdominal wall weakness is lower.

Usually there are two rows of perforators, medial and lateral. Medial perforators usually perfuse further over the midline, but they can perfuse zone 2 weaker on the entry side. Lateral perforators have the advantage that they keep the medial muscle undamaged during harvesting.

! Patients after pregnancy often have a diastasis of the rectus muscles. This divergence of the muscles causes the lateral perforators to appear wide laterally and they can inadvertently be coagulated or not be included in the flap.

For a TRAM-flap several perforators should be included. This can be done en bloc without defined dissection of individual perforators, or the fascia can be incised along the perforators. The less fascia removed, the more stable the abdominal wall.

Incision of fascia/rectus sheath: The fascia is incised with a knife. Cut around the area of fascia that is integrated into the flap. Usually it is a rectangle that measures 3–4 cm per side. Alternatively, incision is made along the perforators of a row. The incision can be extended caudally. The central rectus muscle that carries the vessels can then be caudally completely resected. Laterally and medially one can usually still leave 1–1.5 cm of muscle. The deep inferior epigastric vessels enter the muscle caudally/laterally. They should be clipped. The rectus sheath incision is then also extended cranially just as far as the rectus muscle has to be dissected. You can now see the cranial muscle, which is dissected from the rectus sheath ventrally. The rectus muscle can now be carefully detached from its bed medially, laterally and dorsally. The further one gets cranially, the more vessels emerge laterally from the muscle. These should be clipped or coagulated. The dissection can be done simply by taking the flap in the left hand and dissecting the muscle with the right hand. This way you always have some traction on the tissue and can dissect more easily. An assistant holds up the abdominal wall with a Langenbeck or liver hook. During the preparation it can be tested again and again how far the rectus muscle has to be exposed cranially. During preparation, the superior epigastric vessels are not visible. They remain hidden in the muscle.

If the flap is sufficiently mobile, it can be pulled through the tunnel into the chest. In this case, the fatty tissue of the lower abdomen is usually rotated through 180° into the thoracic site. When pulling through, care must be taken that the muscle/fascia/perforator unit does not shear off and that the vessels are torn off due to too much tension.

If possible, the rectus sheath is closed primarily. We use an interrupted suture (Vicryl) to adapt the fascia coarsely; above this the closure is made with a double-armed, barbed-hook suture (e.g. Quill). In the cranial area, the fascial suture should not restrict the muscle turnover and thus blood circulation. Below this, the rectus sheath should be securely closed. If the sutures distort the umbilicus towards the harvest side, the opposite fascial side should also be gathered with the same suture.

If no primary suture of the rectus sheath is possible, a mesh is used. A mesh made of Vicryl and Prolene (Vypro) has proven here. It is partially resorbable. If possible, the mesh edges are placed in the rectus sheath and attached there with non-resorbable sutures. This means that at least the edges of the mesh cannot be felt through the skin.

After a drain is inserted the abdominal wall closure can take place. For this purpose, the patient is placed in the beach chair position. Immediately caudally of the umbilicus, a Vicryl suture (3–0) is placed at the fascia of the linea alba. This suture serves as fixation for the umbilicus and the flap that is crated later. The ends can be clamped together with the stay suture of the umbilicus. The cranial and caudal abdominal wound margin can now be approximated. First, Scarpa's fascia is adapted with strong interrupted sutures (e.g. Vicryl). Subcorial suturing is then performed with Monocryl or Vicryl (e.g. 3–0) using the interrupted single stiches. The skin is closed with a running intracutaneous suture.

Before the abdomen is completely closed, the position of the umbilicus should be determined. In order to improve the positioning, the skin should already be adapted centrally. Over the umbilicus, a caudally pedicled U- or V-shaped flap in the width of the navel is then incised. The incision is performed in all layers. The umbilicus is then pulled out through the resulting hole with the stay suture. Fat resection around the incision and flap area can improve the optical result. The umbilicus is now fixed cranially to the abdominal skin. The portion corresponding to the U-flap is resected from the umbilicus. The flap is then sutured to the umbilicus with the provided Vicryl sutures. This results in a three-point fixation of the caudal umbilicus and the cranial flap to the rectus sheath on the linea alba. This allows an aesthetic umbilical shaping. The remaining suture can be done intracutaneously with resorbable suture material (e.g. Monocryl 4–0).

■■ Special Cases

If there are fewer or only poor perforators on the planned side, a contralateral flap can also be used during the operation. Fitting through the tunnel is slightly more difficult due to the rotation.

Another technique that is still occasionally propagated is the so-called delay operation. In a first operation, the caudal perfusion of the TRAM-flap is ligated. Both the two superficial and the two deep inferior epigastric vessels are ligated in this operation. The complete caudal incision can also be performed in the operating theatre. After at least 2 weeks, the cranially pedicled flap can then be harvested in the second operation. This delay technique is intended to condition perfusion via the superior epigastric artery. From our point of view, this is a procedure that has only very rare indications.

11.2.6.3 "Supercharged" or "Turbocharged" Flap

The following techniques should be mentioned, although they have only few indications. The TRAM-flap is transposed into the breast on the superior epigastric artery. If more volume is required at the breast and normal DIEP-flap surgery alone is not possible (e.g. in the case of coagulation disorders), the ipsilateral caudal portion of the rectus muscle with the deep inferior epigastric artery can be included in the flap in selected indications – like with DIEP-flap surgery. These vessels can then be additionally connected to the IMA, their perforators or even axillary (◘ Fig. 11.10). Occasionally, this surgery with pedicled and free flap technique is described as "supercharged" TRAM (◘ Figs. 11.10, 11.11, and 11.12).

If, in addition to the single-sided rectus muscle pedicle via the superior epigastric vessels, the contralateral rectus muscle with the inferior epigastric vessels is included and connected microsurgically to the breast, this is described as "turbocharged" TRAM. Instead of the inferior epigastric vessels, the superficial inferior epigastric vessels (SIEA) can of course also be used.

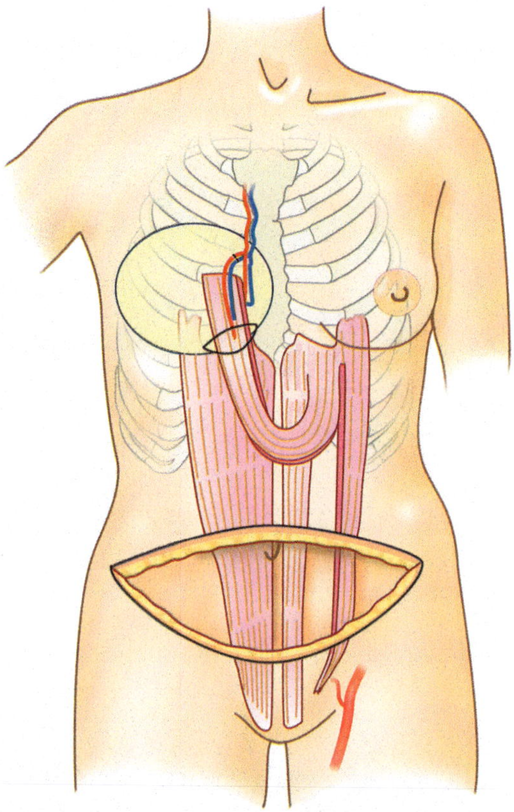

◘ **Fig. 11.10** Harvesting of the contralateral TRAM-flap on the cranially pedicled rectus muscle. Cranial of the entry of the perforators from the muscle into the subcutaneous fatty tissue, an incision of the anterior rectus sheath is sufficient. The tissue of the lower abdomen is transposed into the breast via a tunnel in the medial IMF. In this case, the inferior epigastric vessels are also connected to the IMA, resulting in a "supercharged" TRAM-flap

These procedures naturally increase morbidity and should only be used for a given indication.

11.2.6.4 Shaping and Inset of the Flap; Buried Flap

Not required parts should be resected; not required skin should be de-epithelialized. Leaving the dermis keeps the subdermal vascular plexus intact, and perfusion is not harmed. Flap inset should follow the breast shape. Shaping the TRAM-flap is less flexible than with a DIEP-flap due to the fixed pedicle. The contralateral breast should be the breast that indicates the shape, or a contralateral mastopexy/reduction or even augmentation is planned. If the breasts have a ptosis or are large, this has to be integrated into the reconstructive algorithm. If unsafe parts of the

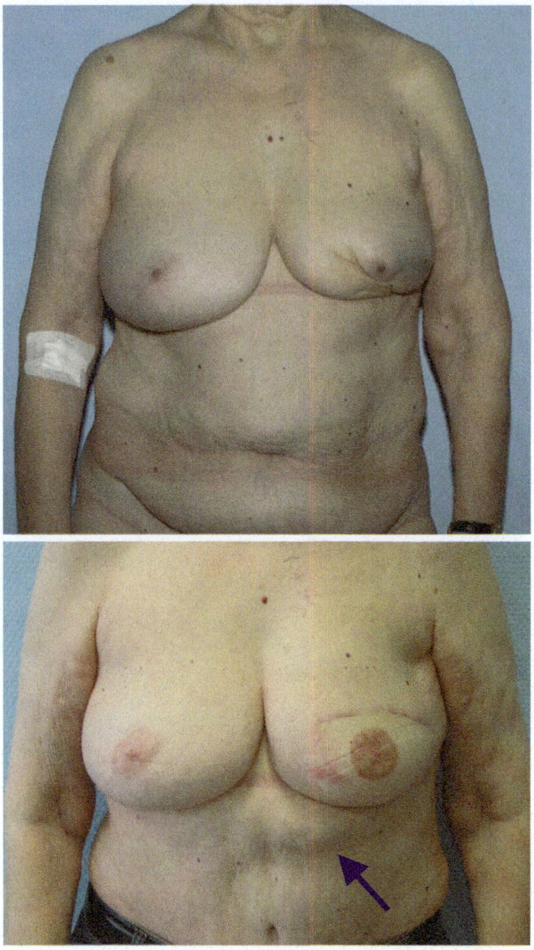

Figs. 11.11 and 11.12 Patient with recurrence after BCT and radiation, left side. Due to a homozygous factor V disorder (Leiden mutation), the reconstruction was performed as a pedicled TRAM-flap with additional anastomosis of the epigastric vessels to the IMA. After 1 year, the pivot/rotation point (arrow) of the muscle is still visible and palpable

flap are not removed, they should be placed laterally or caudally, where they can be better removed than in the décolleté of the breast.

> **Areas of a flap that are not adequately perfused or show a venous congestion should not be transplanted but removed beforehand, even if the flap should become smaller than desired. Subsequent augmentation with a lipofilling or a small implant is better than a fat necrosis and/or revision operation resulting from the perfusion disorder.**

Shaping can also be done actively. Parts that are not needed can be removed; surplus fat underneath Scarpa's fascia can be removed with respect to the perforators, which allows better transition from thoracic tissue to the flap. Coning sutures can be applied to achieve projection. However, the sutures should not impair perfusion and thus cause fat necrosis.

In secondary reconstructions with a transverse scar, the scar is excised and the cranial part is elevated from the muscle. It can be done with the lower part too. The flap is the placed into this pocket. The skin island in this case is ellipsoid. If the skin is altered from radiation, the TRAM-flap needs a long time to sag in its natural position. Especially in ptotic contralateral breasts, it is better to remove the caudal skin from the thoracic wall from the mastectomy scar to the IMF. The TRAM-flap is then de-epithelialized cranially, placed into the cranial pocket and sutured with the abdominal skin left in place to the IMF. The décolleté has its original skin, and caudally the TRAM-flap is naturally shaped without any restrictions from scars or skin problems. This inset follows the aesthetic units of the breast. Unfavourable is the different colour of the abdominal skin compared to the original breast skin.

There are many concepts regarding the flap sutures. We think that the flap should at least be fixed medially and in the IMF to avoid dents and malposition and allow smooth transitions. However, as the TRAM-flap is pedicled, it has some medial fixation. Cranially and laterally sutures should be applied if the flap is better positioned and shaped. To avoid fat necrosis, the flap should only be fixed at the Scarpa's fascia or the dermis.

Bringing the patient into a sitting position intraoperatively can help to estimate the amount of needed skin, and its position on the flap in secondary reconstructions thus facilitates symmetry. If the mastectomy skin flap is not well perfused or cannot be assessed properly, the abdominal skin can be left on the flap. The mastectomy flap is placed over the flap. The flap is now buried. After some days viability of the mastectomy skin can be assessed. If the mastectomy skin has survived, the abdominal skin is removed in a short second operation; if not the mastectomy skin can be replaced by flap skin.

11.2.7 Monitoring

In the case of complication-free mastectomy or secondary reconstruction, a decision must be made whether to use flap skin. If this is the case, a flap monitoring can be done. If no skin island is required, no active monitoring is required.

If the perfusion of the skin of the mammary gland in a SSM or NSM cannot be clearly assessed intraoperatively, the skin can be completely left on the flap. With this buried flap technique, it is possible to wait up to 5 days until the status is determined. If parts of the mastectomy skin still have to be removed because of reduced perfusion, the resulting defects can be replaced in a second operation with the skin of the flap.

11.2.8 Aftercare, Complications and Additional Surgery

Aftercare follows the scheme for DIEP-flap surgery. Complications are also the same; however, due to the harvest of the entire muscle donor site, morbidity is increased. The different perfusion leads to more fat necrosis, and the flap itself is less robust. Corrective surgery can also be performed in the same way as DIEP-flap surgery.

Conclusion

The pedicled TRAM-flap is nowadays a backup procedure that can be used in the few patients for whom microvascular flap surgery is not possible. The abdominal wall morbidity is higher; the quality of the reconstruction is less excellent than with DIEP-flaps. Nevertheless, the TRAM-flap is a technique that can deliver good results and should be mastered if indicated.

Literature

Latissimus Dorsi Flap

1. Hamdi M, Van Landuyt K, Hijjawi JB, Roche N, Blondeel P, Monstrey S. Surgical technique in pedicled thoracodorsal artery perforator flaps: a clinical experience with 99 patients. Plast Reconstr Surg. 2008;121:1632–41.
2. Heitmann C, Pelzer M, Kuentscher M, Menke H, Germann G. The extended latissimus dorsi flap revisited. Plast Reconstr Surg. 2003a;111:1697–701.
3. Heitmann C, Guerra A, Metzinger SW, Levin LS, Allen RJ. The thoracodorsal artery perforator flap: anatomic basis and clinical application. Ann Plast Surg. 2003b;51:23–9.
4. Olivari N. The latissimus flap. Br J Plast Surg. 1976;29:126–8.

Pedicled Transverse und Vertical Rectus Abdominis Muscle-Flap (TRAM/VRAM-Flap)

5. Fansa H, Schirmer S, Frerichs O, Gehl HB. Significance of abdominal wall CT-angiography in planning DIEA perforator flaps, TRAM flaps and SIEA flaps. Handchir Mikrochir Plast Chir. 2011;43:81–7.
6. Knox AD, Ho AL, Leung L, Tashakkor AY, Lennox PA, Van Laeken N, Macadam SA. Comparison of outcomes following autologous breast reconstruction using the DIEP and pedicled TRAM flaps: a 12-year clinical retrospective study and literature review. Plast Reconstr Surg. 2016;138:16–28.
7. Levine SM, Patel N, Disa JJ. Outcomes of delayed abdominal-based autologous reconstruction versus latissimus dorsi flap plus implant reconstruction in previously irradiated patients. Ann Plast Surg. 2012;69:380–2.
8. Macadam SA, Zhong T, Weichman K, Papsdorf M, Lennox PA, Hazen A, Matros E, Disa J, Mehrara B, Pusic AL. Quality of life and patient-reported outcomes in breast cancer survivors: a multicenter comparison of four abdominally based autologous reconstruction methods. Plast Reconstr Surg. 2016;137:758–71.
9. Spear SL, Ducic I, Cuoco F, Hannan C. The effect of smoking on flap and donor-site complications in pedicled TRAM Breast reconstruction. Plast Reconstr Surg. 2005;116:1873–80.
10. Wu C, Clayton JL, Halvorson EG. Racial differences in ischemic complications of pedicled versus free abdominal flaps for Breast reconstruction. Ann Plast Surg. 2014;72:S172–5.

Secondary Reconstruction of Partial Defects

H. Fansa, C. Heitmann, *Breast Reconstruction with Autologous Tissue*,
https://doi.org/10.1007/978-3-319-95468-4_12

Partial defects can occur after BCT or oncoplastic operations. They can be primarily corrected (see ► Chaps. 4 and 5) or treated secondarily. These defects can be pure volume defects, i.e. the breast has less volume than the opposite side. Or removal of breast tissue and skin leads to a combined volume and skin deficit, which changes the breast shape. This also manifests itself in the asymmetry of the breasts. However, the removal of the skin causes a change in the shape of the breast and usually a distortion of the NAC. The reconstruction of these breasts is difficult. A further complication is that the breasts are usually irradiated as part of oncological therapy. The tissue of these patients in particular is usually somewhat firmer and less elastic. In addition, interventions after radiation can lead to increased wound-healing disorders.

For the treatment of partial defects, some techniques are available, which are explained elsewhere in this book. With one exception, this chapter deals with the appropriate strategy for correcting partial defects.

12.1 Do Nothing

If the defect is small and the asymmetry is not pronounced, it must be evaluated whether an additional intervention is necessary at all. Possibly the risks to be accepted are higher than the benefits. Patients' expectations can also be high.

12.2 Contralateral or Bilateral Mastopexy and Reduction Mammaplasty

In the case of partial defects of large breasts or breasts with ptosis, it should be considered whether a reduction and mastopexy on the contralateral side or both sides would solve the problem better than a reconstruction of the original condition. In this way, both volume and skin deficits can be elegantly compensated after BCT. This is the best choice for suitable patients, as standardized techniques and predictable results can be achieved. In principle, these patients should be offered a BCT with oncoplastic techniques and an adjustment of the opposite side in the first place (see ► Chap. 5).

12.3 Volume with Lipofilling: Scar Correction

In the case of defects where only volume but no skin is missing, the reconstruction can be attempted by lipofilling. The indication and technique are described in ► Chap. 13. It is important to explain to the patients that several interventions may be necessary to achieve the goal. If there is a combination of volume deficit and retracted scar, surgical scar correction can be attempted as a first step. Alternatively, during lipofilling, the scar can be injected and slightly loosened, and the final scar correction is carried out as a final step. The procedure should depend on how adherent the scar is. If it is too sticky, no improvement will be achieved by lipofilling alone.

12.4 Implants for Partial Reconstruction

Pure volume reconstructions can also be performed with implants. However, the difficulty here is that most patients have received radiation therapy with BCT. Implant failure and capsular contracture are clearly increased here. In addition, the deficit can be so small that no commercially available implant is available.

12.5 Local Flaps for Partial Reconstruction

Defects that affect skin and volume and cannot be solved by lipofilling or reduction surgery require local flap surgery. Below are brief descriptions of the possible flaps. These are usually individual solutions with a small number of cases. In more obese patients and patients with a smoking history, local perforator flap plastics are associated with increased wound–healing disorders.

12.5.1 Latissimus Dorsi Muscle Flap

Latissimus muscle flap or the use of the flap as perforator flap (TDAP, ► Sect. 11.1) is a classical technique for volume and skin reconstruction. Especially defects in the two outer quadrants or between NAC and IMF can be well substituted with this flap. The additional scars on the back are a disadvantage.

12.5.2 Parascapular Flap

The parascapular flap is an important flap for microsurgical reconstruction of the extremities. The anatomy and its perfusion area are always constant. It can be used as a pedicled flap to fill defects in the upper outer quadrant and lateral thorax/axilla. Because no muscle is affected by the operation, there is almost never a postoperative limitation of movement. Local transposition can result in a dog-ear that may have to be removed in another operation.

Overview Parascapular Flap

Indication:
- Defects in the upper outer breast pole, lateral breast

Skin island:
- Fasciocutaneous flap without muscle.
- Vertical position along the anterior edge of the latissimus dorsi muscle.
- Size: up to 30 cm long and 7–10 cm wide, depending on the pinch test; the harvesting area is primarily closed.
- Skin thickness, approx. 2–3 cm.

Pedicle:
- Superficial circumflex scapular artery; it runs through the lateral, triangular, space formed by the triceps, teres major and minor muscles. The space can always be palpated.
- Originates from the subscapular artery (from which the thoracodorsal artery also originates)
- Easy to locate with the Doppler
- Length: approx. 5–6 cm

Caveat: After axillary operations, the subscapular artery may be damaged.

Operation:
- Surgery in lateral position, like a latissimus flap.
- The triangular space is the pivot point. Usually this is about 2 cm cranial and lateral of the dorsal axillary fold at 90° abducted arm.
- As a pedicled flap, the dissection only needs to be done as far as necessary.

12.5.3 Intercostal Perforator Flaps and Thoraco-epigastric Flaps

Smaller defects in the outer and lower poles of the breast can be reconstructed with local perforator flap from the intercostal area, the intercostal artery perforator or ICAP. In the inframammary fold and caudal thereof are the anterior intercostal perforators. This anterior intercostal flap has been de facto described by Bohmert as a thoraco-epigastric flap with medial pedicle; the main perforators are found in the IMF and caudal thereof between the 5th and 7th ICR. The harvesting area is closed by mobilizing the abdominal wall cranially.

Lateral intercostal perforators, LICAP, are located in the transition from the breast to the lateral thoracic wall. These perforators are located in extension of the IMF towards the lateral midaxillary line, i.e. between the lateral breast border and the anterior edge of the latissimus dorsi muscle. The characteristics of the perforators are individual, so that a Doppler examination is recommended in advance.

Both flap types are only suitable for patients who have excess skin in the harvesting area, so that the donor's site can be closed tension-free. The scars of the anterior ICAP flap can often be hidden in the IMF. The scars of LICAP run laterally from the chest into the thoracic wall and the back (◘ Fig. 12.1).

Overview Intercostal Perforator Flaps (ICAP)

Indication:
- Defects in the lower and lateral breast poles

Skin island:
- Perforator flaps without muscle.
- Anterior ICAP: horizontal position along and caudal of the IMF; size: up to 10 cm long and 5–7 cm high, depending on the pinch test; the donor site is closed primarily.
- Lateral ICAP: horizontal) position lateral to the IMF, midaxillary line; size: up to 20 cm long and 5–10 cm high, depending on the pinch test; the donor site is closed primarily.

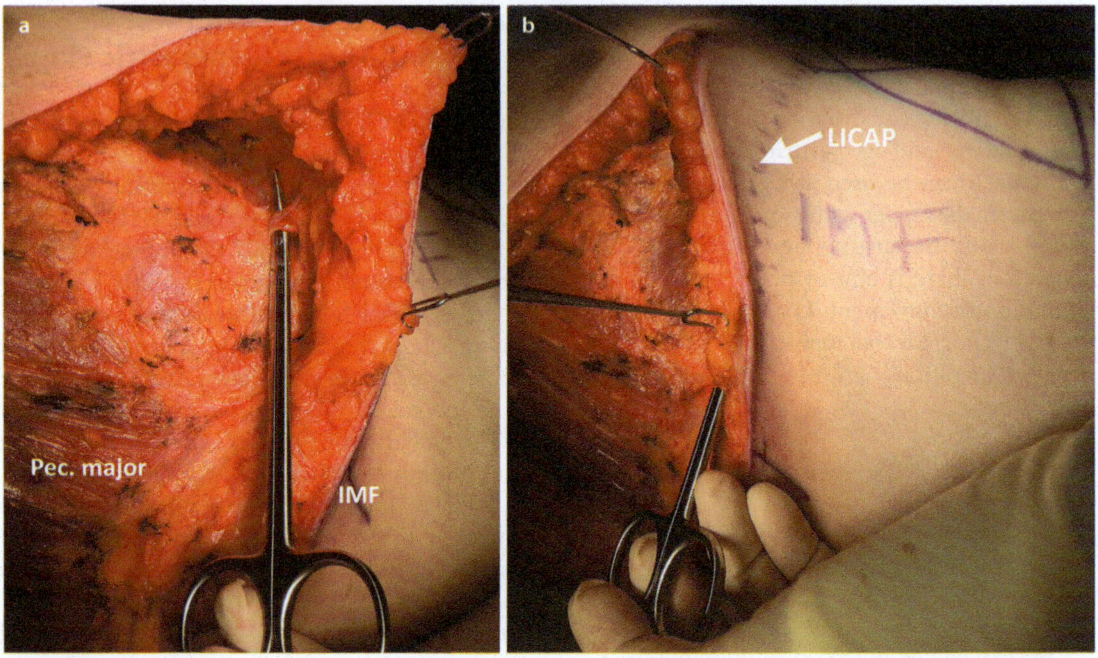

Fig. 12.1 **a** Lateral intercostal perforator (LICAP). The perforator (marked with the scissors) in a mastectomy site exits at the level of the IMF lateral from the breast. **b** Dotted line shows the extension of the IMF to lateral. The scissors indicate the LICAP

Vascular pedicle:

- Intercostal perforators from the IMA and the superior) epigastric artery and the posterior intercostal artery
- Powerful perforators in 4th to 7th ICR
- Easy to locate with the Doppler

Operation:

- Surgery for the anterior flap in supine position; for the lateral ones in lateral position, as with the latissimus flap.
- As a pedicled flaps, the dissection only needs to be done as far as necessary.

12.6 Microsurgical Flaps for Partial Reconstruction

If a partial defect cannot be reconstructed with local flap after a BCT, partial reconstruction with a free flap can also be performed with given oncological safety. However, it should be carefully considered whether the remaining breast tissue should be left or resected, as microsurgical reconstruction is performed mostly only once. The flaps from the lower abdomen (DIEP/SIEA) and the inner thigh (IT-flap) are used (see ► Sects. 10.1, 10.2 and 10.3) (Figs. 12.2 and 12.3).

12.7 Complete Reconstruction

In some cases the partial defect cannot be reconstructed with local techniques, the local flaps are not possible or different therapies have to be combined with great effort. This can be, for example, after locally treated recurrences and renewed radiation therapy with large skin deficits and malposition of NAC and breast itself. Even if it seems radical, it usually makes sense to perform a complete mastectomy and reconstruction with autologous tissue. The shape of the mastectomy and its structure must then be planned individually (► Chap. 10). However, it is important that implant reconstruction is rather contraindicated in such cases after radiation, since implants after radiation can lead to a high rate of implant failure. Autologous tissue is the key to success.

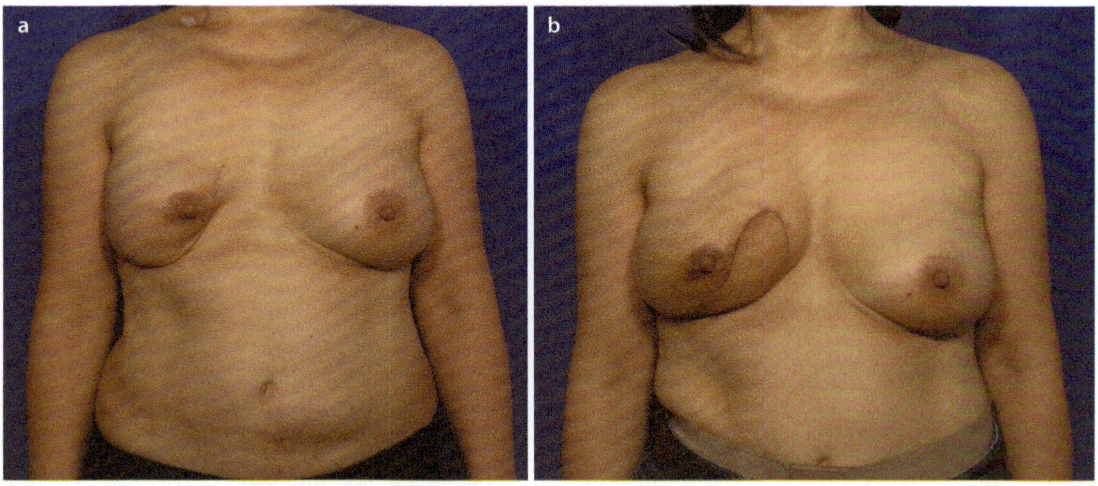

Fig. 12.2 **a** Patient after mastectomy right and DIEP reconstruction (elsewhere). Resection of a local medial recurrence with removal of the medial DIEP-flap. Patient desired a medial breast reconstruction. Despite the resection of the medial DIEP-flap, the lateral DIEP remained well perfused and soft. **b** Reconstruction of the medial breast with a IT-flap from the opposite side. Anastomosis to the IMA cranial of the first DIEP anastomosis. Results after 3 weeks

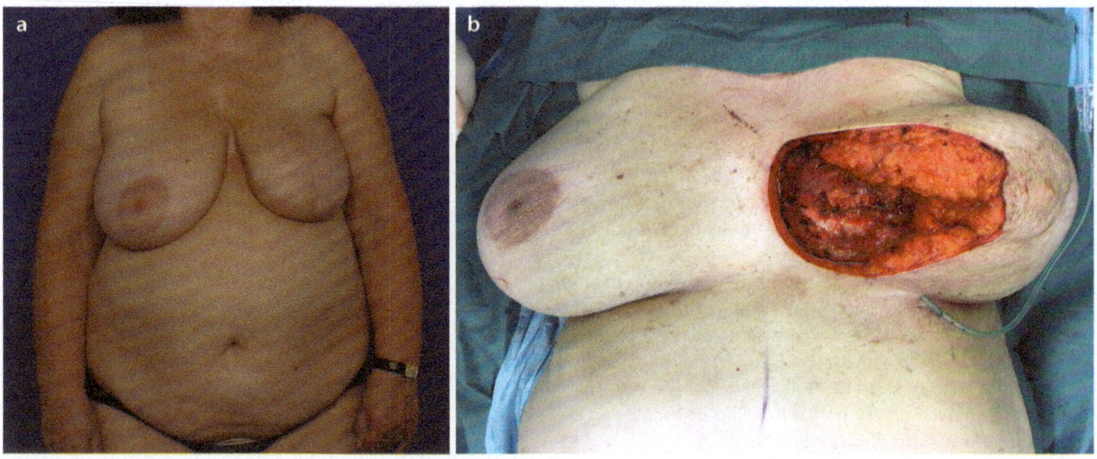

Fig. 12.3 **a** Patient with recurrence (DCIS) after BCT 6 years ago. The recurrence is close to the sternum. **b** Resection and resulting defect. **c** Harvested SIEA-flap. **d** Anastomosis to a IMAP. **e** Result after 1 week

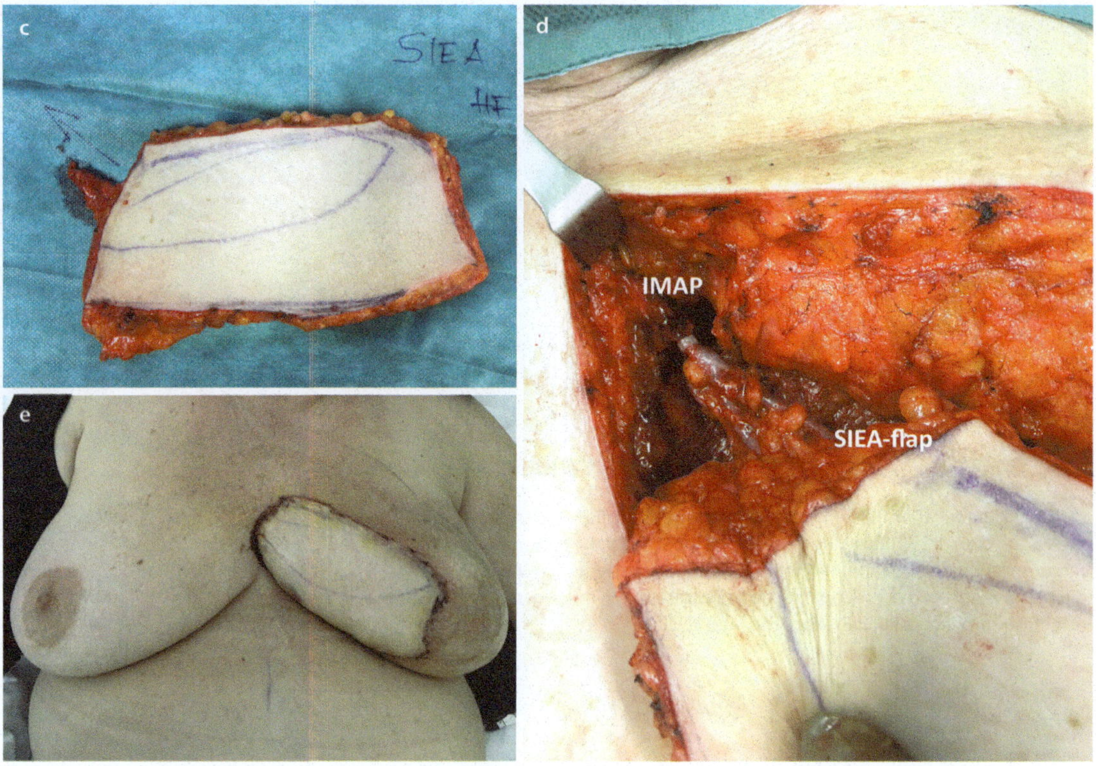

Fig. 12.3 (continued)

Literature

1. Bohmert H. Experience in breast reconstruction with thoraco-epigastric and advancement flaps. Acta Chir Belg. 1980;79:105–10.
2. Chetta MD, Aliu O, Zhong L, Sears ED, Waljee JF, Chung KC, Momoh AO. Reconstruction of the irradiated breast: a national claims-based assessment of postoperative morbidity. Plast Reconstr Surg. 2017;139:783–92.
3. Hakakian CS, Lockhart RA, Kulber DA, Aronowitz JA. Lateral intercostal artery perforator flap in breast reconstruction: a simplified pedicle permits an expanded role. Ann Plast Surg. 2016;76(Suppl 3):S184–90.
4. Hamdi M, Van Landuyt K, de Frene B, Roche N, Blondeel P, Monstrey S. The versatility of the inter-costal artery perforator (ICAP) flaps. J Plast Reconstr Aesthet Surg. 2006;59:644–52.
5. Jeon EY, Cho YK, Yoon DY, Seo YL, Lim KJ, Yun EJ. Angiographic analysis of the lateral intercostal artery perforator of the posterior intercostal artery: anatomic variation and clinical significance. Diagn Interv Radiol. 2015;21:415–8.
6. Mirzabeigi MN, Lanni M, Chang CS, Stark RY, Kovach SJ, Wu LC, Serletti JM, Bucky LP. Treating breast conservation therapy defects with brava and fat grafting: technique, outcomes, and safety profile. Plast Reconstr Surg. 2017;140:372e–81e.
7. Persichetti P, Tenna S, Brunetti B, Aveta A, Segreto F, Marangi GF. Anterior intercostal artery perforator flap autologous augmentation in bariatric mastopexy. Plast Reconstr Surg. 2012;130:917–25.

Reconstruction Using Lipofilling/Fat Grafting

H. Fansa, C. Heitmann, *Breast Reconstruction with Autologous Tissue*,
https://doi.org/10.1007/978-3-319-95468-4_13

Lipofilling is the injection of aspirated fat from the same patient, which is specially prepared. Fat transplantation, autologous fat grafting (AFG) and lipofilling are synonyms.

The technique was first described in the late nineteenth century. Since the procedure was not yet mature, healing rates and results left much to be desired. Coleman and others reintroduced lipofilling to clinical practice, and the process became popular again in the late 1980s. Coleman initially used it only as a filler substance in the face; the other indications were slowly added. Today, it is hard to imagine reconstructive surgery without lipofilling, although there are still many uncertainties.

There is currently no prospectively randomized study on the best sampling methods, the healing effects and possible breast cancer inductions. Everything we currently know we know from clinical observations. What is becoming increasingly clear, however, is that patients who have received lipofilling to improve breast symmetry after breast cancer-related procedures have a better quality of life. In this way, however, we can offer patients a good surgical technique with few complications.

13.1 Indications

Lipofilling can be used wherever an age-related loss of fat tissue occurs. But also disease-related fat loss is an indication. In addition to these physiological or pathological atrophies, lipofilling can also be used for contour defects, dents, scars or thinned out subcutaneous fat tissue after the treatment of breast cancer. The euphoria of the treatment of radiation-induced changes has subsided, as has the de novo reconstruction of the breast after ablation only by autologous fat. Although this indication is offered in special cases, it currently remains a niche market due to the multiple interventions and the not always predictive successes.

From our point of view, the indication is mainly the compensation of contour irregularities and dents, asymmetries and scars. It is also possible to reline the subcutaneous fat layer, e.g. after a mastectomy. Also autologous flaps can be improved with lipofilling especially in the transition zones between mastectomy skin and the flap or in augmenting the flap with lipofilling.

13.1.1 Safety

Lipofilling is safe when applied to healthy tissue according to the current state of knowledge. Questions arose after lipofilling was used to fill defects according to BCT whether this would induce a local recurrence. In animal studies, the stem cells present in the lipoaspirate have been able to induce a malignancy. Clinically, these fears have not yet been confirmed.

In Germany, there is an S2 k guideline for autologous fat transplantation. This recommends caution with lipofilling if the patient has a proven genetic predisposition (e.g. BRCA1) or a positive family history. Also, after a BCT in DCIS or invasive carcinomas, lipofilling is recommended only after "2 years recurrence-free period" after initial surgical treatment. There should be no contraindication after SSM. Until a prospective multicentre study is available, which may provide clear indications and contraindications, we are dependent on clinical observations.

! Lipofilling is safe according to the current state of knowledge. The indications should follow the current guidelines for autologous fat transplantation.

13.1.2 Contraindications

In addition to the above-mentioned concerns about genetic breast cancer disposition, active breast cancer is a contraindication. Inflammatory events in the donor or recipient area or necessary anticoagulation are also unsuitable. A disease-related or drug-related immunosuppression and a strong smoking abuse and malnutrition (also through diets) are a relative contraindication.

13.1.3 Healing and Frequency of Surgery

The injected fat must revascularize in the recipient bed if it is to survive permanently. The surgeon taking into account the parameters listed below can hardly influence this process. A certain immobilization and the avoidance of tension due to too much fat in the recipient region may contribute to a better healing. A balanced perioperative diet and smoking restriction can have a positive influence on the healing process. However, it can be the case that only 30–50% of the injected fat heals. If this is not enough, the procedure must be repeated. In our experience one should wait 3–6 months between the interventions. This fact that fat might not heal must be discussed with the patients in advance.

13.2 Physiology

The fat is aspirated under sterile conditions at one part of the body, decanted and concentrated and then injected into the desired region. In order not to damage the cells during suction, suction should be performed gently, i.e. with a reduced vacuum. The fat is then decanted, i.e. freed of detritus, tumescent solution and oil. It is then sterile injected. Since the fat only survives if it revascularizes in the recipient area, the injection should be fan-shaped. An injection as a bolus is unsuitable, as only a fat necrosis or oil cysts develop. The type of injection, pressure, distribution and the recipient bed determines healing. Too high injection volumes increase tissue tension and reduce capillary perfusion and thus healing. When vital cells reach the recipient bed, they survive there by diffusion until revascularization, which should take place by the fifth postoperative day at the latest. Stem cells contained in fat are also involved in the healing process.

13.3 Informed Consent

The disclosure of general and special risks should be documented with standardized and evaluated forms. Infection, hematoma and wound healing complications can occur. Dents, asymmetries and skin changes can occur in the donor area. The non-healing of the injected fat and asymmetries in the recipient area should also be mentioned. In very rare cases, the fat can calcify, be converted into cysts and result in a second operation. Reoperation may be required if the desired effect is not achieved. Radiological checks are possible after half a year, but patients should point out the lipofilling to the radiologist, since fat necrosis, cysts or calcifications occur after lipofilling and can be confused with malignant findings.

Also planned second interventions should always be mentioned in advance. Any information and discussion about the risks of the operations should be documented in writing. Telephone calls (as telephone notes) or e-mails should also be included in the patient file.

! The non-healing of fat and asymmetries in the recipient area and in the donor area should also be mentioned. Reoperations may be necessary.

13.4 Technique

Lipofilling is a simple technique but also an operation that requires a lot of material. The operation is performed under sterile conditions. First, the fat is aspirated at the previously agreed location. We prefer either the conventional tumescence technique, in which the tumescent solution is first infiltrated, and then suction can be performed following. Alternatively, the water jet-assisted technique can be used, in which the fat is simultaneously aspirated, while the water jet helps to dissolve the fat.

The operation can be performed under local or general anaesthesia, as an outpatient or inpatient, depending on the effort involved. The positioning on the operation table depends on the removal and recipient areas.

13.4.1 Tumescence Solution

The solution consists of lidocaine and adrenaline in 0.9% saline solution. According to Pace et al., bicarbonate is not necessary as a buffer because it does not buffer sufficiently in the used concentration, but there is a risk of precipitation.

The infiltration solution consists of lidocaine 0.05% with adrenaline 1:1.000.000; this corresponds to 1000 ml 0.9% saline solution with 50 ml 1% lidocaine and 1 ml adrenaline 1:1000. A maximal dose of 35 mg per kgBW is recommended (Table 13.1) [5].

13.4.2 Aspiration and Preparation

The donor area depends on the agreement with the patient. The areas on the flanks, the abdomen and the inner and outer thighs are common. If diet-resistant fat deposits are used as a donor site, the result of the healing is considered to be

Table 13.1 Maximal infiltration amount of tumescence solution with respect to body weight. For example, in a 70 kg patient, a maximum dosage of 35 mg/kg allows a maximum infiltration of 2450 mg lidocaine. With a 0.05% lidocaine solution, a maximum amount of 4900 ml would be safe [5]

Body weight (kg)	Max. infiltration (litre)
50	3.5
60	4.2
70	4.9
80	5.6
90	6.3
100	7.0

slightly better. If desired, the aspiration for the lipofilling can be combined with an aesthetic suction. However, additional information on the risks should be provided. The needles are inserted via small incisions.

Suction is performed after infiltration or together using the water jet infiltration. Suction should not exceed 500 mbar; otherwise the cells are endangered in their vitality. The aspiration cannula should not be smaller than 2 mm in diameter. There is evidence that longer cannulas may damage more cells. The skin should not be damaged during suction, and dents and asymmetries should be avoided. In this context, reference is made to textbooks on plastic surgery. The skin is closed with non-absorbable suture material (nylon 5–0 or 6–0).

13

Once the fat has been aspirated, the excess solution can be decanted. This can be done by centrifugation or simply by letting it stand. The fat "swims" on top of the tumescent solution. The oil is on top of the fat. Depending on the process, the decanted fat can now be transferred into syringes via a filter that takes out the detritus. Due to current legal regulations (in Germany), the removed tissue is not to be stored but must be used immediately. When adding platelet-rich plasma (PRP), the necessary legal requirements must be observed.

13.4.3 Filling and Transplantation

The success of the injection depends on several factors: the type and diameter of the cannulas, the type and volume of the syringe, the application technique and the anatomical situation. For injection at the breast, 3, 5 and 10 ml syringes with Luer Lock are suitable. The pressure used to inject the fat should not be too strong, as otherwise the cells can die during injection. The needles should not be too long and blunt at the front. Too long, too bent and too thin cannulas can impair the result. Cannula thickness should be between 1 mm and 3 mm. Application aids are also offered. All cannulas are now also available as disposable needles.

The needle is inserted through a puncture incision with an 11-blade or 18-gauge cannula. The puncture sites, especially after a cannula puncture, usually leave no scars. The injection must be homogeneous in small portions; a bolus must be avoided as it is not revascularized. The simplest applications are fan-shaped applications in several tunnels in which ideally a fat strand is placed in the tissue no thicker than 3 mm (Figs. 13.1, 13.2, 13.3, and 13.4). This offers the chance to be revascularized from all sides. In a fan-shaped injection with injection channels offset at 90° to each other, a 3D structure of fat strands can thus

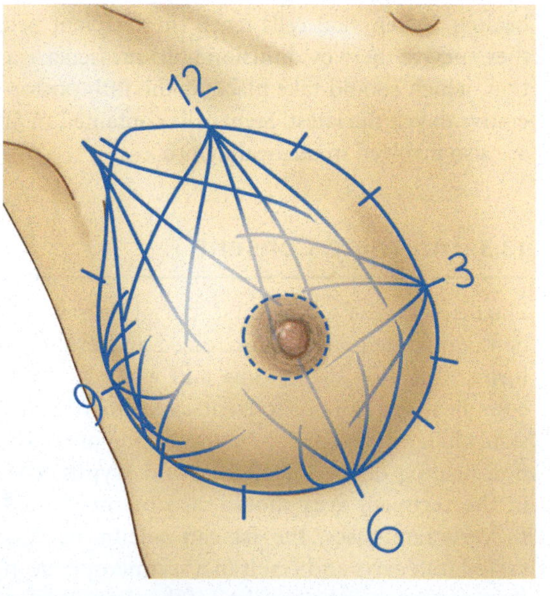

Fig. 13.1 Planning of lipofilling on the right breast modified according to Khouri Jr and Khouri [5]. A clockwise distribution facilitates documentation and avoids double injections. The fan-shaped injection in thin strands allows optimal revascularization. The injection is performed in the base of the breast and also from periareolar into the subcutaneous breast skin. The movement from periareolar to the thoracic wall is easier than from the base to apical. When using long cannulas, the application must be carried out carefully to prevent injuries to the thorax

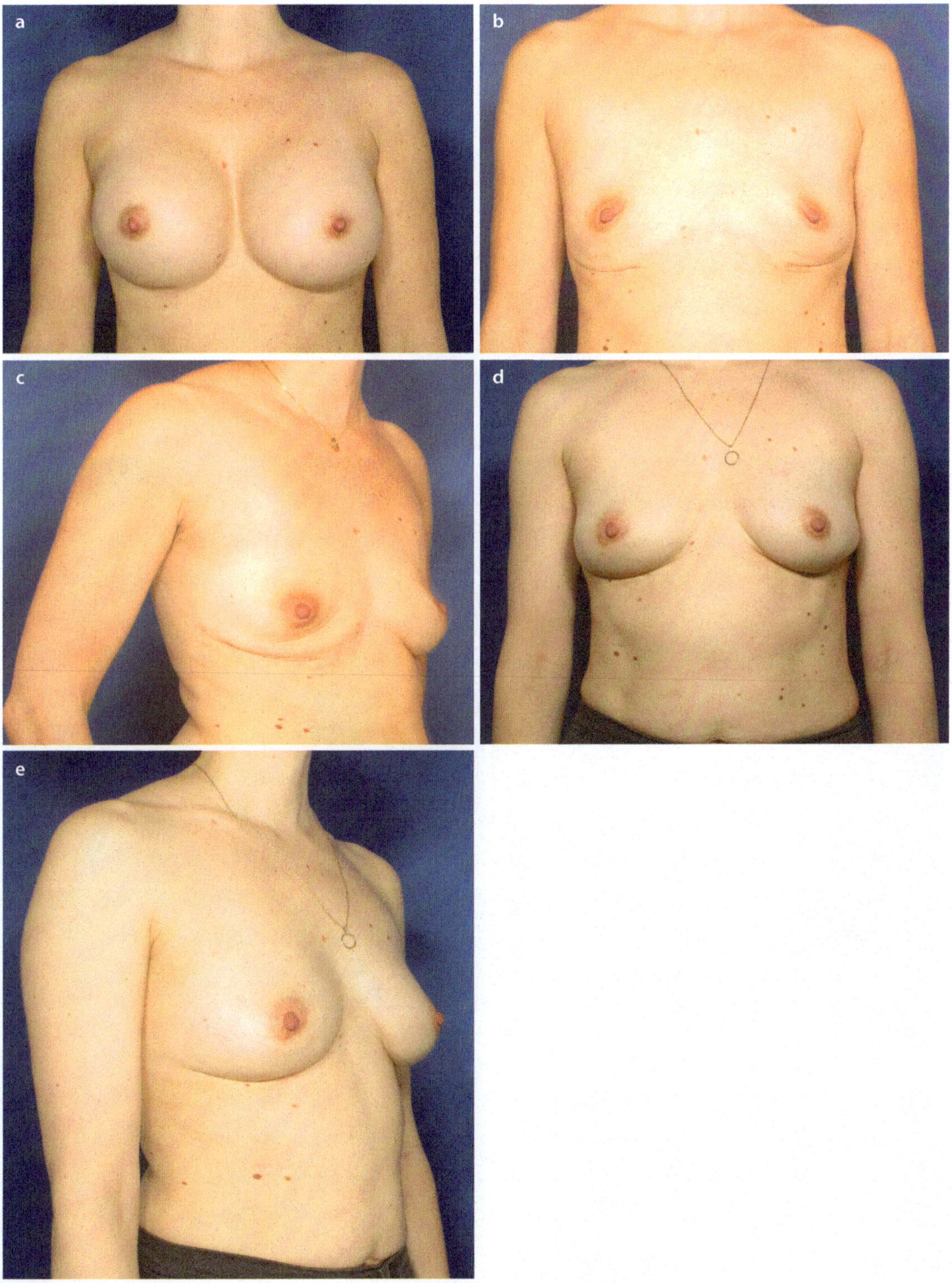

Fig. 13.2 **a** Example of a patient with capsular contracture. She wanted the implants removed without any further measures. **b, c** After removal, the breast was ptotic. A lipofilling session was then performed, in which 200 ml per breast were injected. **d, e** Result after 6 months. A further lipofilling was no longer desired

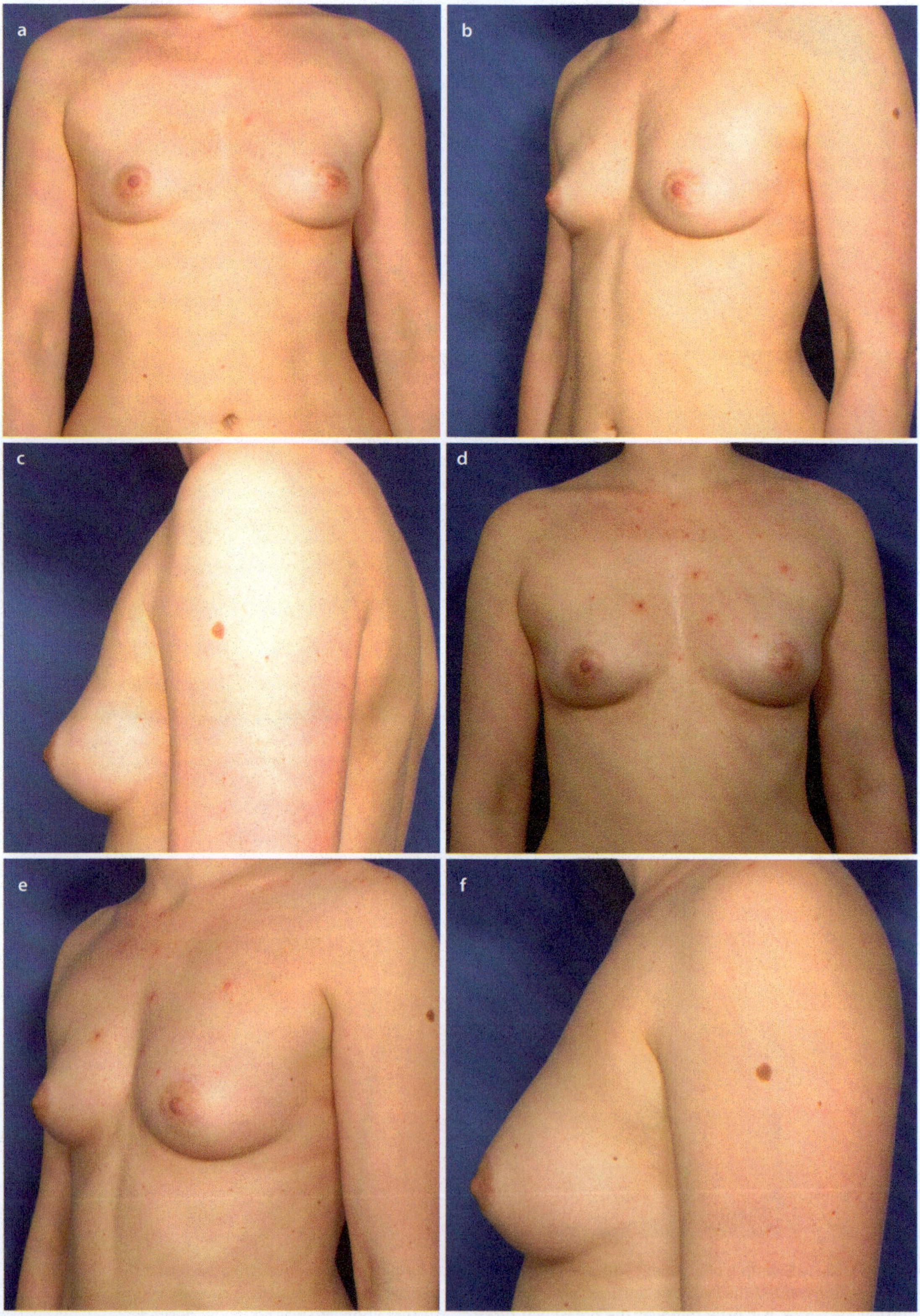

Fig. 13.3 **a–c** Example of a patient with hypoplastic and asymmetrical breasts. An implant was rejected. Lipofilling was performed, in which about 200 ml was injected on the right and about 150 ml on the left. **d–f** Result after 6 months. The volume could be filled in all parts; a slight reduction of the too high IMF on the right was also possible

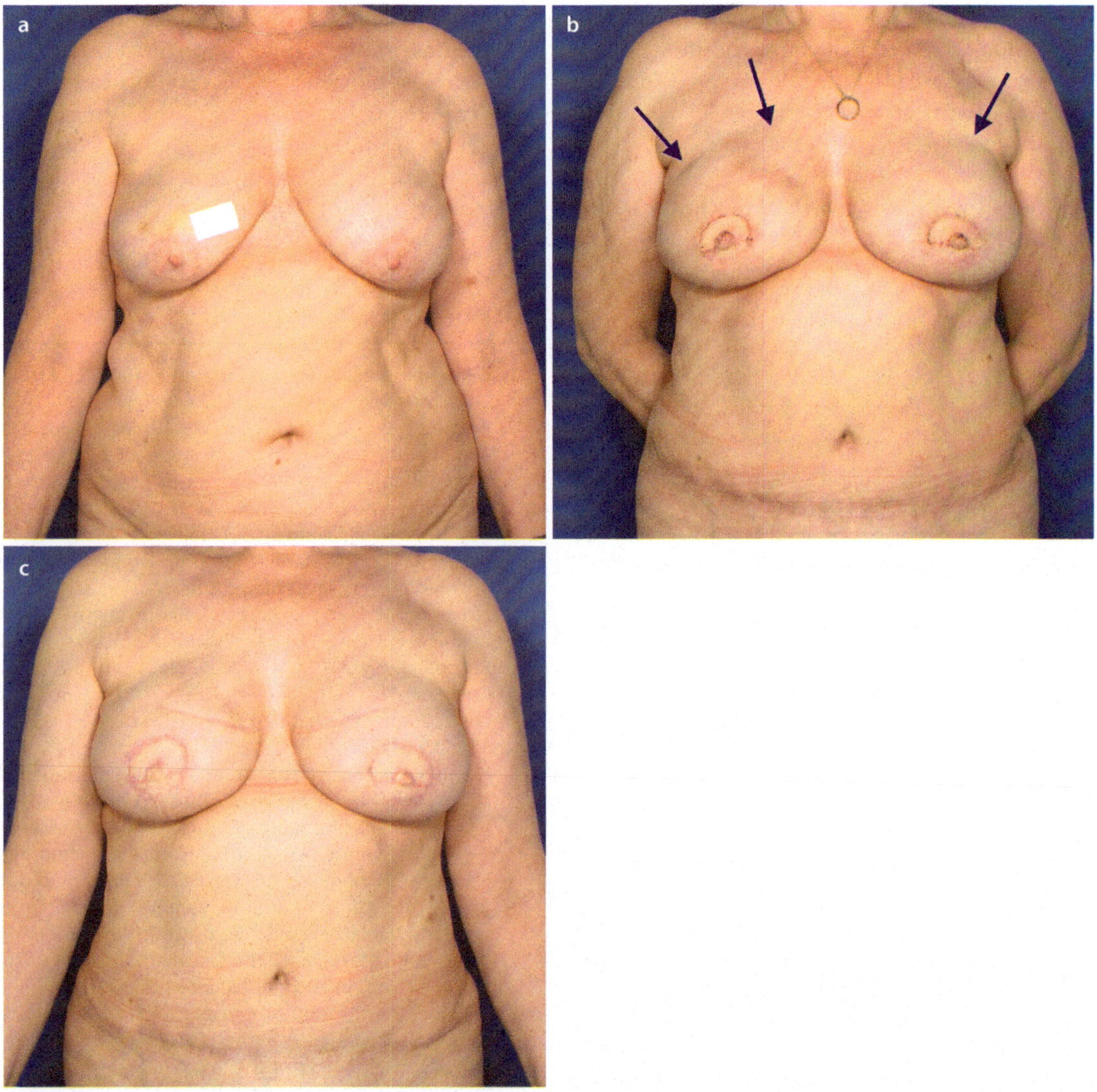

■ **Fig. 13.4** **a** Patient with breast carcinoma (right) and prophylactic mastectomy (left). **b** SSM on both sides with DIEP flap and subsequent nipple reconstruction. The patient wanted to improve the transition zone between the flap and the cranial thoracic skin. **c** Six months after lipofilling, the situation improved, more on the right than on the left side

be produced. Injection can be done from basal to ventral. Direct injection into glandular tissue should be avoided. Otherwise, injections can easily be placed in muscle, in perimuscular tissue subcutaneously or in autologous reconstructed tissues. Lipofilling between implant and skin is a special feature. Care must be taken not to damage the implant during the injection. If lipofilling is performed as part of an implant change, it can be injected either with the old implant/expander in place or after removal of the old implant and before the new implant is positioned. The tissue can be held under tension with a Kocher forceps so that it can be injected more easily.

With scars, advancing the cannula can be difficult. Such resistance should not be overcome with force, as slipping of the cannulas into the thorax can be a serious complication. In such cases, an attempt can be made to make the tissue slightly more receptive with a kind of subcutaneous scar release through an 18-gauge cannula ("Rigottomies", named after the Italian surgeon Gino Rigotti and the suffix -tomy). The cannula is inserted through the skin and used like an inner blade. Scars are released, and an inner mesh/expansion is created that can accommodate more fat. However, such a scar release can also impair the revascularization of the fat.

Key Techniques According to Khouri Jr and Khouri [5]
- No injection without motion
- Injection/motion rate <0.1 ml
- Sprinkle with precision
- Smaller syringe → greater precision
- No two motions in the same direction

13.4.4 After Treatment

Compression garments have been proven for at least 2 weeks in the donor sites to avoid seromas and shearing and to support the skin in shrinking. Manipulation should be avoided in the recipient area. Ideally, the area should be immobilized with a bra or a soft plaster bandage, for example. Smoking, dieting or exercising should be avoided in the first few weeks. In the first few days, the recipient area may swell and turn red. Here, a natural inflammatory reaction must be distinguished from an infection.

13

13.5 Complications

The surgical complication rate is low if the procedure is carried out properly. Larger haematomas can occur in the donor site, depending on the area. These are usually treated conservatively. Nerve injuries are extremely rare. A permanent loss of sensitivity should be examined. Abdominal injuries due to the aspiration in that area were described, but overall they are extremely rare. If there is a suspicion, a general surgeon must be called immediately. In the case of extensive aspiration or poor skin quality, a dimpling of the skin may occur, which may result in subsequent lifting operation. Asymmetries that have to be corrected can also occur. It is important to point this out in advance in the case of existing preoperative asymmetries. Wound healing disorders are very rare in sterile procedures. A very rare complication is necrotizing fasciitis, which requires immediate revision by experienced plastic surgeons and intensive treatment.

In the recipient area, the fat cannot heal at all or even asymmetrically. Conversions of fat into fat necrosis, oil cysts or calcification can occur. Few case reports have described the formation of a carcinoma after lipofilling. If an unclear tumour is suspected, a quick diagnostic clarification and therapy is recommended.

Literature

1. German guidelines autologous fat grafting: http://www.awmf.org/leitlinien/detail/ll/009-017.html
2. Bennett KG, Qi J, Kim HM, Hamill JB, Wilkins EG, Mehrara BJ, Kozlow JH. Association of fat grafting with patient-reported outcomes in postmastectomy breast reconstruction. JAMA Surg. 2017; https://doi.org/10.1001/jamasurg.2017.1716.
3. Cohen O, Lam G, Karp N, Choi M. Determining the oncologic safety of autologous fat grafting as a reconstructive modality: an institutional review of breast cancer recurrence rates and surgical outcomes. Plast Reconstr Surg. 2017;140:382e–92e.
4. Coleman SR. Long-term survival of fat transplants: controlled demonstrations. Aesthet Plast Surg. 1995;19:421–5.
5. Khouri RK Jr, Khouri RK. Current clinical applications of fat grafting. Plast Reconstr Surg. 2017;140:466e–86e.
6. Luan A, Zielins ER, Wearda T, Atashroo DA, Blackshear CP, Raphel J, Brett EA, Flacco J, Alyono MC, Momeni A, Heilshorn S, Longaker MT, Wan DC. Dynamic rheology for the prediction of surgical outcomes in autologous fat grafting. Plast Reconstr Surg. 2017;140:517–24.
7. Mazzola RF, Mazzola IC. The fascinating history of fat grafting. J Craniofac Surg. 2013;24:1069–71.
8. Mirzabeigi MN, Lanni M, Chang CS, Stark RY, Kovach SJ, Wu LC, Serletti JM, Bucky LP. Treating breast conservation therapy defects with brava and fat grafting: technique, outcomes, and safety profile. Plast Reconstr Surg. 2017;140:372e–81e.
9. Pace MM, Chatterjee A, Merrill DG, Stotland MA, Ridgway EB. Local anesthetics in liposuction: considerations for new practice advisory guidelines to improve patient safety. Plast Reconstr Surg. 2013;131:820e–6e.
10. Petit JY, Maisonneuve P, Rotmensz N, Bertolini F, Rietjens M. Fat grafting after invasive breast cancer: a matched case-control study. Plast Reconstr Surg. 2017;139:1292–6.
11. Serra-Mestre JM, Fernandez Peñuela R, Foti V, D'Andrea F, Serra-Renom JM. Breast cleavage remodeling with fat grafting: a safe way to optimize symmetry and to reduce intermammary distance. Plast Reconstr Surg. 2017;140:665e–72e.
12. Sinno S, Wilson S, Brownstone N, Levine SM. Current thoughts on fat grafting: using the evidence to determine fact or fiction. Plast Reconstr Surg. 2016;137:818–24.
13. Spear SL, Coles CN, Leung BK, Gitlin M, Parekh M, Macarios D. The safety, effectiveness, and efficiency of autologous fat grafting in breast surgery. Plast Reconstr Surg Glob Open. 2016;4:e827.

Reconstruction of the Nipple Areola Complex (NAC)

H. Fansa, C. Heitmann, *Breast Reconstruction with Autologous Tissue*,
https://doi.org/10.1007/978-3-319-95468-4_14

The reconstruction of the nipple-areola complex (NAC) should be the last step in breast reconstruction. Asymmetric placement can affect the aesthetic result. Therefore, reconstruction should only be performed in exceptional cases during the volume reconstruction. In the case of bilateral reconstructions, the nipple reconstruction should also be performed on one side at most during the volume reconstruction. Whether a NAK reconstruction is to be carried out is determined by the patient. The ideal time is 3–6 months after completion of the volume reconstruction.

A distinction must be made between the reconstruction of the nipple and the areola. The reconstruction of the nipple is the first step.

14.1 Position

In single-sided reconstructions and symmetrical breasts, the position can be easily determined by orienting oneself to the contralateral side. As always, the marking is done with the patient in upright position with hanging arms. The jugular notch-nipple distance, the nipple-sternum distance and the midline of the breast serve as orientation. The nipple should always be marked in front of a mirror together with the patient before the operation in order to avoid incorrect positions. Patients can also apply a round ECG pad to the desired position. This almost always gives an exact and consented position (◘ Figs. 14.1 and 14.2).

It becomes more difficult if the healthy opposite side is not symmetrical. If the patient wants to have an alignment operation on the healthy side (tightening/reduction/augmentation), first wait for the volume correction and later reconstruct the nipple. If she does not want an operation on the opposite side and if positioning in orientation to the opposite side is not possible, e.g. due to a ptosis, the nipple should be oriented on the reconstructed breast.

In the case of bilateral reconstructions, position determination after completion of the volume reconstruction is usually possible without any problems.

14.2 Nipple Reconstruction

14.2.1 Pigmentation

If the patient does not want an elevated nipple, the nipple can be optically reconstructed in 3D technique as part of the areola pigmentation. This procedure is inexpensive and avoids new scars.

14.2.2 Nipple Sharing

In this technique, a portion of the opposite side is removed and grafted to the desired position as a free graft like a full-thickness skin graft. This method is particularly suitable for large nipples. We prefer nipple sharing from the lower part of the healthy nipple. The upper part is then folded to a caudal closure (◘ Fig. 14.3). The scar

14

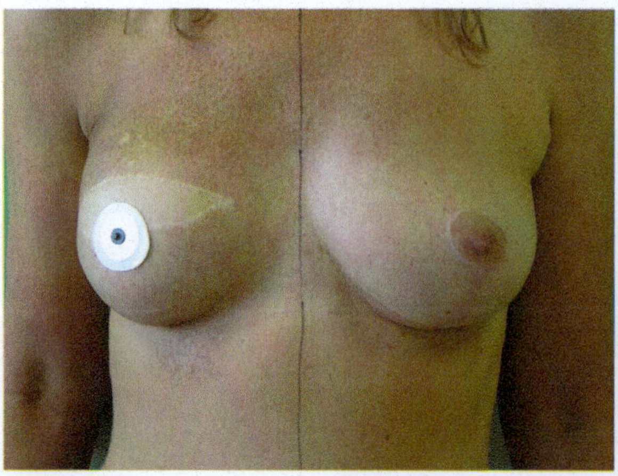

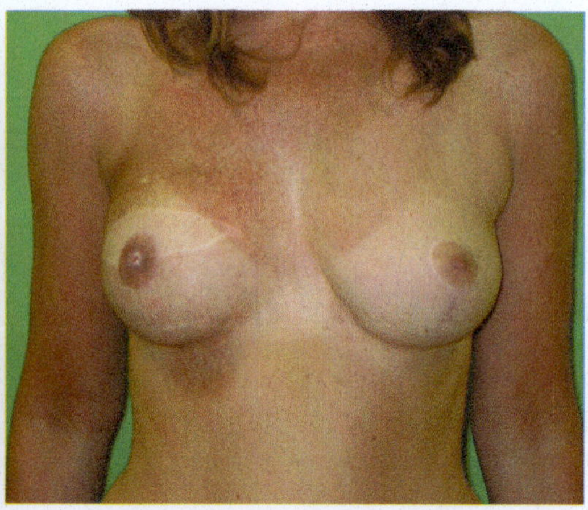

◘ **Figs. 14.1 and 14.2** Patient with secondary DIEP after radiation therapy. The ECG pad was stuck in front of the mirror by the patient herself. The nipple (here nipple sharing) is placed exactly at this position

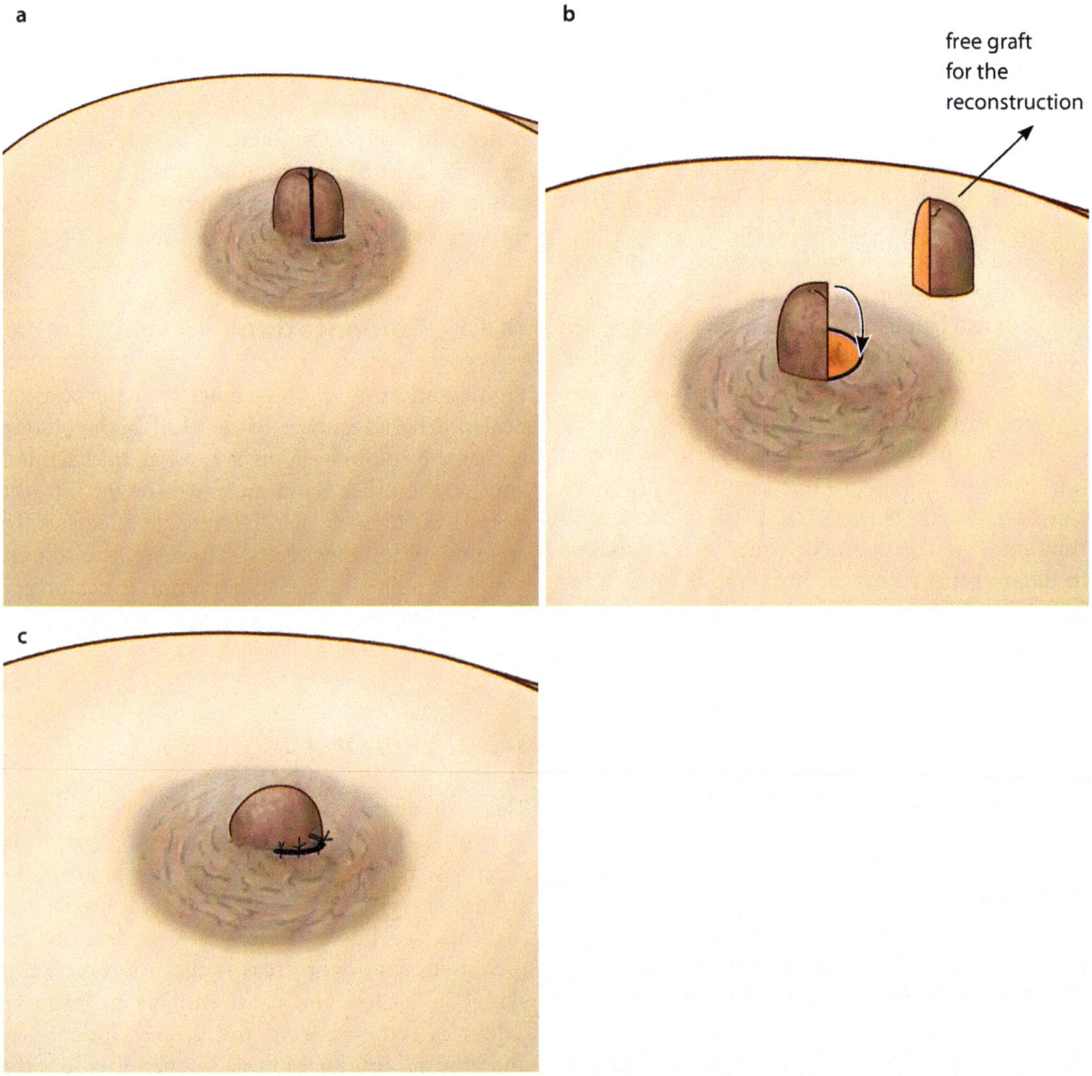

Fig. 14.3 **a, b** In nipple sharing, the lower third/half of the healthy nipple is resected under local anaesthesia. **c** The cranial part of the nipple is sutured caudally with single interrupted sutures. The resected part is grafted to its new position after de-epithelialization of the new position. The sutures should be done in single interrupted technique (5–0 or 6–0). A compression dressing with a fatty gauze or PU foam provides the necessary compression. The dressing should be left in place for about 5 days

is not very visible. The advantage of this nipple reconstruction is the similar texture and colour of the new nipple. Disadvantageous is a possible loss of sensitivity of the donor nipple and a possible depigmentation in healing disorders (Fig. 14.3).

The operation can be performed under local anaesthesia. The donor nipple is anaesthetised, the lower part is resected and folding down the cranial part of the nipple closes the nipple. The new position is de-epithelialized and the nipple sutured. The suture should be made with non-absorbable material (e.g. Ethilon 5-0 or 6-0). The dressing is done with a fatty gauze and a pressure bandage on top.

14.2.3 Reconstruction of the Nipple with Local Flaps

Local flaps can reconstruct an elevated nipple. Due to scars, tension and pressure, the new nipple always loses about 50% of its projection, depending on the technique. This should be taken into account during planning. Patients should also be informed. Some patients want a big nipple, and others want a low one. The fact that reconstructed nipples are always upright should also be discussed.

The techniques depend on the scars present. There are many different techniques. Usually two standard techniques are sufficient.

The modified star-flap (also called "angel-flap" or C-U or C-V-flap) uses a centrally and cranially pedicled trilobed flap. The sides are harvested either as V or as U, mobilized and sutured together. The C component serves as a cover. The donor site is primarily closed (▫ Figs. 14.4 and 14.5).

The M-Dot flaps allow the integration of existing scars into the flap so that perfusion problems can be avoided (▫ Fig. 14.6). Here two counter-rotating flaps are planned, which are M-shaped in the part that forms the nipple roof. Due to the M shape, they interlock. The wider the base of the flaps, the safer the perfusion, but the nipple becomes more oval.

The operation can be performed under local anaesthesia. The suture is made with resorbable or non-resorbable material (e.g. Monocryl or Ethilon 5-0 or 6-0). The dressing is applied around the new nipple in such a way that it is omitted and supported. Compression on the nipple is avoided.

The complication rate is low if the procedure is carried out properly. Complete or partial necrosis of the reconstructed nipple is possible. Wound-healing disorders during nipple sharing and areola reconstruction with skin grafts can also occur. In most cases a conservative approach is sufficient. Careful debridement and PVP-iodine dressings in the initial phase and dressings with soft polyurethane foam dressing in the healing phase can usually achieve a good result.

Corrections of the nipple shape or over-projecting nipple may occasionally become necessary after healing. This can be done under local anaesthesia. The lack of projection remains a problem that is difficult to solve. This can be concealed somewhat by adequate pigmentation. Many techniques for increasing the projection were described, for example, fat and cartilage, and also various filler substances, primarily hyaluronic acid, were applied to increase the projection. All this has not turned out to be permanent in our hands.

14.3 Areola

The areola is restored either by pigmentation or by skin transplantation. The primary goal is to restore the colour. This should be oriented to the opposite side. The pigmentation differs from the tattoo in that the colour is introduced into the deep epidermis, but not into the dermis.

14.3.1 Pigmentation

Pigmentation should take place after the scar has healed. The advantage of medical pigmentation is that the colours are on the one hand harmless and on the other hand are not brought into the dermis. As a result, hardly any side effects of the colours are to be expected. However, the colours may fade a bit earlier. Pigmentation is performed on an outpatient basis and, if necessary, under local anaesthesia.

14.3.2 Skin Grafting

The areola can also be restored by skin grafting. The skin is taken as full-thickness skin graft from areas which have approximately the colour of the areola. The groin or the contralateral areola and the upper eyelids are suitable. A prerequisite for the latter two donor areas is that there is excess skin. The easiest and most suitable in terms of colour is removal from the groin. Under local anaesthesia (or anaesthesia, depending on the extent of the operation), a full-thickness skin graft measuring about 40–45 mm in diameter is removed. To close the defect, the resection should be marked ellipsoid. The donor site can be closed primarily with resorbable material. A special after-treatment is not necessary.

The resected skin is cleaned from fatty tissue; hair follicles can be removed by pulling them out with a forceps. The skin where the new areola is planned is de-epithelialized with a knife or scissors. Since the full-thickness skin still shrinks slightly, the areola can be planned slightly larger than the opposite side. The circumference can be circular or in the sense of a running-W. The suturing is done continuously with non-absorbable suture material.

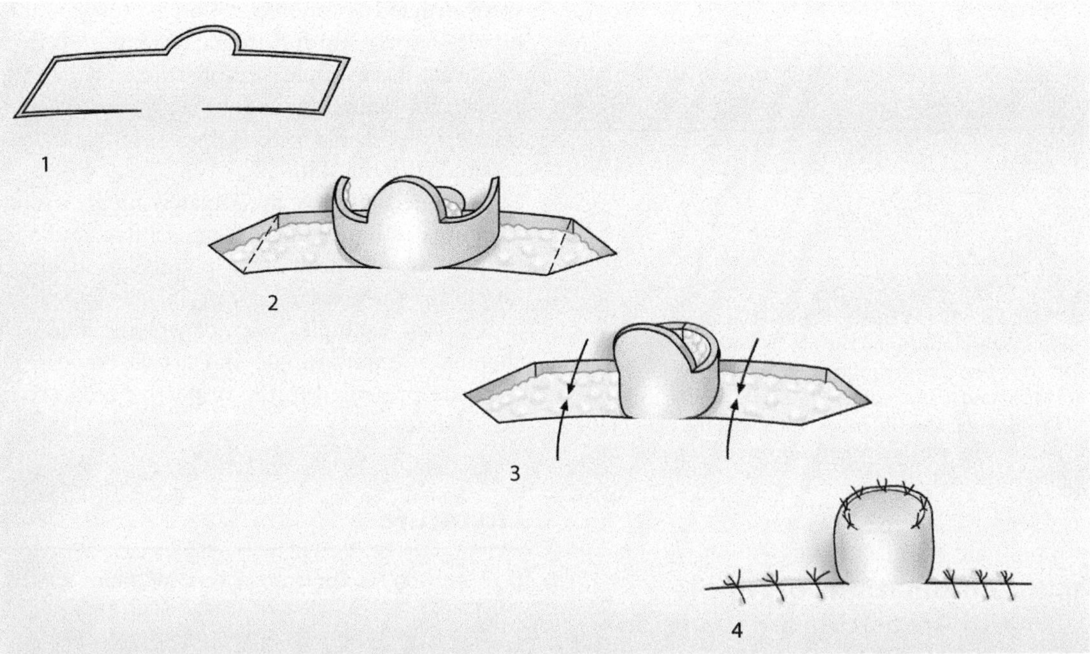

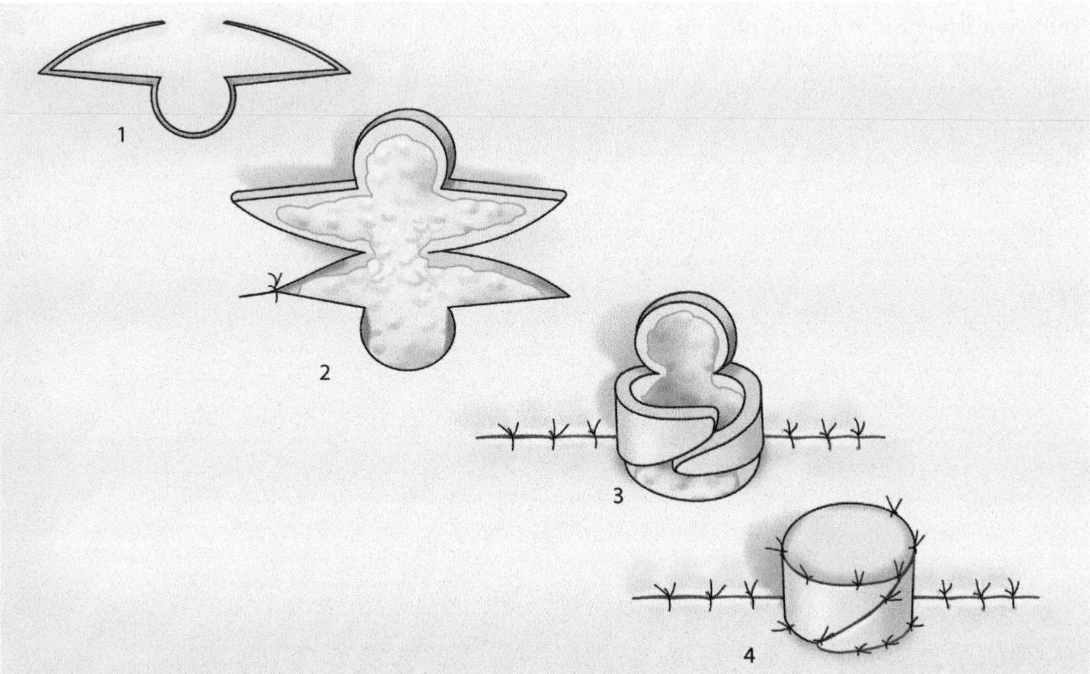

Figs. 14.4 and 14.5 A central and cranial pedicle is used for this C-U-shaped trilobed flap for nipple reconstruction. The sides are elevated either as V or as U, mobilized and sutured together. The use of the U-shape should allow more permanent projection. For better closure of the donor site, the U-component is converted into a triangle. If the flap is pedicled cranially, the scars remain caudal and so little visible. The C component serves as a cover. The donor site is primarily closed. The larger the C, the wider the nipple; the higher the V/U lobe, the higher the nipple. The planning should always include existing scars in order to avoid perfusion disorders

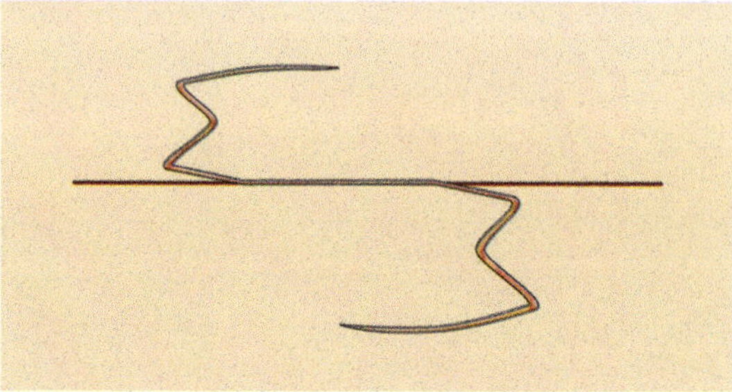

Fig. 14.6 The M-Dot flaps allow the integration of existing scars (horizontal line in this example) into the flap. Here two counter-rotating lobes are placed, which are M-shaped in the part that forms the nipple roof. Due to the M shape, they interlock. The wider the base of the flaps, the safer the blood perfusion, but this makes the nipple more oval

14.4 Combinations of Nipple and Areolar Reconstructions

The reconstruction of the nipple and the areola can be done together or separately. Certain processes can preferably be combined with each other. One technique in which everything is reconstructed in one operation is, for example, nipple sharing and full-thickness skin graft from the groin. If the nipple is reconstructed with a flap and a full-thickness skin graft is planned, the new nipple must also be de-epithelialized and then covered with the skin.

An alternative is the isolated nipple reconstruction, as nipple sharing or as a flap, and after the wound has healed the pigmentation of the nipple and the areola.

Clinical examples are not presented in this chapter, as many nipple and areola reconstructions are presented in the respective reconstruction chapters.

Literature

1. Halvorson EG, Cormican M, West ME, Myers V. Three-dimensional nipple-areola tattooing: a new technique with superior results. Plast Reconstr Surg. 2014;133:1073–5.
2. Kroll SS, Reece GP, Miller MJ, Evans GR, Robb GL, Baldwin BJ, Wang BG, Schusterman MA. Comparison of nipple projection with the modified double-opposing tab and star flaps. Plast Reconstr Surg. 1997;99:1602–5.

Aplasia

H. Fansa, C. Heitmann, *Breast Reconstruction with Autologous Tissue*,
https://doi.org/10.1007/978-3-319-95468-4_15

Breast aplasia may be congenital or may occur after surgery. A known genetic aplasia is the Poland syndrome: usually the breast and the pectoral muscles are missing (◘ Figs. 15.1, 15.2, and 15.3). In rare cases, changes in the arm and hand (symbrachy-phalangia) may occur. Poland syndrome is more frequently localized on the right side and more frequently in men than in women. Exact data is missing. In Poland syndrome, not only the missing breast but often also the missing contour of the pectoralis muscles, i.e. the anterior border of the axilla, is disturbing for the patients. The extent can vary.

Iatrogenic aplasia can occur if the mammary gland is damaged prepubertally. During cardiac and thoracic surgery in children, the gland can be damaged if the incision is made at breast level. However, this usually only becomes apparent when breast growth begins and the affected side does not develop.

Burns during childhood can also damage the skin and the gland to such an extent that growth does not occur. The gland itself may have been damaged, or the scar contracture resulting from the burn or its treatment hinders the development and growth of the gland.

15.1 Therapy

The reconstruction uses all the techniques described so far and must be discussed individually with the patient and, if necessary, her parents.

If the breast is not at all developed, not only the breast volume but also the breast skin must be reconstructed. Of course, the skin can also be reconstructed by flap surgery. This can be the method of choice, especially after burn scars. However, the resulting scars and the different skin colour can impair the acceptance of the reconstruction.

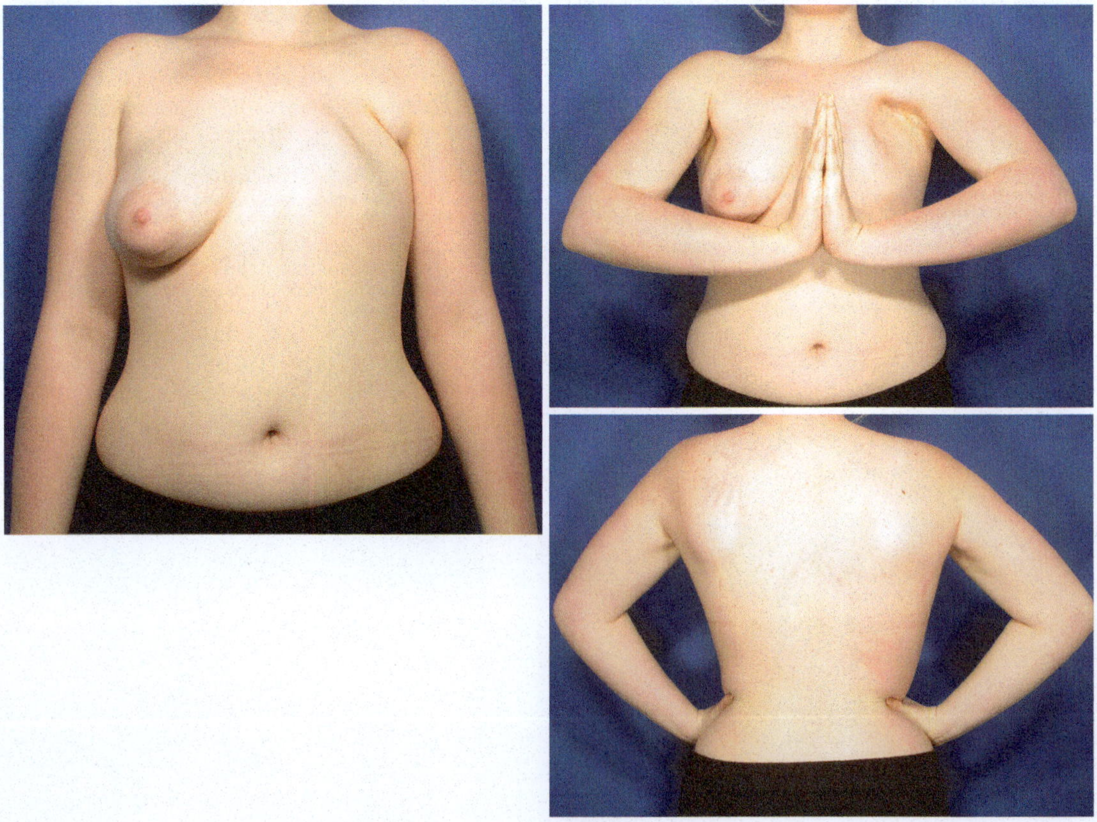

◘ **Figs. 15.1–15.3** Poland syndrome with thoracic deformity, aplasia of the breast with missing nipple and missing pectoralis major/minor muscle on the left. Muscle contraction of the pectoral muscles shows that the anterior axillar border is completely missing. The malformation of the entire left shoulder girdle can also be seen from dorsal

15.2 Time Line

Both breast growth and thoracic growth should be completed in these extensive reconstructions; otherwise chest deformities or aesthetically inadequate results may occur. Breast growth is often completed before the patients become adults. The exact time of reconstruction should be discussed with the patient and the parents.

15.3 Techniques

15.3.1 Expander

In aplasia, it is necessary to reconstruct the breast skin first. With the new, anatomically shaped and fixable expanders with integrated port, the reconstruction is much more reliable than with conventional round expanders.

The selection of the expander depends on the healthy breast. If this is very large, the reconstruction concept can include a reduction (as last step) of the healthy side.

When an expander is inserted, the future borders of the breast must be defined medially and in the IMF. In addition, it can become difficult to caudalize the nipple, which is usually positioned more cranially and laterally. Here a later operation may be necessary, during which the NAC is transposed or freely grafted.

The position of the expander should be epimuscular when stretching the skin. A submuscular position is possible, but due to the ventral muscle tension, it can lead to deformity of the rib cage if the ribs are pressed towards the thorax especially in younger patients. Such deformity does not lead to breathing problems but reduces the projection of future breast reconstructions by the extent of the "dent". The incision should be made in the future IMF and should be oriented to match the healthy breast.

15.3.2 Reconstruction

The reconstruction of the volume and the shape can be carried out after completion of the expansion, either with autologous tissue or implants, possibly combined with lipofilling. In very slender patients with little donor tissue, an implant can be inserted first, which is later converted into an autologous tissue reconstruction. The advantages and disadvantages of the respective procedures are to be discussed with the patient and, if necessary, her parents.

In addition to the insertion of regular implants, custom-made implants can also be used after expansion. However, these usually have a higher complication rate with regard to encapsulation and dislocation.

The incision should follow the expander incision. If the pectoral muscle is present, the implant can be placed in the cranial part submuscularly or epipectorally with the appropriate skin thickness. In the case of aplasia of the muscle, it is located under the skin. If a transposition of the latissimus muscle is planned, the implant position is below the muscles and the skin island.

A reconstruction of the pectoralis muscle contour, i.e. the frontal axillary fold, is only possible with autologous tissue. This usually requires an additional axillary incision. The transposed latissimus dorsi muscle can reconstruct the contour. In this technique, the tendinous insertion of the latissimus muscle is used to imitate the ventral pectoralis contour. To maintain the posterior contour of the axilla, however, the teres major muscle, which runs together with the latissimus dorsi muscle, should be retained.

Another form of contour reconstruction of the pectoralis is the IT-flap (◘ Figs. 15.4, 15.5, 15.6, 15.7, 15.8, 15.9, 15.10, 15.11, 15.12, and 15.13). The fat of the thigh serves the volume reconstruction; the *M. gracilis* can restore the contour. Bilateral IT-flaps can also be used for one breast. The anastomosis is then made at the IMA or its perforators for the breast volume or in the axilla at the subscapular vessels for the axillary contour or volume compensation of the thorax. Some groups suggest a neurotization of the gracilis muscle. Branches of the pectoral nerves (if present) or intercostal nerves may be used for this purpose. End-to-side coaptation to the thoracodorsal nerve has also been described. Whether this neurotization improves, the outcome cannot be assessed on the basis of the few case numbers.

In addition to reconstructions with autologous tissue from the thigh, other autologous tissue reconstructions such as DIEP flap surgery or gluteal flap surgery for volume reconstructions are also possible.

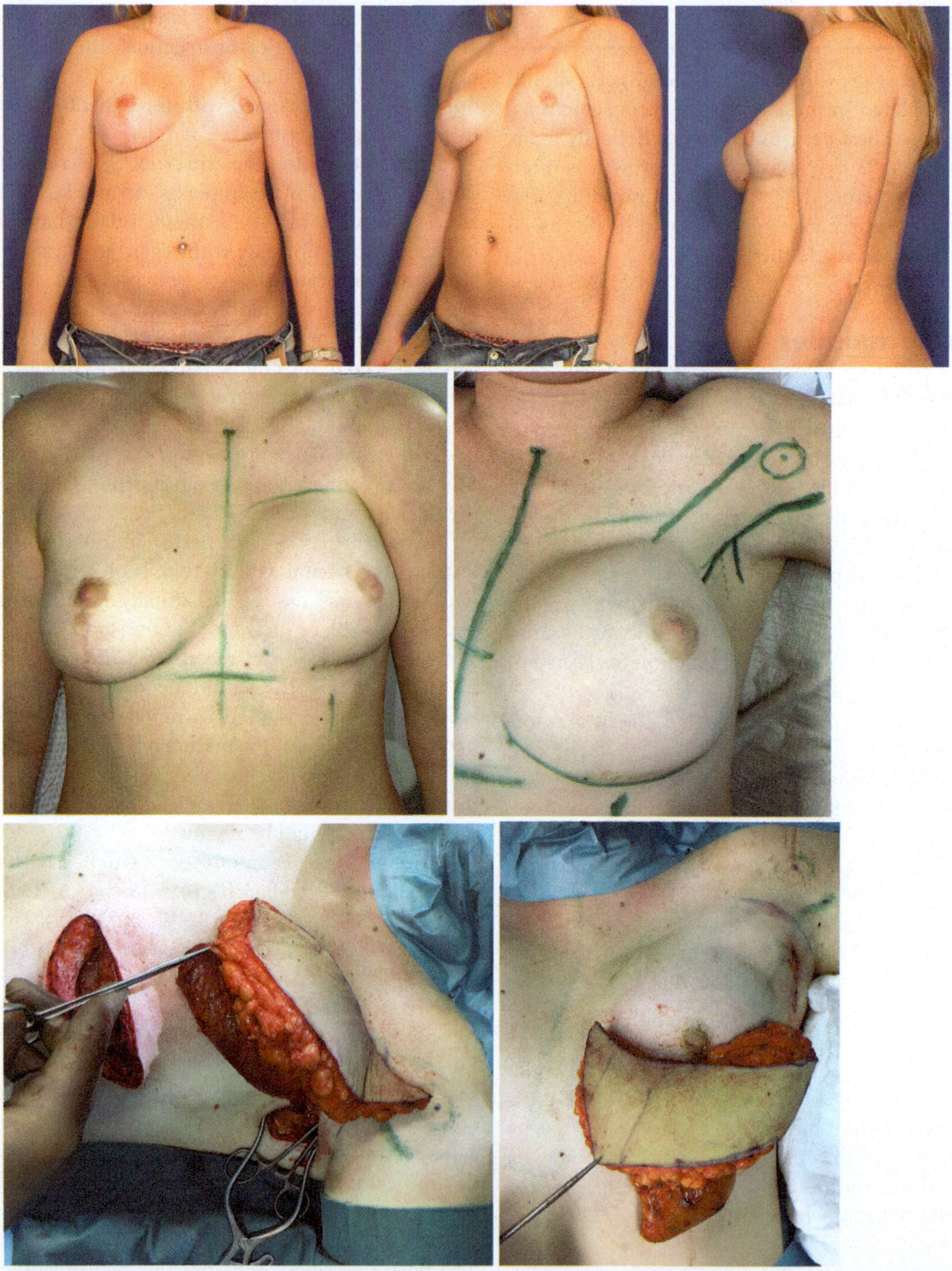

Figs. 15.4–15.13 (4–6) Poland syndrome left with existing nipple after expander and implant reconstruction in a 28-year-old patient; a total of more than seven previous operations, including reduction mammoplasty of the right breast. Existing, rock-hard capsular contracture (4° according to Baker) with typical cranial/lateral malposition of the nipple. (7) Planned implant and capsule removal and simultaneous reconstruction with two IT-flaps. Preoperative marking of IMF and breast midline. (8) Marking of the anterior axilla border and incision in the axilla for anastomosis of one flap. The point at the top right of the shoulder marks the planned fixation of the gracilis muscle to reconstruct the anterior axillary line. (9) The ipsilateral IT-flap is used for the cranial/lateral contour. The pedicle can thus be anastomosed elegantly in the axilla on the subscapular vascular tree. (10) The contralateral IT-flap is used for the actual breast reconstruction. The anastomosis is performed at the IMA and IMV.

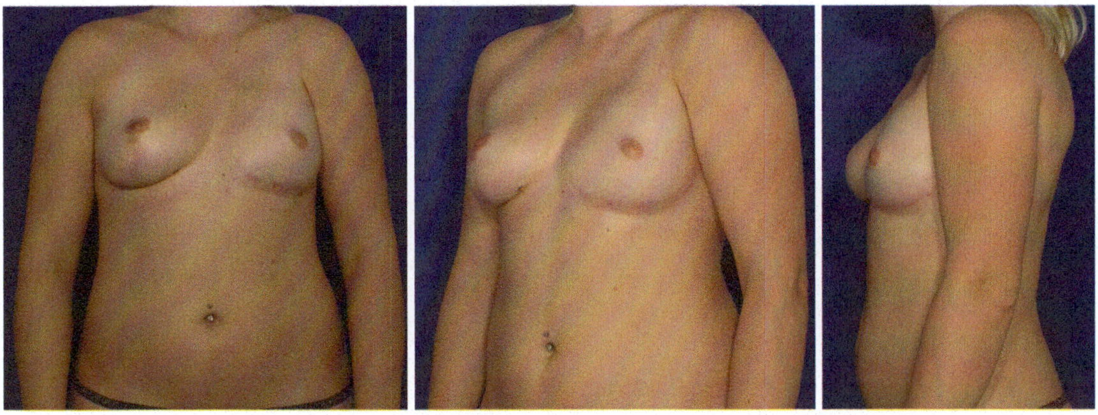

Figs. 15.4–15.13 (continued) (11–13) Result after 6 weeks. The volume and contour reconstruction has taken place successfully. The right side still requires an additional reduction. The position of the NAC is acceptable

15.3.3 Lipofilling

The de novo reconstruction of a completely aplastic breast with lipofilling is usually lengthy and usually means several operations. On the other hand, lipofilling is an inexpensive, low-scarring method of generating volume. However, lipofilling together with more traditional methods such as implants and flaps is certainly a good reconstruction technique.

15.3.4 NAC

The NAC position should be corrected as the last step of the reconstruction. If the patient is satisfied with the position of the NAC, no correction should be forced.

Often the nipple-areola complex is localized too far cranially and rather laterally due to the missing breast volume and skin. If it has not been possible to bring the NAC to the correct, symmetrical position with the initial expansion, this can be attempted secondarily. It should be evaluated whether it is a relative or absolute malposition. With a relative one, the NAC appears mispositioned if, for example, the volume is inadequate or the distance between nipple and IMF is too short or too long. With an absolute malposition of the NAC, the distance between the cranial border of the breast and NAC is too short. Also in the vertical level the NAC can lie too far laterally or also medially.

The positioning of an NAC that is too cranial is usually difficult, because if the skin is too high, there is hardly any displaceable skin between the clavicle and the base of the breast. Colwell et al. [1] have proposed to insert an expander between the chest and clavicle for correction. The skin is to be stretched, and the relative position of the MAK corrected.

In addition to S-shaped or double-U named flaps, a V-Y flap was also described (Fig. 15.14). These flaps must be harvested gently, especially if an implant has been used for volume reconstruction. In these cases, the incision should end at the implant capsule. Alternatively, direct removal and free grafting or resection and de novo reconstruction of the NAC are possible. All techniques leave scars in the area where the NAC is resected. They can become conspicuous due to the downward pull of the breast. This situation has to be discussed with the patients in advance.

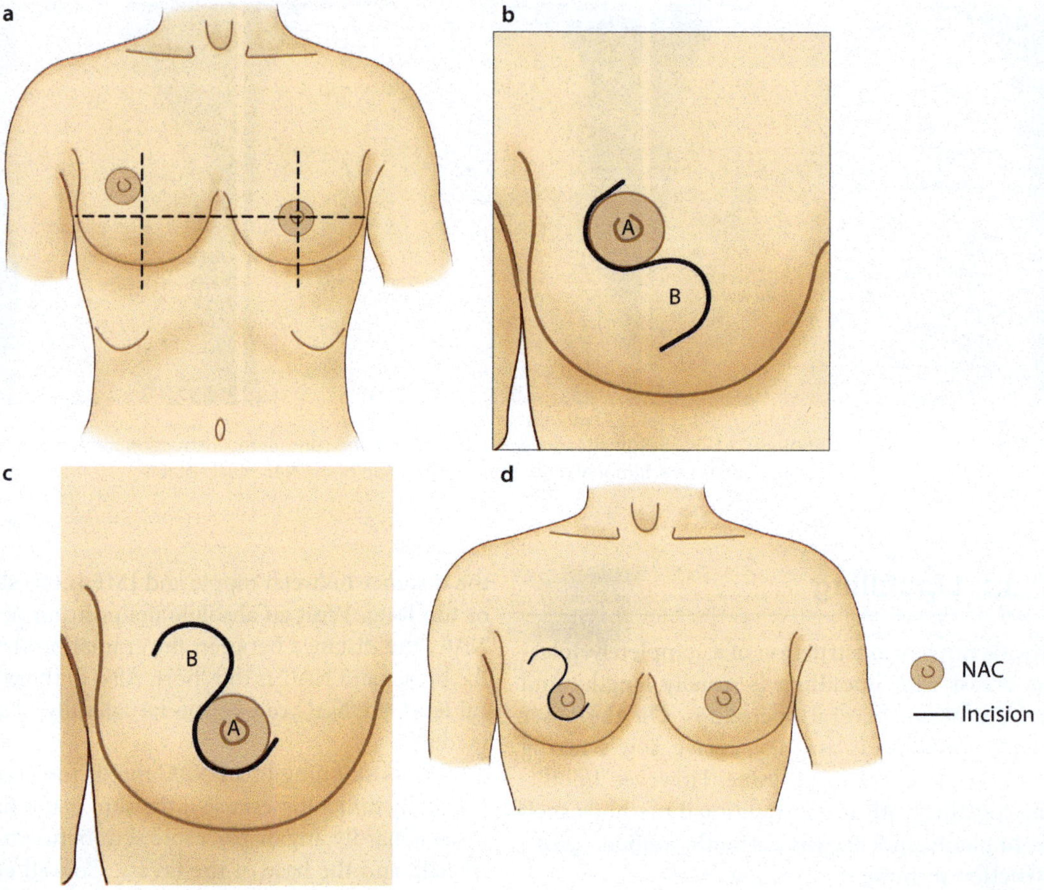

Fig. 15.14 The position of the NAC that is too high/laterally can only be corrected with difficulty. **a** A technique according to Mohmand and Naasan [4] and Spear and Albino [6] is the replacement of flap A and B by S-shaped flaps. **b** The S leaves the NAC cranially pedicled. **c** The flaps are exchanged. As a rule, dog ears are formed at the ends of the flaps. These should only be corrected later. Scars appear in the former location of the NAC. Mobilization must take place in all layers in order not to endanger the perfusion of the NAC. With an implant in place, the dissection stops on the implant capsule. **d** Result after flap replacement

15

Literature

1. Colwell AS, May JW Jr, Slavin SA. Lowering the post-operative high-riding nipple. Plast Reconstr Surg. 2007;120:596–9.
2. Derder M, Whitaker IS, Boudana D, Marchac A, Hivelin M, Mattar N, Lepage C, Claude O, Benjoar MD, Bosc R, Lantieri L. The use of lipofilling to treat congenital hypoplastic breast anomalies: preliminary experiences. Ann Plast Surg. 2014;73:371–7.
3. Huemer GM, Puelzl P, Schoeller T. Breast and chest wall reconstruction with the transverse musculocutaneous gracilis flap in Poland syndrome. Plast Reconstr Surg. 2012;130:779–83.
4. Mohmand H, Naasan A. Double U-plasty for correction of geometric malposition of the nipple-areola complex. Plast Reconstr Surg. 2002;109:2019–22.
5. Seyfer AE, Fox JP, Hamilton CG. Poland syndrome: evaluation and treatment of the chest wall in 63 patients. Plast Reconstr Surg. 2010;126:902–11.
6. Spear SL, Albino FP. Management of the high-riding nipple after breast reduction. Clin Plast Surg. 2016;43:395–401.

Supplementary Information

H. Fansa, C. Heitmann, *Breast Reconstruction with Autologous Tissue*,
https://doi.org/10.1007/978-3-319-95468-4

Index

G

H

I

S

T

V

W

The manufacturer's authorised representative in the EU is Springer Nature Customer Service Centre GmbH, Europaplatz 3, 69115 Heidelberg, Germany. If you have any concerns regarding our products, please contact ProductSafety@springernature.com

Printed and bound by CPI Group (UK) Ltd, Croydon, CR0 4YY
22/09/2026
02221056-0011